Applied Psychology for NURSES

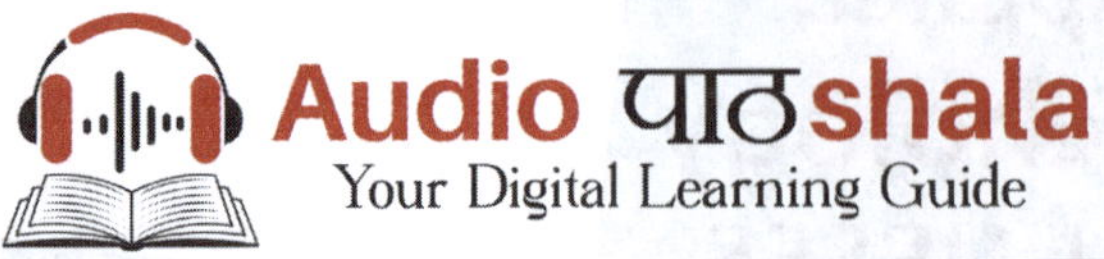

Audio पाठShala seamlessly integrates audio lessons, offering a comprehensive learning experience. Audio पाठShala not only fosters a deeper understanding of subjects but also caters to diverse learning styles, making education more inclusive and enjoyable.

Topics for Audio पाठShala

1.	Introduction to Psychology
2.	Body-Mind Relationship
3.	Developmental Psychology
4.	Personality
5.	Attention
6.	Perception
7.	Intelligence
8.	Learning
9.	Memory
10.	Thinking
11.	Aptitude
12.	Motivation
13.	Emotions
14.	Stress and Adaptation
15.	Attitude

Applied Psychology for NURSES

As per the Revised INC Syllabus of BSc Nursing

Semester I

SIXTH EDITION

R Sreevani PhD (Psychiatric Nursing)
Professor and Head
Department of Psychiatric Nursing
Dharwad Institute of Mental Health and
Neurosciences (DIMHANS)
Dharwad, Karnataka, India

Foreword
K Reddemma

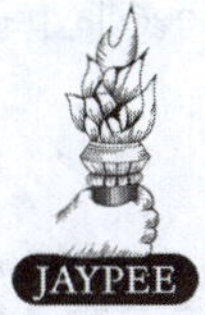

JAYPEE BROTHERS MEDICAL PUBLISHERS
The Health Sciences Publisher
New Delhi | London

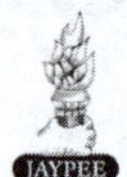

Jaypee Brothers Medical Publishers (P) Ltd

Headquarters
EMCA House
23/23-B, Ansari Road, Daryaganj
New Delhi 110 002, India
Landline: +91-11-23272143, +91-11-23272703
+91-11-23282021, +91-11-23245672
E-mail: jaypee@jaypeebrothers.com

Corporate Office
Jaypee Brothers Medical Publishers (P) Ltd.
4838/24, Ansari Road, Daryaganj
New Delhi 110 002, India
Phone: +91-11-43574357
Fax: +91-11-43574314
E-mail: jaypee@jaypeebrothers.com

Overseas Office
JP Medical Ltd.
83, Victoria Street, London
SW1H 0HW (UK)
Phone: +44-20 3170 8910
E-mail: info@jpmedpub.com

EU GPSR Authorised Representative
Logos Europe, 9 rue Nicolas Poussin
17000, La Rochelle, France
Phone: +33 (0) 6 67 93 73 78
E-mail: Contact@logoseurope.eu

Website: www.jaypeebrothers.com

Website: www.jaypeedigital.com

© 2025, Jaypee Brothers Medical Publishers

The views and opinions expressed in this book are solely those of the original contributor(s)/author(s) and do not necessarily represent those of editor(s) and publisher of the book.

All rights reserved. No part of this publication may be reproduced, stored or transmitted in any form or by any means, electronic, mechanical, photocopying, recording or otherwise, without the prior permission in writing of the publishers.

All brand names and product names used in this book are trade names, service marks, trademarks or registered trademarks of their respective owners. the publisher is not associated with any product or vendor mentioned in this book.

Medical knowledge and practice change constantly. This book is designed to provide accurate, authoritative information about the subject matter in question. However, readers are advised to check the most current information available on procedures included and check information from the manufacturer of each product to be administered, to verify the recommended dose, formula, method and duration of administration, adverse effects and contraindications. It is the responsibility of the practitioner to take all appropriate safety precautions. Neither the publisher nor the author(s)/editor(s) assume any liability for any injury and/or damage to persons or property arising from or related to use of material in this book.

This book is sold on the understanding that the publisher is not engaged in providing professional medical services. If such advice or services are required, the services of a competent medical professional should be sought.

Every effort has been made where necessary to contact holders of copyright to obtain permission to reproduce copyright material. If any have been inadvertently overlooked, the publisher will be pleased to make the necessary arrangements at the first opportunity.

Inquiries for bulk sales may be solicited at: jaypee@jaypeebrothers.com

Applied Psychology for Nurses

First Edition: 2009
Second Edition: 2013
Reprint: 2015
Third Edition: 2018
Fourth Edition: 2022
Fifth Edition: 2024
Revised Reprint: 2024
Sixth Edition: **2025**
Reprint : 2026

ISBN: 978-93-6616-588-2

Printed in India by K.K. Printers, Kundli, Haryana-131 028.

Dedicated to

My Husband

Foreword

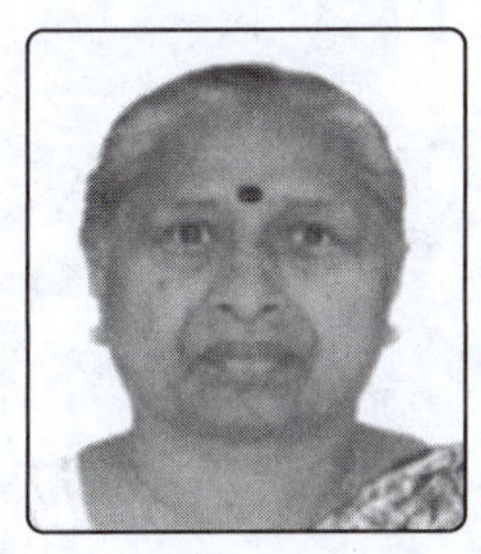

It is a matter of immense pleasure that Dr R Sreevani has again put her efforts together for the student community by compiling a comprehensive textbook titled *Applied Psychology for Nurses* and requested me to write foreword for the same. Her previous publication *A Guide to Mental Health and Psychiatric Nursing* has been a phenomenal success and gained much recognition with the student community in particular.

The present book broadly covers fundamentals of psychological concepts for the undergraduate and graduate nurses with special focus on nursing implications making it unique. The text is presented in line with the revised nursing syllabus for GNM, BSc (N) and PC BSc (N) students.

The author has used simple language and presented the subject in her own lucid style. A right mix of tables, flowcharts and figures has been used to make the concept comprehensible and aid learning. Units on Sensation and Perception, Learning, Memory, Thinking, Intelligence, Motivation, Emotions, Attitudes, Personality, Developmental Psychology, Social Psychology, Guidance and Counseling and Psychological Assessment have been dealt with in-depth and incorporated nursing implications making it a must-buy for the nursing community.

I wish her success in all her future endeavors.

K Reddemma
Nodal Officer
National Consortium for PhD in Nursing
St John's College of Nursing
Bengaluru, Karnataka, India
Indian Nursing Council
Formerly
Dean, Behavioral Sciences
Professor, Department of Nursing
National Institute of Mental Health and Neurosciences (NIMHANS)
Bengaluru, Karnataka, India

Preface to the Sixth Edition

The concept of psychology in nursing education is by no means "new". Despite coming from a different discipline, psychology has a huge relevance to nursing practice. For those aspiring nurses who have ever wondered the need for them to devote hours in studying psychology, they have not probably realized that both are interrelated with each other. If you are still wondering how a nursing career is related to psychology, think about a time you have ever had a nurse tend to you. If you felt that your nurse was caring, compassionate, and good at making you feel comfortable, then your nurse was using psychology. Without it, there is no trust and no bond created, which can sometimes be the difference between a patient healing and getting worse.

Nurses work in a setting where they are required to interact with other professionals and caregivers in an effort to bring the best quality care for their patients. While managing patients, they are not only required to understand the physical pain associated with the illness but also change their thoughts and attitudes to improve the well-being. They need to fully understand how other people behave and act in certain situations—this is where psychology comes into play. Nurses who study psychology extensively are trained to understand a wide range and depth of emotions and what those emotions can cause in an ill or injured patient. It is the knowledge of psychology that enables nurses to gain the trust of their patients and learn how to interact with patients based on different factors such as gender and age. For instance, during an illness, young patients experience greater fear than adults. They may have difficulties in understanding their illness. A nurse can apply her knowledge of child development and psychology and relate to the young patients in a way their apprehensions are alleviated. Thus, psychology can help improve the nurse-patient relationship. As the nurses perform under unthinkable stress, they also need to use psychology on themselves so as to navigate through all the emotions of a patient. Without psychology and nursing careers coming together, it would be hard for a nurse to do her job.

It is a matter of great pleasure that the sustained interest and enthusiasm that students and faculty have evinced in fifth edition of "*Applied Psychology of Nurses*" has prompted the publishers to request for a subsequent edition. The sixth edition as the previous one is strictly aligned as per the revised Indian Nursing Council (INC) syllabus. While retaining the strengths of the fifth edition, an effort has been made to give the latest edition a new look and make it more student friendly. I have gone through the entire text thoroughly and revised the content with simpler language where necessary. A few illustrations have been modified to engage the reader more effectively. Also, a digital learning guide "*Audio* पाठ Shala" has been provided with this textbook to enable easy learning and recall.

Each chapter is followed by a synopsis to give a bird view of the important aspects dealt with in the respective chapter. Long essays, short essays, short notes, and MCQs have been included at the end of each chapter to serve as an active learning exercise. An exhaustive glossary of various terms used has also been provided at the end of the textbook to gain a broad understanding of the subject.

Students of general, BSc, MSc Nursing, and other health professionals interested in getting an overview of psychology may also find the textbook useful. All constructive suggestions from readers in making this edition more valuable and useful will be earnestly solicited. I am confident that this new edition reflects what instructors want and need, a book that motivates students to understand and apply psychology to their own lives as well.

R Sreevani

Preface to the First Edition

As per the Indian Nursing Council (INC) syllabus for GNM, BSc (N), PC BSc (N) students, psychology is prescribed as a subject in their academic curriculum. During my teaching experience I have always found that though many books have been published on the subject they do not really cater to the specific needs of the student community, nurses in particular. The students have often sought recommendations for a publication which caters to their complete syllabus. For lack of such a textbook there was always a high demand for prepared notes which they could use during their examinations. This edition is a genuine effort to mitigate their hardship and also to stimulate academic interest and build an appreciation of the relevance of psychology, motivating and engaging the students.

This edition of *Psychology for Nurses* though will add to the Psychology section in the book shelves, it will definitely be a special one for the nurse community. In this edition a concerted effort has been made to cover the basic principles of psychology and also focus on applied topics in units such as Sensation and Perception, Learning, Memory, Thinking, Intelligence, Motivation, Emotions, Attitudes, Personality, Developmental Psychology, Social Psychology, Guidance and Counseling and Psychological Assessment. The matter has been produced in a simple language with tables, figures and flowcharts so as to directly support learning, easy understanding and retention of the concept. Learning new concepts and theories is of no much value unless the same can be put to use in real-life situations. In a unique effort to bridge the gap between theory and practice, special care has been exercised to incorporate Nursing Implications at all appropriate places, providing ample opportunity for the intelligent nurse to conceptualize her role.

An exhaustive glossary has been provided at the end of the text to aid the student nurse understand the meaning of the keywords and their usage. To facilitate the students from examination point of view, a set of review questions—long essays, short essays and short answers type have been included at the end of each unit. To assess the level of understanding gained on various topics, a unit-wise question bank (objective) has been provided at the end of the text.

I will be deriving immense satisfaction if the nursing personnel apply psychological principles described in the textbook in their day-to-day learning and practice. I am confident that this book will provide good teaching material for the instructor and moreover motivate the students towards understanding and applying psychology in their job and personal lives as well. Suggestions for improvement will be gratefully acknowledged.

R Sreevani

Acknowledgments

I would like to begin by thanking the Almighty God, who bestowed upon me the spiritual strength and perseverance to make it all happen.

I would like to thank the publishers M/s Jaypee Brothers Medical Publishers (P) Ltd, New Delhi, for being supportive all through. I would like to extend my special thanks to Shri Jitendar P Vij (Group Chairman), Mr Ankit Vij (Managing Director), and Mr MS Mani (Group President) for continuing to repose strong faith in me.

Nobody has been more important to me in the pursuit of this title than the members of my family. I would like to thank my grandparents, parents, and in-laws, whose love and guidance are with me in whatever I pursue. They are the ultimate role models. While I wish to thank my loving and supportive husband Mr Giridhar who has been a source of constant support, I would also like to specially acknowledge the contribution made by my elder son Master Pranith Ambati in organizing and conceptualizing the visual material and reading through the complete text during the manuscript preparation and proofing stage. A word of appreciation is due to my younger son Master Daivik Ambati for exhibiting keen interest in the complete process from beginning to end.

I extend my sincere thanks to Dr Madhu Choudhary (Director–Educational Publishing), Ms Pooja Bhandari [Director–Production (Books and Journals)], Ms Sunita Katla (Executive Assistant to Group Chairman and Publishing Manager), Mr Ajay Kumar Sharma [DGM–Production (Books and Journals)], Ms Samina Khan (Executive Assistant to Director–Educational Publishing),Ms Alisha Talwar (Team Lead–Nursing), Mr Vijay Kumar Bhatia (Manager–Production), Ms Seema Dogra (Cover Visualizer), Ms Neha Verma (Graphic Designer–Cover), Ms Geeta Rani (Proofreader), Ms Uma Adhikari (Typesetter), Mr Ratan Lal (Graphic Designer), and their team members for the wonderful back office support.

I wish to present my special thanks to Mr Venugopal (Regional Head-Business Development, DigiNerve) for his small talks which have been a huge inspiration in over a decade of association with him.

Applied Psychology Syllabus

PLACEMENT: I semester

THEORY: 3 credits (60 hours)

DESCRIPTION: This course is designed to enable the students to develop understanding about basic concepts of psychology and its application in personal and community life, health, illness and nursing. It further provides students opportunity to recognize the significance and application of soft skills and self-empowerment in the practice of nursing.

COMPETENCIES: On completion of the course, the students will be able to:

- Identify the importance of psychology in individual and professional life.
- Develop understanding of the biological and psychological basis of human behavior.
- Identify the role of nurse in promoting mental health and dealing with altered personality.
- Perform the role of nurses applicable to the psychology of different age groups.
- Identify the cognitive and affective needs of clients.
- Integrate the principles of motivation and emotion in performing the role of nurse in caring for emotionally sick client.
- Demonstrate basic understanding of psychological assessment and nurse's role.
- Apply the knowledge of soft skills in workplace and society.
- Apply the knowledge of self-empowerment in workplace, society and personal life.

COURSE OUTLINE

T – Theory

Units	Time (hours)	Learning outcomes	Contents	Teaching/ learning activities	Assessment methods
I	2 (T)	Describe scope, branches and significance of psychology in nursing	**Introduction** ◆ Meaning of psychology ◆ Development of psychology—scope, branches and methods of psychology ◆ Relationship with other subjects ◆ Significance of psychology in nursing ◆ Applied psychology to solve everyday issues	Lecture-cum-discussion	◆ Essay ◆ Short answer
II	4 (T)	Describe biology of human behavior	**Biological basis of behavior** ◆ Introduction ◆ Body mind relationship ◆ Genetics and behavior ◆ Inheritance of behavior ◆ Brain and behavior ◆ Psychology and sensation – Sensory process – Normal and abnormal	◆ Lecture ◆ Discussion	◆ Essay ◆ Short answer

Contd...

Contd...

Units	Time (hours)	Learning outcomes	Contents	Teaching/ learning activities	Assessment methods
III	5 (T)	Describe mentally healthy person and defense mechanisms	**Mental health and mental hygiene** ◆ Concept of mental health and mental hygiene ◆ Characteristic of mentally healthy person ◆ Warning signs of poor mental health ◆ Promotive and preventive mental health strategies and services ◆ Defense mechanism and its implication ◆ Frustration and conflict—types of conflicts and measurements to overcome ◆ Role of nurse in reducing frustration and conflict and enhancing coping ◆ Dealing with ego	◆ Lecture ◆ Case discussion ◆ Role play	◆ Essay ◆ Short answer ◆ Objective type
IV	7 (T)	Describe psychology of people in different age groups and role of nurse	**Developmental psychology** ◆ Physical, psychosocial and cognitive development across life span—prenatal through early childhood, middle to late childhood through adolescence, early and mid-adulthood, late adulthood, death and dying ◆ Role of nurse in supporting normal growth and development across the life span ◆ Psychological needs of various groups in health and sickness—infancy, childhood, adolescence, adulthood and older adult ◆ Introduction to child psychology and role of nurse in meeting the psychological needs of children ◆ Psychology of vulnerable individuals—challenged, women, sick, etc. ◆ Role of nurse with vulnerable groups	◆ Lecture ◆ Group discussion	◆ Essay ◆ Short answer
V	4 (T)	Explain personality and role of nurse in identification and improvement in altered personality	**Personality** ◆ Meaning, definition of personality ◆ Classification of personality ◆ Measurement and evaluation of personality—Introduction ◆ Alteration in personality ◆ Role of nurse in identification of individual personality and improvement in altered personality	◆ Lecture ◆ Discussion ◆ Demon-stration	◆ Essay and short answer ◆ Objective type

Contd...

Contd...

Units	Time (hours)	Learning outcomes	Contents	Teaching/ learning activities	Assessment methods
VI	16 (T)	Explain cognitive process and their applications	**Cognitive process** ◆ Attention—definition, types, determinants, duration, degree and alteration in attention ◆ Perception—meaning of perception, principles, factor affecting perception ◆ Intelligence—meaning of intelligence—effect of heredity and environment in intelligence, classification, introduction to measurement of intelligence tests—mental deficiencies ◆ Learning—definition of learning, types of learning, factors influencing learning—learning process, habit formation ◆ Memory—meaning and nature of memory, factors influencing memory, methods to improve memory, forgetting ◆ Thinking—types, level, reasoning and problem solving ◆ Aptitude—concept, types, individual differences and variability ◆ Psychometric assessment of cognitive processes—introduction ◆ Alteration in cognitive processes	◆ Lecture ◆ Discussion	◆ Essay and Short Answer ◆ Objective Type
VII	6 (T)	Describe motivation, emotion, attitude and role of nurse in emotionally sick client	**Motivation and emotional processes** ◆ Motivation—meaning, concept, types, theories of motivation, motivation cycle, biological and special motives ◆ Emotions—meaning of emotions, development of emotions, alteration of emotion, emotions in sickness—handling emotions in self and other ◆ Stress and adaptation—stress, stressor, cycle, effect, adaptation and coping ◆ Attitudes—meaning of attitudes, nature, factor affecting attitude, attitudinal change, Role of attitude in health and sickness ◆ Psychometric assessment of emotions and attitude—introduction ◆ Role of nurse in caring for emotionally sick client	◆ Lecture ◆ Group discussion	◆ Essay and short answer ◆ Objective type

Contd...

Contd...

Units	Time (hours)	Learning outcomes	Contents	Teaching/ learning activities	Assessment methods
VIII	4 (T)	Explain psychological assessment and tests and role of nurse	**Psychological assessment and tests** ◆ Introduction ◆ Types, development, characteristics, principles, uses, interpretation ◆ Role of nurse in psychological assessment	◆ Lecture ◆ Discussion ◆ Demon-stration	◆ Short answer ◆ Assess-ment of practice
IX	10 (T)	Explain concept of soft skill and its application in work place and society	**Application of soft skill** ◆ Concept of soft skill ◆ Types of soft skill—visual, aural and communication skill ◆ The way of communication – Building relationship with client and society – Interpersonal relationships (IPR): Definition, types, and purposes, interpersonal skills, barriers, strategies to overcome barriers ◆ Survival strategies—managing time, coping stress, resilience, work—life balance ◆ Applying soft skill to workplace and society – Presentation skills, social etiquette, telephone etiquette, motivational skills, teamwork, etc. ◆ Use of soft skill in nursing	◆ Lecture ◆ Group discussion ◆ Role play ◆ Refer/ complete soft skills module	Essay and short answer
X	2 (T)	Explain self-empower-ment	**Self-empowerment** ◆ Dimensions of self-empowerment ◆ Self-empowerment development ◆ Importance of women's empowerment in society ◆ Professional etiquette and personal grooming ◆ Role of nurse in empowering others	◆ Lecture ◆ Discussion	◆ Short answer ◆ Objective type

CONTENTS

CHAPTER

1 Introduction to Psychology

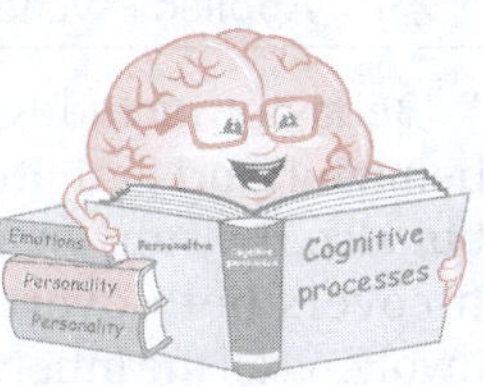

CHAPTER OUTLINE

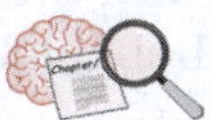

- Development of psychology
- Nature of subject psychology
- Scope of psychology
- Methods of psychology
- Relationship of psychology with other subjects
- Significance of psychology in nursing
- Applied psychology to solve everyday issues

Psychology is an offspring of subject philosophy. Psychology is derived from two Greek words, 'psyche' and 'logos'. 'Psyche' means 'mind, soul or spirit' and 'logos' means the 'study of' or 'knowledge'—study of soul. The word soul was used vaguely and there were many interpretations that could be given to it. Later on, William James used the term 'mind', which replaced 'soul'. As years went by the meaning of psychology changed. Those who studied what was called 'mind' found that they could neither see it nor understand it. Seeing what it did meant they had to study the activities of human beings. The influence of physiology made some scientists like Wilhelm Wundt of Germany define psychology as the study of 'consciousness'. However, this was also discarded in the course of time and the current definition of psychology as the systematic study of human and animal 'behavior' came to be accepted **(Flowchart 1.1)**.

MEANING OF BEHAVIOR

'Any manifestation of life is activity' and behavior is a collective name for these activities. The term behavior includes the following:

- Motor or conative activities (walking, swimming, dancing, etc.)
- Cognitive activities (thinking, reasoning, imagining)
- Affective activities (feeling happy, sad, angry, etc.)

Flowchart 1.1: Evolution of meaning of psychology

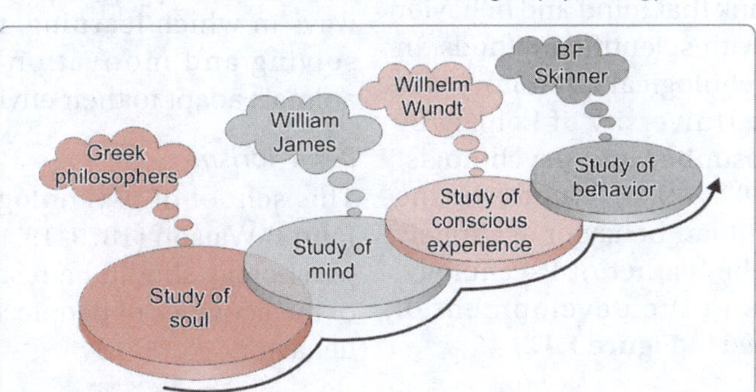

Behavior includes not only the conscious behavior and activities of the human mind but also the subconscious and unconscious. It covers both overt and covert behaviors involving all the inner experiences and mental processes.

In a nutshell the term behavior refers to the activities and experiences of a living organism over its life time.

DEFINITIONS OF PSYCHOLOGY

- Psychology is the science of human and animal behavior. It includes the application of behavioral science to human problems.
- Psychology is the science of human behavior.

  —Walter Bowers Pillsbury (1911)
- Psychology is a science which aims to give us better understanding and control of the behavior of the organism as a whole.

  —William McDoughall (1949)
- Psychology is the scientific study of activities of the individual in relation to his environment.

  —Woodworm and Marquis
- Psychology is the investigation of human and animal behavior and of the mental and physiological processes associated with the behavior. **—Jackson (1976)**

DEVELOPMENT OF PSYCHOLOGY

Psychology as a separate area of study split away from philosophy a little over 100 years ago. The successes of the experimental method in the physical sciences encouraged some philosophers to think that mind and behavior could be studied with scientific methods. In 1879, the first psychological laboratory was established at the University of Leipzig by the German philosopher and psychologist Wilhelm Wundt (1832–1920). Wundt was the first to measure human behavior accurately and is known as the 'Father of Psychology'. Major landmarks in the development of psychology are listed in **Figure 1.1.**

Schools of Psychology

William James, Wilhelm Wundt and other psychologists of the time thought of psychology as the study of mind. In the first decades of the twentieth century, psychologists came to hold quite different views about the nature of mind and the best way to study it. Schools of thought formed around these psychologists. These schools of thought are known as the schools of psychology.

Structuralism

This early school of psychology grew up around the ideas of Wilhelm Wundt in Germany and was established by one of Wundt's students, Edward B Titchener (1867–1927). The goal of the structuralist was to find the units or elements which make up the mind. The main method used to discover these elementary units of mind was introspection.

Gestalt Psychology

This school of psychology was founded in Germany around 1912 by Max Wertheimer (1880–1943) and his colleagues. These psychologists felt that structuralists were wrong in thinking of the mind as being made up of elements. They argued that mind could be thought of as resulting from the whole pattern of sensory activity and the relationships and organizations within this pattern.

Functionalism

Functionalists such as John Dewey (1873–1954), James R Angell (1869–1949) and Harvey Carr (1873–1954) proposed that psychology should do 'what mind and behavior do'. The functionalists performed experiments on the ways in which learning, memory, problem solving and motivation help people and animals adapt to their environments.

Behaviorism

This school of psychology originated with John B Watson (1879–1958). He insisted that psychology should be restricted to the study of the activities of people and animals—their behavior.

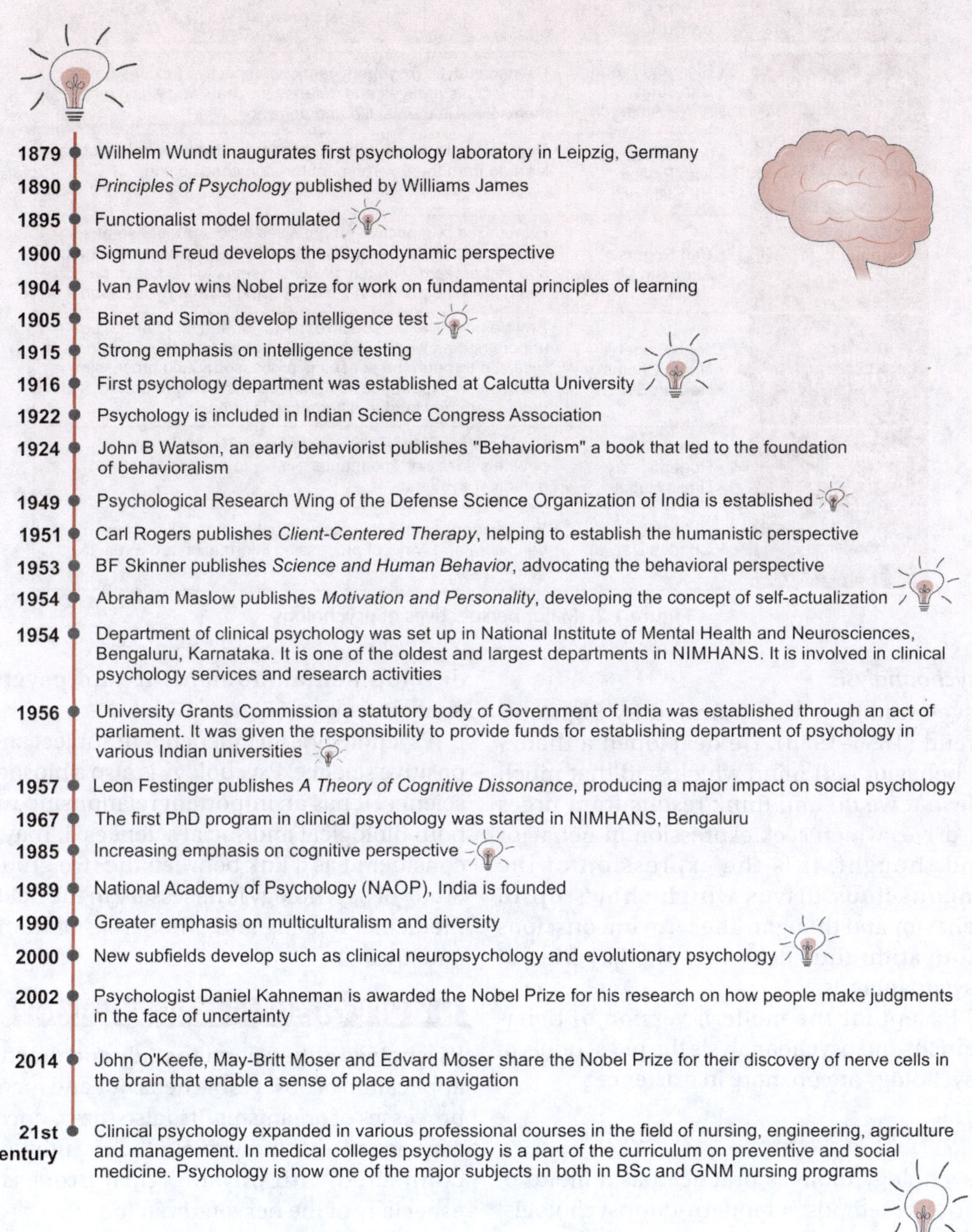

Figure 1.1: Major landmarks in the development of psychology

Perspective	Principal contributors	Basic premise
Psychoanalytic perspective	• Sigmund Freud • Carl Jung • Alfred Adler	• Psychoanalytic (psychodynamic) perspective focuses on the unconscious motives and defense mechanisms which manifest themselves in mental life and behavior
Behavioral perspective	• John B Watson • Ivan Pavlov • BF Skinner	• Psychologists with a behavioral perspective view behavior as learned from the environment through conditioning
Humanistic perspective	• Carl Rogers • Abraham Maslow	• Humanistic perspective emphasizes a person's sense of self and each individual's attempts to achieve personal competence and self-esteem. The aim of humanism is to help each person attain his full potential in life or become all that he is capable of
Cognitive perspective	• Jean Piaget • Noam Chomsky • Herbert Simon	• From a cognitive perspective, behavior and mind are to be understood as ways in which information from the environment received through the senses is processed. Such processing is the basis of experience. Differences in the way information is processed may lead to differences in behavior
Biological perspective	• James Olds • Roger Sperry • David Hubel	• Psychologists with a biological perspective try to relate people's behavior and mental events to their nervous and glandular systems
Evolutionary perspective	• Charles Darwin	• Evolutionary perspective assumes that many of our core behaviors and ways of processing information are a result of evolution

Figure 1.2: Major perspectives of psychology

Psychoanalysis

Psychoanalysis was founded by Sigmund Freud (1856–1938). He developed a theory of behavior and mind which said that much of what we do and think results from urges or drives which seek expression in behavior and thought. It is the expression of the unconscious drives which shows up in behavior and thought. The term unconscious motivation thus describes the key idea of psychoanalysis.

Except for the modern version of behaviorism and psychoanalysis the old schools of psychology are no more in existence.

Major Perspectives of Psychology

Psychology today is practiced as a blend of various methods. A modern-day psychologist leans towards using one of the methods more than the other but depends on all that has been developed in the past. Various viewpoints about what is important in understanding mental life and behavior characterize the present outlook. Among these perspectives are the behavioral, biological, cognitive, social, developmental, humanistic and psychoanalytic aspects **(Figure 1.2)**.

Psychology is an independent subject and a positive science. Psychology is also a biosocial science. It has an important relationship with both biological and social sciences. It may be considered as a link between the two groups. Study of psychology is necessary in the field of medicine, nursing and other areas of human endeavor.

NATURE OF SUBJECT PSYCHOLOGY

Psychology is the scientific study and practical application of observable behavior and mental processes of organisms. It is also the science of experience of an individual which is intimately connected with physiological processes, especially of the nervous system.

- **Psychology uses scientific methods:** Almost all the methods of psychology are more or less scientific in their nature. Out of these the experimental method is the most scientific. Modern psychology widely uses this method in all its branches. In experimental method both dependent and independent variables are distinguished. While the dependent variables are controlled, the effect of independent variables is observed. Thus, in the experiment the psychologist observes a certain phenomenon in strictly controlled situations. The psychological laboratories are continuously developing and new and more exact instruments being constantly put to use. With these instruments psychologist observes the phenomenon, records, compares, classifies and discovers various principles through generalization.

- **Psychology is factual:** Psychology studies facts of behavior by observation and experiments, not by values.
- **Laws of psychology are universal:** The laws of psychology are found to be the same at all times and places under similar conditions.
- **Laws of psychology are verifiable:** By verification and reverification psychological principles have been found to be true everywhere. They can be verified by any one.
- **Psychology discovers the cause-effect relationship in human behavior:** Psychology not only observes behavior but also finds out cause-effect relationship in it. For example, psychology has discovered why and in what circumstances a child becomes a delinquent or a degenerate. These findings have been put to use and found to be correct. Thus psychology discovers the 'how' of behavior together with its 'what'.
- **Psychology predicts human behavior:** By discovering the cause-effect relationship psychologists are also able to accurately predict human behavior. In modern progressive countries appointments to various government posts are being made based on the predictions coming out of psychological tests.

From the above characteristics it can be deduced that the nature of psychology is scientific **(Figure 1.3)**.

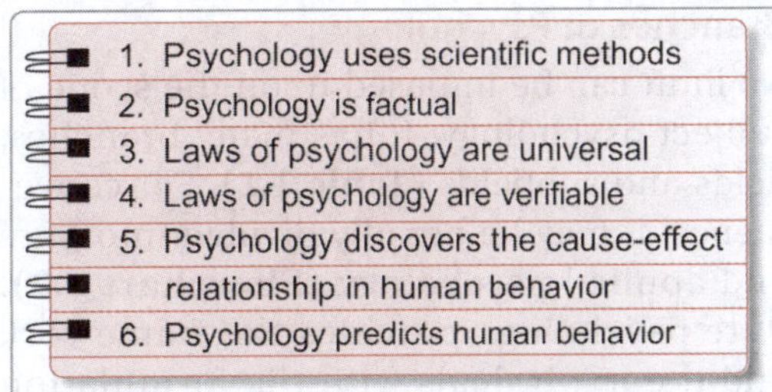

Figure 1.3: Nature of subject psychology

SCOPE OF PSYCHOLOGY

The scope of a subject can usually be discussed under the following two headings:

1. Limits of its operations and applications.
2. Branches, topics and subject matter with which it deals.

Limits of Operations and Applications

The field of operation and application of subject psychology is too vast.

- It studies, describes and explains the behavior of living organisms.
- It describes all types of life activities and experiences—whether conative, cognitive or affective, implicit or explicit, conscious, unconscious and subconscious of a living organism.
- It studies not only human behavior but also human experience, language and other forms of communication. Psychologists are interested in individual differences which can either be genetically determined or occurring as a result of learning. They study how individuals and society interact and behave as members of small and large groups.
- It is applicable to all the living creatures created by the almighty irrespective of their species, caste, color, age, sex, mental or physical state. Thus normal, abnormal, children, adolescents, youth, adults, elderly persons, criminals, patients, workers, officials, students, teachers, parents, consumers, etc., are all studied in subject psychology.
- It also studies the behavior of animals, insects, birds and plant life.

Branches of Psychology

No limit can be imposed upon the scope of subject psychology. It has many branches, fields and subfields **(Table 1.1)**. For convenience, it may be broadly divided into pure and applied psychology **(Flowchart 1.2)**. Pure psychology provides the framework and theory. It deals with the formulation of psychological principles and theories. It suggests various methods and techniques for the analysis, assessment, modification and improvement of behavior.

In applied psychology the theory generated through pure psychology finds its practical shape. Here ways and means of the application of psychological rules, principles, theories and techniques with reference to the real practical life situations are discussed.

Branches of Pure Psychology

1. **General psychology:** General psychology deals with the fundamental rules, principles and theories of psychology in relation to the study of behavior of a normal adult.
2. **Abnormal psychology:** Abnormal psychology deals with the behavior of individuals who are unusual. It studies mental disorders, their causes and treatment.
3. **Social psychology:** Social psychology deals with the group behavior and interrelationships of people with others (how an individual is influenced by others and how an individual influences others behavior). It studies various types of group phenomena such as public opinion, attitudes, beliefs and crowd behavior. Social psychologists study the ways in which individuals are affected by other people.
4. **Physiological psychology:** This branch of psychology describes and explains the biological and physiological basis of behavior. It concerns the structure and functions of sense organs, nervous system, muscles and glands underlying all behavior. It emphasizes on the influence of bodily factors on human behavior.

Table 1.1: Major subfields of psychology

Subfields	Description
Biopsychology	Biopsychology examines how biological structures and functions of the body affect behavior
Clinical neuro-psychology	Clinical neuropsychology unites the areas of biopsychology and clinical psychology, focusing on the relationship between biological factors and psychological disorders
Cognitive psychology	Cognitive psychology focuses on the study of higher mental processes
Counseling psychology	Counseling psychology focuses primarily on educational, social and career adjustment problems
Cross-cultural psychology	Cross-cultural psychology investigates the similarities and differences in psychological functioning and across various cultures and ethnic groups
Environmental psychology	Environmental psychology considers the relationship between people and their physical environment, how the physical environment affects emotions and the amount of stress experienced in a particular setting
Evolutionary psychology	Evolutionary psychology deals with the influence of genetic inheritance from ancestors on behavior
Experimental psychology	Experimental psychology studies the processes of sensing, perceiving, learning and thinking about the world
Forensic psychology	Forensic psychology focuses on legal issues and helps determine the root cause of criminal behavior. It evaluates criminals and attempts to understand their mindset and motives while the crime was being committed
Health psychology	Health psychology explores the relationship between psychological factors and physical ailments or diseases
Personality psychology	Personality psychology focuses on the consistency in people's behavior overtime and the traits that differentiate one person from another
School psychology	School psychology is devoted to counseling elementary and secondary school children with academic or emotional problems
Sport psychology	Sport psychology applies psychology to athletic activity and exercise

Flowchart 1.2: Branches of psychology

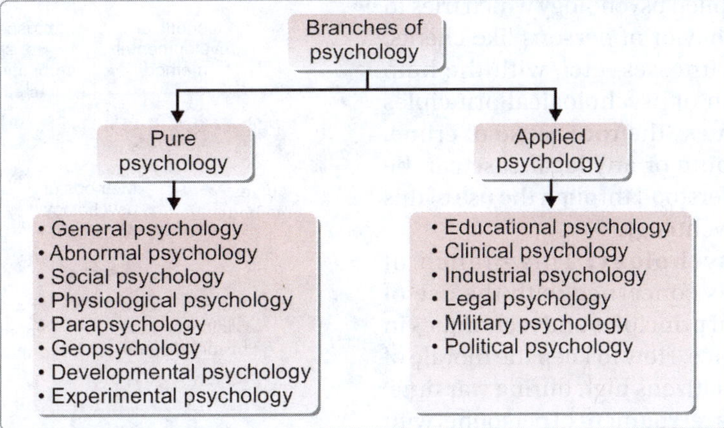

5. **Parapsychology:** Parapsychology deals with extrasensory perceptions, causes of rebirth, telepathy and allied problems.
6. **Geopsychology:** This branch of psychology describes and explains the relationship of physical environment particularly weather, climate and soil with behavior.
7. **Developmental psychology:** This branch of psychology describes the processes and factors that influence growth and development in relation to the behavior of an individual from birth to old age. It is further subdivided into branches like child psychology, adolescent, adult and geriatric psychology. Development psychologists try to understand complex behaviors by studying their beginning and the orderly ways in which they change or develop over the life span.
8. **Experimental psychology:** This branch of psychology studies the ways and means of carrying out psychological experiments using scientific methods. Experimental psychologists do basic research in an effort to discover and understand the fundamental and general causes of behavior. They study basic processes such as learning, memory, sensation, perception and motivation.

Branches of Applied Psychology

1. **Educational psychology:** Educational psychology is that branch of applied psychology which tries to apply psychological principles, theories and techniques to human behavior in educational situations. The subject matter of this branch covers psychological ways and means of improving all aspects of the teaching/learning process. Educational psychologists are most often involved in the increase in efficiency of learning in schools by applying psychological knowledge related to learning and motivation.
2. **Clinical psychology:** This is the largest subfield of psychology. This branch of applied psychology describes the causes of mental illness, abnormal behavior of a patient and suggests treatment and effective adjustment of the affected person in the society.
3. **Industrial psychology:** This branch of applied psychology seeks the application of psychological principles, theories and techniques for the study of human behavior in relation to industrial environment. Industrial psychologists apply psychological principles to assist public and private organizations with their hiring and placement programs, training and supervision of personnel and improvement of communication within the organization. They also counsel employees within the organization who need help with their personal problems.

4. **Legal psychology:** Legal psychology is that branch of applied psychology which tries to study the behavior of persons like clients, criminals, witnesses, etc., with the help of application of psychological principles and techniques. The root cause of crime, offence, dispute or any legal case can be properly understood through the use of this branch of psychology.
5. **Military psychology:** This branch of psychology is concerned with the use of psychological principles and techniques in military science. How to keep the morale of soldiers and citizens high during war time, how to secure recruitment of personnel with good leadership and fighting capacities, etc., are the various topics that are dealt within this branch of psychology.
6. **Political psychology:** This branch of psychology relates itself with the use of psychological principles and techniques in studying politics and deriving political gains.

METHODS OF PSYCHOLOGY

Psychology is termed as the scientific study of human behavior. Special tools and procedures help us in gathering and organizing its subject matter and essential facts about behavior. These procedures termed as methods help in studying human behavior **(Figure 1.4)**. They are as under:

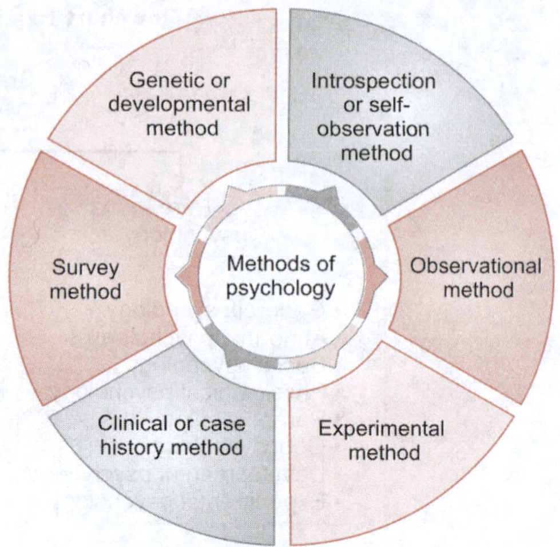

Figure 1.4: Methods of psychology

1. Introspection or Self-observation Method

Introspection also known as self-observation method is one of the oldest methods of psychology which means 'to look within'. It is defined as the process of directly examining one's own conscious mental states such as thoughts and feelings.

As it is not possible to understand the inner feelings and experiences of other persons, the subject is asked to systematically observe his own behavior and report the same which is later analyzed to understand behavior. This characteristic of the introspection method is not available to other natural sciences.

Steps in Introspection Method

The steps involved introspection are presented in **Figure 1.5**.

1. **Look within:** The psychologist encourages the individuals to look within and describe his thoughts, feelings and experiences.
2. **Begin to question:** The individual begins to question the working of his own mind processes by trying to look within and recall what happened and how he is feeling.

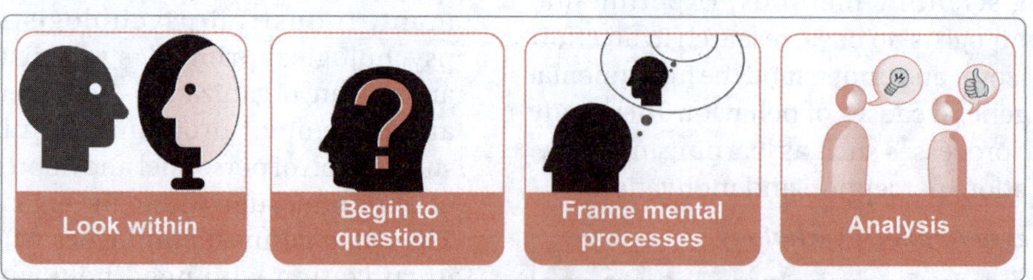

Figure 1.5: Steps in introspection method

3. **Frame mental processes:** The individual consolidates knowledge about his mental processes and reports. During this step the subject gets direct, immediate and intuitive knowledge about the mind.
4. **Analysis:** The psychologist analyses and interprets information. This helps in advancement of scientific knowledge.

For example, a patient after an operation may be asked to report how he feels. The patient will try to look within and recall what happened and how he is presently feeling. The patient then reports his mental processes. This report will help in improving the treatment modality.

Merits

- Introspection is a fundamental method of psychology. Observation and experimentation are based upon introspection.
- Introspection gives us direct, immediate and exact knowledge of our own mental processes.
- It enables us to fully understand the behavior of an individual.
- This method does not require any apparatus or laboratory, is inexpensive and easy.

Demerits

- This method is not applicable for children, animals or mentally retarded people as they lack introspection.
- It is purely a private affair and cannot be verified by other observers.
- In many cases the patients may not have the insight to know their condition or language to describe it accurately.
- Introspection involves attention to a mental process. When we attend to the mental process we withdraw attention from the object and no sooner we do so the mental process vanishes making introspection impossible.
- It is logically defective because one and the same person is the experimenter and observer. It is not possible for the same individual to act as an experimenter as well as an observer.

Difficulties in introspection can be overcome by habit and discipline of mind. It requires the power of abstraction and mental alertness.

2. Observational Method

Observation is the objective method of studying the behavior of individuals. It is defined as the systematic observation of an individual's behavior under natural or controlled condition, analyzed and interpreted by the observer.

It is essentially a way of perceiving the behavior as it is. In this method the observer observes and collects the data, analyzed and interpreted according to the perception of the observer. This method becomes more objective when it is done in a systematic way with a predetermined criterion.

Steps in Observation Method

Steps involved in observation method are presented in **Figure 1.6**.

1. **Observation of behavior:** The observer, observes the behavior in a natural setting

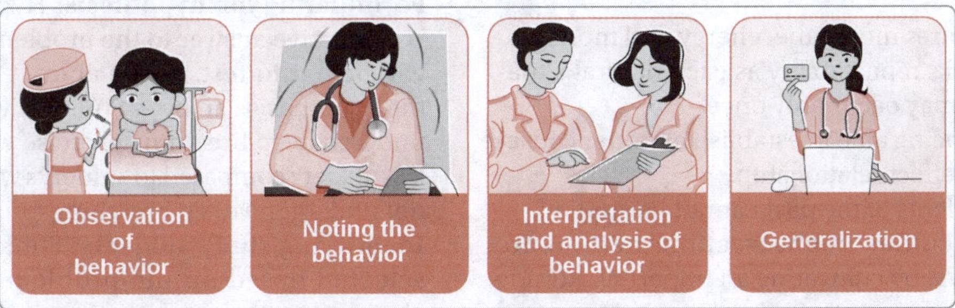

Figure 1.6: Steps in observation method

or in a controlled environment. Here the behavior is perceived as it is.
2. **Noting of behavior:** It deals with recording the information/behavior according to the perception of the observer.
3. **Interpretation and analysis of behavior:** Recorded information is analyzed objectively and scientifically to interpret the behavior patterns.
4. **Generalization:** Based on analysis and interpretation it is possible to make certain generalizations.

For example, a researcher wants to observe the activities of nurses in an intensive care unit. He can use either direct or indirect observation technique using observational checklist to assess the activities of nurses. In another example, chronic ward nurse wants to use observational method to observe the behavioral problems of severely mentally ill individuals. The nurse can use direct observational checklist to assess the behavioral problems.

Merits

- Economical, natural and flexible
- Data can be analyzed, measured, classified and interpreted
- The results can be verified and relied
- Can be used on animals, children, mentally ill and unconscious patients
- Observation method is quite suitable for observing developmental characteristics like children's habits and interests.

Demerits

- Chances of subjective reporting and prejudices of observer creeping in are many.
- Requires more time, energy and money.
- It lacks repeatability as each natural situation may occur only once.
- Not being able to establish a proper cause-and-effect relationship.
- Problems of the past cannot be studied.

Difficulties in observation method are overcome by cultivating an impartial attitude of mind by constructive imagination and cautious observation.

3. Experimental Method

Experimental method is considered as the most scientific and objective method of studying behavior. The word experiment comes from a Latin word meaning 'to try', 'put to test'. Therefore, in experimentation we try or put to test the material or phenomenon, the characteristics of consequences of which we wish to ascertain. The use of this method has raised psychology to the status of an experimental science like physics, chemistry and physiology.

Experimental method studies the cause and effect relationship between the variables of human behavior such as effect of anxiety on intake of alcohol. To study the cause and effect relationship, psychologists use objective observations under controlled conditions to observe actions or behaviors of individuals. From these observations certain conclusions are drawn and theories or principles established.

Essential Features of Experimental Method

- Requires two persons, the experimenter and the subject (the person whose behavior is being observed).
- Experiments are conducted on living organisms.
- All experiments are conducted under controlled conditions.

Steps in Experimentation

- **Stating the problem:** The first step in an experiment is stating the problem. For example, to study the effects of deep breathing exercise on reducing anxiety among students.
- **Formulating the hypothesis:** Hypothesis is a tentative answer to the problem which will be put to test. In the above example the hypothesis can be—'Students who will undergo deep breathing exercise will have less anxiety compared to students who have not undergone deep breathing exercises.'
- **Identifying study subjects:** Subjects are selected based on the problem. In the above example, students form the study subjects. After finalizing the subjects, the

researcher identifies the dependent and independent variables. The independent variable stands for the cause and the dependent variable is characterized as the effect of the cause. In the above example 'anxiety' is the dependent variable while deep breathing is the independent variable.

- **Allotting subjects to experimental (treatment) and control groups:** Generally, the subjects in the experiment are divided among two groups, one control and the other experimental. In this step, the researcher allots students to experimental and control group. Experimental group students will undergo deep breathing exercise program while the control group students will not receive any intervention.
- **Measuring the dependent variable:** In a controlled environment the variables are observed and measured objectively. In the above example, anxiety of students among both the groups is measured. While experimenting, it is important that only the specified independent variables be allowed to change. Factors other than the independent variable must be held constant.
- **Comparing the results of two groups:** The dependent variables of experiment and control group subjects are compared statistically. For example, experimental and control group students' anxiety scores can be compared. Based on the results the hypothesis may be proved or disproved. The various steps involved in experimental method are depicted in **Flowchart 1.3**.

Merits
- Scientific method
- Establishes cause and effect relationship
- Maximum control of phenomena
- Repetition is possible

Demerits
- All problems in psychology cannot be studied by this method as some of them may not be subject to experimentation.
- Experimental method is a costly and time consuming method. Moreover, handling of this method demands specialized knowledge and skill. In the absence of such expertise this method is not functional.
- Experimental method fails to study behavior in naturalistic conditions.

Flowchart 1.3: Steps in experimental method

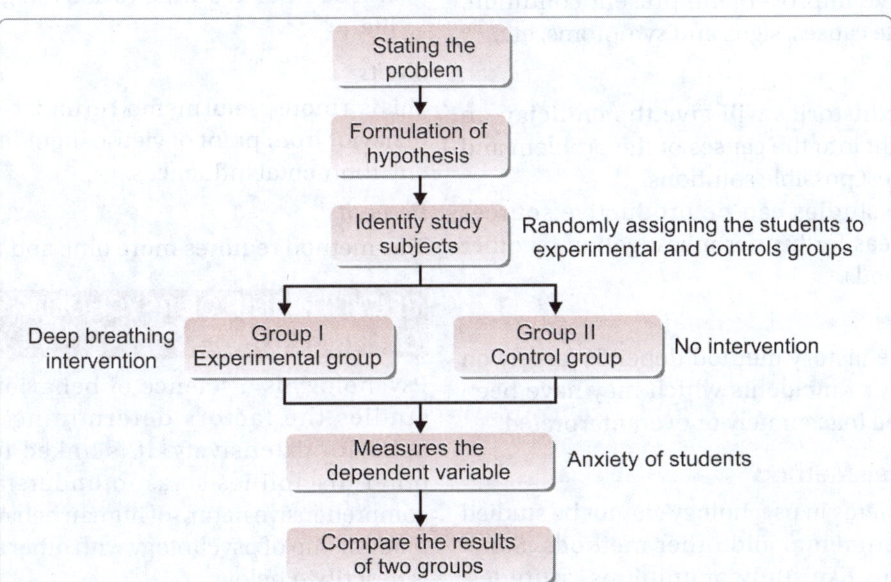

- It cannot always be used especially if the experiment might be dangerous to the subjects.

In spite of various limitations it is a fact that the results obtained by experimental method are reliable, verifiable, definite, precise and capable of quantitative treatment compared to those obtained by other methods.

4. Clinical or Case History Method

This method is used by clinical psychologists, psychiatrists, psychiatric social workers in child guidance clinics or mental hygiene clinics and allied institutions. It aims at studying the cause and basis of people's anxieties, fears and personal maladjustments. A great deal of relevant data is collected using case histories, interviews, home visits and psychological tests to draw valid inferences about the nature of individual's difficulties and problems, the probable origin and course of development. This may suggest some course of action to be pursued in helping the individual.

In this technique, information is collected from the memory of the individual, his parents, family members, friends, teachers and all other available records and reports. Information thus collected includes past history of the disease, treatment already taken, changes if any like improvement, present condition, probable causes, signs and symptoms, etc.

Merits

- Case histories will give the clinician an insight into the causes of the problem and suggest possible solutions.
- Case studies can be productive sources of ideas for further investigation by other methods.

Demerits

The case history method depends largely on memory of incidents which may have been observed inaccurately or over interpreted.

5. Survey Method

All problems in psychology cannot be studied by experimental and other methods. Some problems like study of opinions, attitudes, healthcare needs, etc., need to be studied by means of survey method. This is commonly employed in social psychology.

Survey method involves collection or gathering of information from a large number of people using questionnaires, inventories, checklists, rating scales and interviews.

Merits

A large amount of data can be collected in a short period of time.

Demerits

Behavior is not observed directly.

6. Genetic or Developmental Method

Psychologists study not only the behavior of an individual at a particular time but also his development from birth to death, the influence of heredity and environment in the development of the person and conditions favorable and unfavorable for normal and abnormal behavior. For example, to understand the learning behavior of an adult, the study will have to begin from his childhood. This can be done in two ways:

1. Cross-sectional study wherein children of different age groups will be studied simultaneously.
2. Longitudinal study wherein the same child will be studied during various stages of his life.

Merits

This is a more useful method to understand the behavior from point of view of hereditary and environmental influences.

Demerits

This method requires more time and energy.

RELATIONSHIP OF PSYCHOLOGY WITH OTHER SUBJECTS

Psychology is a science of behavior which studies the factors determining human behavior extensively. It is linked to many other disciplines so as to understand the comprehensive nature of human behavior. The relationship of psychology with other subjects is described below:

In the Field of Education

Theories of learning, motivation and personality, etc., have been responsible for shaping and designing the educational system according to the needs and requirements of the students. Application of psychology in the field of education has helped the learners to learn, teachers to teach, administrators to administer and educational planners to plan effectively and efficiently.

In the Field of Medicine

A doctor, nurse or any person who attends to the patient needs to know the science of behavior for achieving good results. Psychology has contributed valuable therapeutic measures like behavior therapy, play therapy, group therapy, psychoanalysis, etc., for the diagnosis and cure of patients suffering from psychosomatic as well as mental diseases.

In the Field of Business and Industry

It has highlighted the importance of knowledge of consumer's psychology and harmonious interpersonal relationship in the field of commerce and industry.

In the Field of Criminology

It has helped in detection of crimes and in dealing with criminals.

In the Field of Politics

It has aided leaders and politicians in acquiring leadership qualities for leading the masses.

In the Field of Guidance and Counseling

It has provided valuable help in relation to guidance and counseling in educational, personal as well as vocational areas.

In the Field of Military Science

Psychology helps in the selection, training, promotion and classification of defense personnel. In fighting the enemy, the morale of the defense personnel and of citizens must at all costs be high which can only be achieved by providing suggestions, insight and confidence.

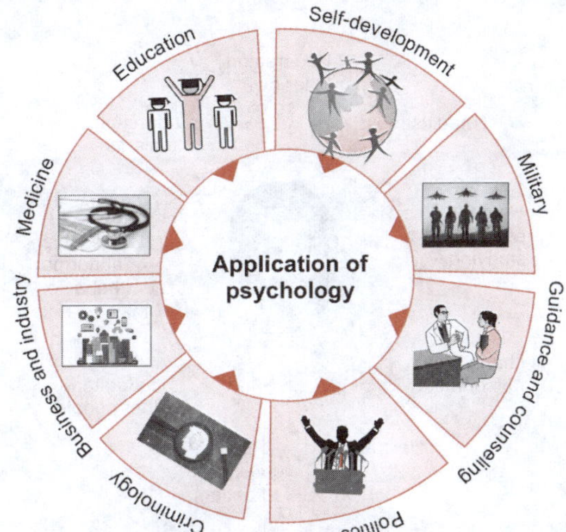

Figure 1.7: Application of psychology in various fields

In the Field of Human Relationship and Self-development

Finally, it has helped human beings to learn the art of understanding their own behavior, seeking adjustment with their self and others and enhancing as well as actualizing their potentialities to the utmost possible **(Figure 1.7)**.

SIGNIFICANCE OF PSYCHOLOGY IN NURSING

While psychology and its applications have become more relevant and respected than any period in the past, they have become an imminent part of every profession including nursing today. This is because of increasing emphasis being laid out on the interplay of body, mind and spirit in the health status of every individual.

The success in life of many people depends on how they get along with others, influence others and react to others. The ability to understand ourselves and others comes from a wise study of psychology. The learning of psychology helps a nurse in the following ways **(Figure 1.8)**:

Understand Her Own Self

The knowledge of psychology allows the nurse to get an insight into her own motives, desires, emotions, feelings, attitudes, personality

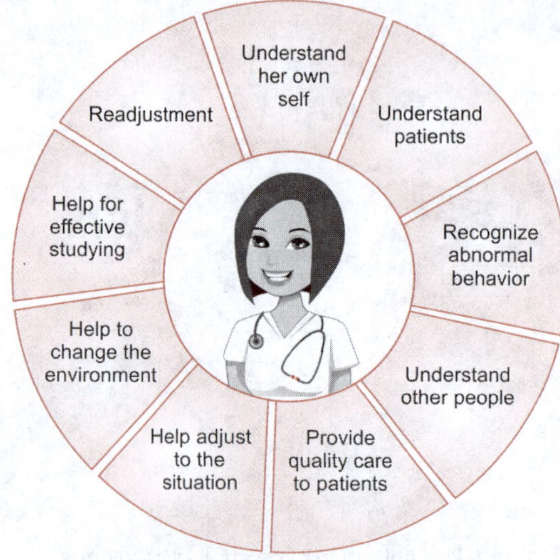

Figure 1.8: Relevance of psychology to nursing

characteristics and ambitions. She realizes that her personality is highly individualistic and complex, and is able to solve her own problems while becoming capable of arriving at major decisions in life. This knowledge also helps her to realize own strengths and weaknesses. By knowing these aspects she can overcome weaknesses that affect her work, develop good personality characteristics, abilities to carry on her responsibilities and perform duties effectively and efficiently. This permits her to direct her own life more productively and relate more easily with others enabling greater control over situations while attaining self-discipline.

Understand Patients

Nurses are professionals meant for providing care to patients. The patient may be male or female, young or old suffering from an acute or a chronic disease and may have come to the hospital with physical or psychological problems. They may also have tensions, worries, pains and many doubts about their illness. The knowledge of psychology will help the nurse to understand the needs and problems of patients and attend to them. She can better understand motives, attitudes, perceptions and personality characteristics of patients. This will help the patient attain quick relief and cure which is the basic motto of a nurse.

Recognize Abnormal Behavior

Psychology is relevant not only in the field of physical health care but also in the field of mental health. Presently more and more people are suffering from mental illnesses. While many of them may be minor in nature some are diagnosed as severe. The knowledge of psychology will help nurses to understand abnormal behaviors and management of mental illnesses. Nurses working in mental hospitals undoubtedly require an adequate knowledge of normal and abnormal psychology.

The knowledge of psychology helps the nurses to recognize mental illnesses at general hospitals and community health centers while providing appropriate guidance to deal with stress, anxiety and other life related problems.

Understand Other People

The student nurse has to study, work and live with other nurses, doctors, patients and their family members. With scientific knowledge on human nature she will understand them better and be more successful in interpersonal relationships. She will learn why others differ from her in their likes and dislikes, interests and abilities and in reactions to others. She will realize how differences in behavior are to a certain extent a result of differences in customs and beliefs or cultural patterns of the groups to which she belongs or the way she has been brought up during her early years.

Provide Quality Care to Patients

A nurse with good knowledge of human psychology can understand the feelings of her patients, their fears and anxieties, what they would like to know and why they behave the way they do.

It will help the nurse to anticipate and meet the requirements of patients and their relatives enabling them to adjust to the unavoidable circumstances in the best possible way. A good understanding by the nurse can lend the patients much necessary support.

Help Patients Adjust to the Situation

Illness and physical handicaps often bring about the need for major adjustments. Many diseases such as heart disease and cancer, etc., require special coping skills and health care. A nurse trained in psychology can be an effective health educator and help in these kind of adjustments.

Help the Student Nurse to Appreciate the Necessity for Changing the Environment or Surroundings

Good nursing care depends upon the ability of a nurse to understand the situations properly and seek the co-operation of other people concerned. The change in environment is sometimes necessary for better adjustment and happiness. For example, a boy who is completely denied the affectionate care of his parents may do better if he is given the care of foster parents.

Help for Effective Studying

A nurse has to learn many new concepts during her training. She has to obtain the correct knowledge of various facts, disease conditions and their treatment. The study of psychology of learning will help the nurse acquire knowledge in an effective way.

Readjustment

Every profession and career requires readjustment. A nurse needs to make the following adjustments for achieving success in her career:

1. Overcoming homesickness and self-reliance are necessary if she has to live hassle free in a hostel or a hospital.
2. Getting used to sick persons who are helpless and desperate and even those who may ventilate their anger by making the nurse a target of their abuses and curses.
3. Try to study and work together.

Knowledge of psychology can be helpful in such efforts as an insight into their emotions will resolve lot of disputes and dilemmas. The wellbeing of a patient is the prime responsibility of a nurse. She must not only treat him physically but also instill confidence in his capacity to improve and recover fully. For this, knowledge of human psychology is essential. The physical and mental wellbeing of a patient mainly depends on the nurse. She has to deal with different people having different problems both physical and mental. To serve them satisfactorily, knowledge of psychology is very essential.

APPLIED PSYCHOLOGY TO SOLVE EVERYDAY ISSUES

Applied psychology is the application of psychological principles and methods to resolve problems of human experience which may be related to health, family, workplace, etc. It is that field of psychology which validates psychological theories and focuses on putting practical research into action to achieve the desired results. The relevance of applied psychology in various walks of life is presented in **Table 1.2**.

Table 1.2: Application of psychology to solve everyday issues

Branch of psychology	Application to solve everyday issues
Educational psychology	• Helps in developing strategies for better teaching approaches • Improves learning environment and gives advice on curriculum formulation • Addresses the needs of students with different abilities and relieves their examination stress
Occupational psychology	• Helps in increasing employee productivity, job satisfaction at work and overall effectiveness of an organization • Aids in organizational functions such as staff recruitment, training, employee relations, performance appraisal, motivation, counseling and maintaining work environment

Contd...

Contd...

Branch of psychology	Application to solve everyday issues
Health psychology	◆ Helps diseased individuals to cope with illness, develop positive attitude, recover from illness and lead quality life ◆ Educates and motivates people to make better health choices, contribute to improving the healthcare system and aid the government in designing healthcare policy
Cognitive psychology	◆ Aids in treating learning disorders, structure the educational curricula to augment learning, and improve decision making ability ◆ Provides help to cope with increased stress levels, memory disorders, brain injury and attentional difficulties
Clinical psychology	◆ Helps in diagnoses, prevention and treatment of emotional disturbances and behavioral problems ◆ Helps the individual to promote wellbeing and personal development
Sports psychology	◆ Helps athletes and sports persons to cope with the intense pressure generated out of competition ◆ Enhances the performance of an athlete, motivates him and hastens the recovery from injuries too ◆ Teaches the common man to enjoy sport and promote wellbeing by sticking to an exercise regimen
Developmental psychology	◆ Aims to resolve individual's issues mostly related to society, school, career, family and health
Criminal psychology	◆ Assists the law enforcement agencies in apprehending criminals ◆ Provides an understanding of will, intention, thoughts, feelings and reactions of criminals with the main goal of reducing crime
Social psychology	◆ Talks about social perceptions and interactions that are key to understanding social behavior ◆ Looks at a wide range of other topics such as leadership, aggression, prejudice, non-verbal behavior ◆ Deals with problems related to social justice, women development, intergroup relations, etc.

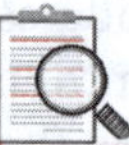

SYNOPSIS

- The term behavior includes motor, cognitive and affective activities.
- Psychology is the science of animal and human behavior.
- Wilhelm Wundt is the father of psychology.
- The nature of subject psychology is scientific as it uses scientific methods.
- The field of operation and application of subject psychology is too vast.
- It studies, describes and explains the behavior of living organisms.
- The branches of pure psychology include general, abnormal, social and physiological psychology. It also includes parapsychology, geopsychology, developmental and experimental psychology.
- The applied branches of psychology include educational, clinical, industrial, legal, military and political psychology.
- The methods of psychology include introspection, observation, experimental, case history and genetic methods.
- Subject psychology is applicable to education, medicine, industry, criminology, political, military and self-development areas.
- The learning of psychology helps a nurse in understand her own self, understand patients, recognize abnormal behavior, understand other people, provide quality care, help patients adjust to the situation, appreciate the environment, help for effective studying and readjustment.
- Applied psychology is the application of psychology principles and methods to resolve problems of human experience.

Review Questions

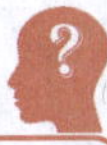

Long Essays

1. Define psychology. Explain methods of observation and case study.
2. Define psychology and explain its nature and scope with special reference to nursing.
3. Critically examine observation method and experimental method.
4. Define psychology. What are the different methods used in the study of psychology? Critically evaluate them.

Short Essays

1. Explain any two branches of psychology.
2. Explain nature of psychology.
3. Describe merits and demerits of experimental method.
4. Explain case study method.
5. Explain the relevance of psychology to nursing.
6. Explain experimental method in psychology.
7. Bring out the similarities and differences between introspection and observation.
8. What is the general importance of psychology? Why should a student nurse study psychology?
9. Scope of psychology.
10. Define introspection method—list the advantages and disadvantages.

Short Notes

1. Write any two definitions of psychology
2. Child psychology
3. Methods of psychology
4. Define any two branches of psychology
5. Case history method
6. List the branches of psychology
7. Behavior
8. Interview method
9. Experimental method
10. Introspection
11. Observation method

Multiple Choice Questions

1. **Psychology is defined as the scientific study of:**
   a. Mental disorders
   b. Mental processes
   c. Human relationships
   d. Human and animal behavior
2. **Which of the following deals with the study of how a person's actions, feelings or thoughts are influenced by others?**
   a. Social psychology
   b. Clinical psychology
   c. Educational psychology
   d. Health psychology
3. **What is general psychology?**
   a. That which deals with fundamental rules and principles of psychology
   b. That which deals with general behavior of people
   c. That which deals with general activities of an organism
   d. That which deals with normal behavior of a person
4. **Behavior includes which of the following 'activities'?**
   a. Motor
   b. Cognitive
   c. Affective
   d. All of the above
5. **Who is the Father of Psychology?**
   a. Sigmund Freud
   b. William James
   c. Ivan Pavlov
   d. Wilhelm Wundt
6. **Understanding subject psychology is important for a nurse because:**
   a. It helps the nurse to understand herself
   b. It helps the nurse to understand others

c. It helps the nurse to improve situations by solving problems
d. All of the above

7. **Which of the following is a scientific method of psychology?**
a. Introspection method
b. Observation method
c. Experimental method
d. Interview method

8. **What is introspection?**
a. Self-motivation
b. Self-observation
c. Self-interest
d. Self-learning

9. **First step of the scientific method involves:**
a. Replication of procedures
b. Formulating an explanation
c. Carrying out research
d. Identifying questions of interest

10. **The purpose of control group in an experiment is to:**
a. Give a comparison that allows the independent variable to be judged
b. Prevent the researcher from cheating
c. Accommodate the extra participants
d. Assist in the design of research project

11. **Scientists who are most likely to study the relationship between stress levels and an individual's likelihood of contracting a disease are _____ psychologists.**
a. Counseling b. Health
c. Cognitive d. Developmental

12. **Mental experiences operate on different levels of awareness. The level that best portrays one's attitudes, feelings and desires is the:**
a. Conscious b. Unconscious
c. Preconscious d. Foreconscious

13. **Wundt described psychology as the study of conscious experience, a perspective he called _____.**

14. **Early psychologists' studied the mind by asking people to describe what they were experiencing when exposed to various stimuli. This procedure is known as _____.**

15. **The statement, 'In order to study human behavior, we must consider the whole of perception rather than its component parts' might be made by a person subscribing to the _____ perspective.**

16. **Which perspective suggests that abnormal behavior is largely the result of unconscious forces?**

17. **'Psychologists should worry only about behavior, i.e. directly observable.' This statement would most likely be made by a person using which psychological perspective?**

18. **The group in an experiment that receives no treatment is called the _____ group.**

19. **_____ psychology describes the relationship of physical environment with behavior.**

20. **_____ psychology explains physiological basis of behavior.**

ANSWER KEY

1. d	2. a	3. a	4. d	5. d	6. d
7. c	8. b	9. d	10. a	11. b	12. b
13. Structuralism	14. Introspection	15. Gestalt	16. Psychodynamic	17. Behavioral	18. Control
19. Geo	20. Physiological				

CHAPTER

2 Biological Basis of Behavior

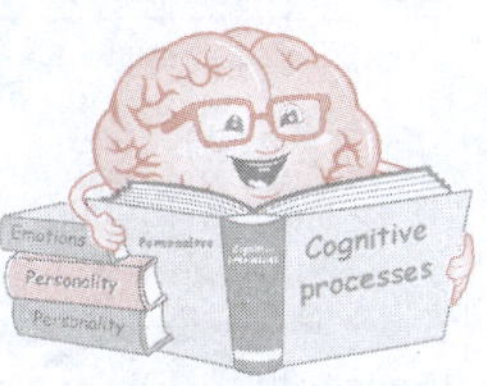

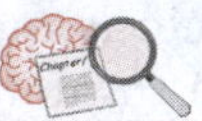

CHAPTER OUTLINE

- Body-Mind relationship
- Genetics and behavior
- Brain and behavior
- Nervous system
- Nature of behavior of an organism
- Psychology and sensation
- Types of sensation and sensory disorders

Biology of behavior is the study of behavioral functions of the nervous system particularly the brain. 'Physiological psychology' is that branch of psychology which seeks to determine how activity in the nervous system is related to both the behavior and the mind.

Many aspects of human behavior and mental functioning cannot be fully understood without some knowledge of the underlying biological processes. Our nervous system, sense organs, muscles and glands enable us to be aware of and adjust to our environment. Our perception of events depends on how our sense organs detect stimuli and how our brain interprets information originating from the senses.

BODY-MIND RELATIONSHIP

- Psychology studies human behavior involving both the body and the mind. They are interrelated and interact upon each other as mental functions and physical states affect each other.
- Body and the mind are two aspects of the living, dynamic and adjusting personality. Mind is regarded as a function of the body and does not exist in isolation from it. It is the sum total of various mental processes such as observing, knowing, thinking, reasoning, feeling, imagining, remembering, judging, etc. Mind also grows just as the body grows.
- Body is represented by physical states and bodily functions. Nervous system and glands are an important part of our body. They are also responsible for ways of thinking, feeling and doing.
- All behaviors have an anatomical and physiological basis. Physiological structures, body fluids, chemicals and mechanical events influence our overt behavior, feelings and experiences. Our mental functions like strong feelings, emotions, attitudes, motives, thinking, etc., influence our bodily activities and processes.
- Emotions are a combination of bodily responses and mental processes. While the body provides energy to fight or cope, mind contributes to the understanding and offers an explanation for one's own actions and that of others. Just as the body produces epinephrine to fight danger, the mind helps to decide whether it is needed or not **(Figure 2.1)**.

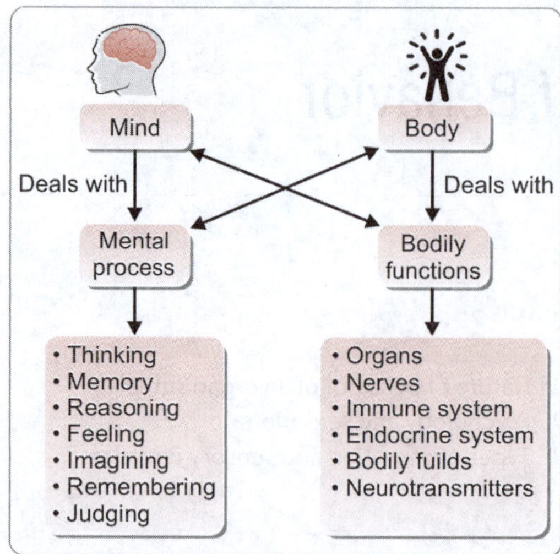

Figure 2.1: Body-mind relationship

Effects of Bodily Conditions on Mental Functioning

- Increased blood pressure causes mental excitement.
- Severe pain reduces the ability to concentrate.
- Chronic illness causes depression.
- Malfunctioning of the endocrine glands may exert full influence on one's personality resulting in lethargy, nervousness, tension, etc.
- Physical fatigue affects our mood and reduces our motivation, interest and concentration.
- Brain injury affects many psychological functions. At the same time well developed brain leads to the development of better intellectual functioning.

Effects of Mental Conditions on Bodily Functioning

- Mental processes are intimately connected to the brain and cortical processes. For example, unpleasant emotions like fear, anger and worry cause irritability, insomnia, headache, etc. Similarly depression affects thinking and memory.
- Emotional conflicts are responsible for peptic ulcer, ulcerative colitis, etc.
- Deep thinking and concentration can cause physical strain.
- According to Franz Alexander repressed feelings of hostility and aggression are expressed through the nervous system causing hypertension and cardiac diseases. Repressed feelings of dependency and wish to receive love affect parasympathetic nervous system resulting in gastrointestinal disorders or respiratory disorders.
- Unconscious motivation and conflicts give rise to many physical complaints and neurotic disorders like conversion disorders.

Relationship between body and the mind has an effect on health and illness. If the relationship is harmonious it leads to good health while an adverse relationship leads to illness. If all the body and mental processes are functioning within normal range the individual will experience good health. Disruption in any one of the processes will lead to illness.

Psychosomatic medicine deals with physical diseases caused by psychological factors. In such cases the patients should be treated for both the body and the mind, e.g., in case of peptic ulcer the treatment is given both by way of drugs and psychotherapy.

While understanding the interrelationship between the body and the mind she should also understand the emotional factors underlying the disease. It is always necessary to study the patient's physical and psychological problems so as to provide comprehensive care.

GENETICS AND BEHAVIOR: HEREDITY AND ENVIRONMENT

Heredity

Heredity is considered as 'the sum total of inborn individual traits'. Biologically, it has been defined as 'the sum total of traits potentially present in the fertilized ovum'. According to Douglas and Holland 'one's heredity consists of all the structures, physical characteristics, functions or capacities derived from parents, other ancestry or species'.

All organisms follow a life cycle which includes growth, development, reproduction and decline. Though there is essential unity in life, the ways in which each organism exercises its capacities is different. These individual qualities of organisms and their basic properties are transmitted by means of heredity.

Mechanism of Heredity and Inheritance of Behavior

The life cycle of an individual begins with the fusion of a sperm and ovum. The origin of every human life can be traced to a single cell called zygote. When a sperm unites with an ovum, zygote is produced. The genes which are the carriers of distinctive traits are present both in the sperm and the ovum. In the fertilized ovum there are 23 pairs of chromosomes, half of which are given by the father and the other half by the mother. While females have 23 pairs of XX chromosomes, males have 22 pairs of XX chromosomes along with two single chromosomes represented by X and Y, the sex chromosomes **(Figure 2.2)**.

Occasionally through some unfortunate bodily error an aberration in chromosomes appears. If an extra chromosome appears making the total 47 rather than the normal 46, mongolism (Down's syndrome or trisomy 21 anomaly) results. A child with Mongolism suffers from deceleration of growth during the prenatal period resulting in a highly complex, multidimensional disorder involving all organs.

When chromosomes are studied under a microscope bands of markings appear

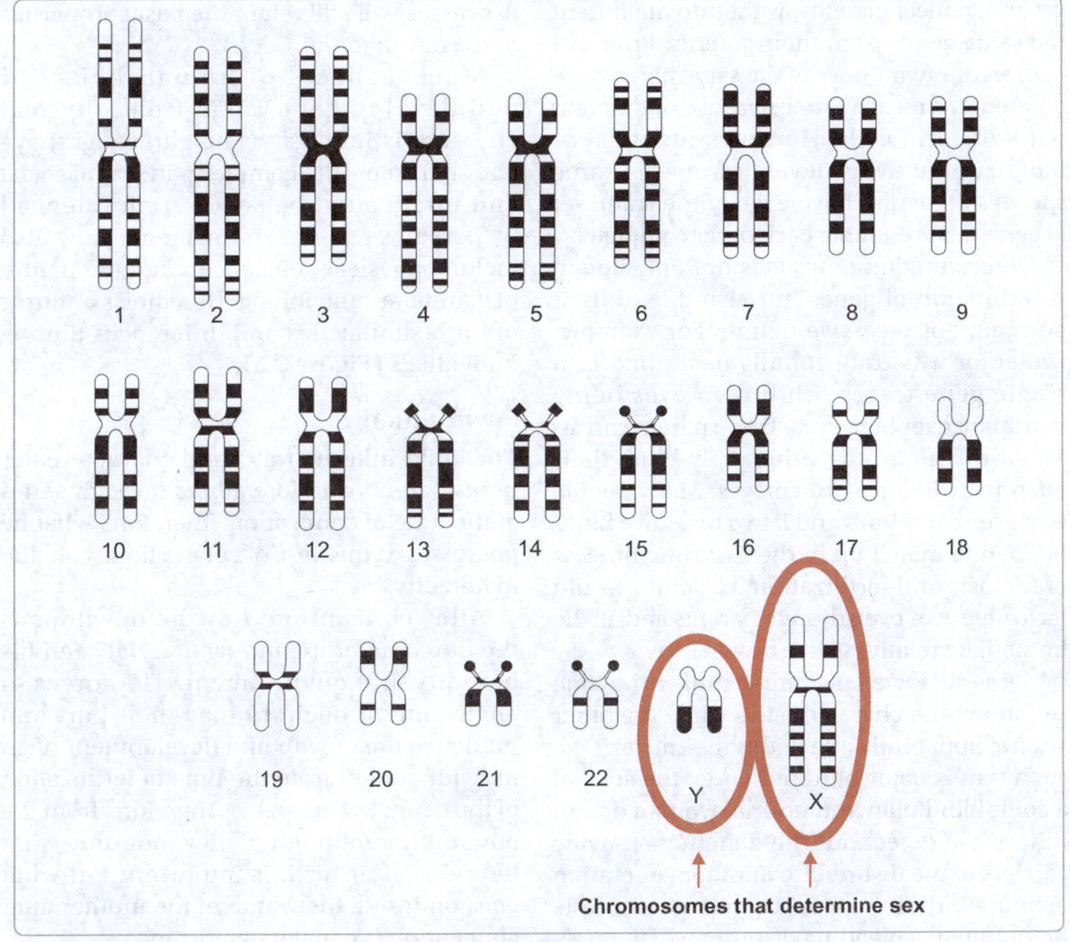

Figure 2.2: Mechanism of heredity

representing an entity called genes which appear to be the actual determiners of traits. Each chromosome is made up of many genes. A man has probably not less than 2,000 and not more than 50,000 genes in the chromosomes. Each gene is the determiner of a specific characteristic such as straight nose or a deep lobed ear. At present, it appears that there is no simple one-to-one relationship between genes and traits, i.e., one gene may influence many characteristics or traits or conversely many genes may combine to determine one characteristic.

Action of the genes on the cytoplasm changes the shape and other characteristics of the cells. The heredity basis of individual differences lies in the unlimited variety of possible gene combinations that can occur. No two siblings get an identical heredity as they do not inherit the same genes from their parents. Fraternal or dizygotic twins born to the same parents are different from each other because of different pairs of germ cells. However, identical or monozygotic twins develop from the same sperm and ovum, have exactly the same set of genes and resemble each other completely.

Determination of traits is not only due to combination of genes but also due to their dominant or recessive nature. For example, eye color was traditionally described as a single gene trait, with brown eyes being dominant over blue eyes. If one parent carries only brown and the other only blue, their offspring will have brown eyes. Many people however, carry both and if two recessive blues happen to match up in the assorting process of meiosis and fertilization, the child would have blue eyes even though parents and all the immediate relatives have brown eyes.

Some characteristics are sex linked, i.e., one sex shows the characteristics while the other sex not apparently affected is the carrier. One such trait is color blindness, e.g., the sons of a color blind man and normal woman do not inherit the defect but the daughters may be carriers of the disorder to another generation of males, their sons. Another example is hemophilia: a bleeding disorder which rarely occurs in women but is transmitted by them to their sons (Stern, 1960).

Occasionally a change occurs in the reproductive cells of a living thing which causes the introduction of completely new traits in the next generation. Such changes are called mutations. Mutant plants and animals might have characteristics that breeders can use to improve existing varieties. In human beings mutations are almost always undesirable. Their causes are not clear but are known to be induced by atomic radiation.

Heredity is the basis for development of human personality. It is like the raw material in the hands of the artist out of which the potter or tailor prepares the specific objects. Any amount of molding and treatment with special processes will still retain the basic properties of the raw material.

Many aspects of human behavior and development range from physical characteristics such as height, weight, eye and skin color. The complex patterns of social and intellectual behavior are influenced by person's genetic endowment. They also include physical deficiencies and the nature of glandular functioning. Heredity is a source of both similarities and differences among individuals **(Figure 2.3)**.

Environment

The child inherits traits and characteristics of his parents and forefathers through genes at the time of conception. Therefore, what he possesses at the time of conception is all due to heredity.

After conception, how he develops is the outcome of the interaction between his heredity and environment. The forces of environment begin to play their part and influence the growth and development of an individual right from the time of fertilization of the ovum by the sperm. Therefore, from the environmental point of view not only what happens after birth is important but what goes on inside the womb of the mother after conception is equally significant.

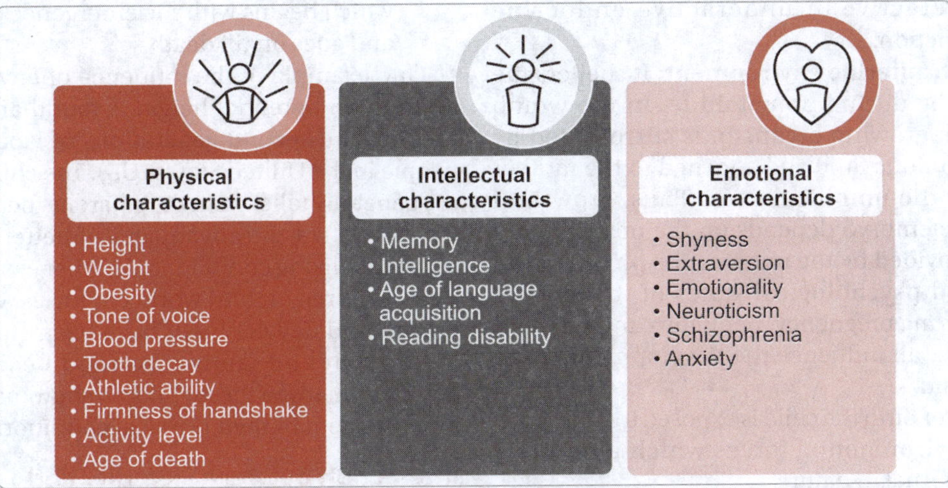

Figure 2.3: Characteristics influenced by genetic factors

Environment covers the social, moral, economical, political, physical and intellectual factors that influence the development of the individual from time to time.

Definitions

- Environment is everything that affects the individual except his genes.
  —Boring, Langfield and Weld
- Environment covers all the outside factors that have acted on the individual since he began life. **—Woodworth**

Types of Environment

There are three types of environment that affect the individual directly or indirectly **(Figure 2.4)**:

1. **Intercellular environment:** It relates to embryonic development. The cytoplasm is in the intercellular environment because the genes surrounded by it are influenced by and in turn influence its characteristics. Endocrine glands and hormones also produce intercellular influence. Many congenital deformities are the result of

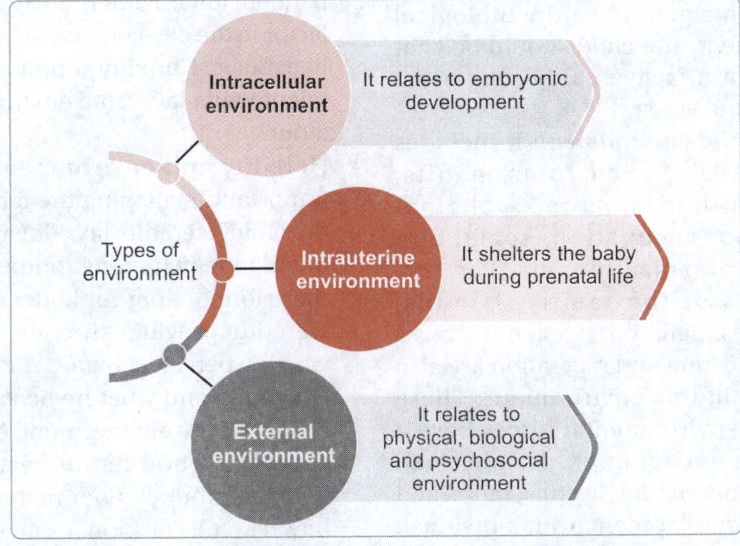

Figure 2.4: Types of environment

overactive or underactive endocrine function.

2. **Intrauterine environment:** It shelters the baby during prenatal life. In the womb the growing organism is surrounded by amniotic fluid and attached to the mother by the umbilical cord. Thus, growth of the embryo depends on the nourishment provided by the mother. The physiological and psychological states of the mother during pregnancy, her habits and interests etc., all influence the development of the child.

   After birth the child is exposed to numerous environmental forces which are purely external in nature.

3. **External environment:** It can be divided into three kinds:
   a. *Physical environment:* Non-living things like water, air, housing, soil, climate, heat, light, radiation, noise, etc., form the physical environment. These affect the body and mind of the growing child. Thus it is necessary to provide a decent home and locality for good physical and mental health of the child.
   b. *Biological environment:* It refers to the living component of man's external environment which consists of plants, animals, insects, bacteria and viruses. It is necessary that the child be allowed to grow in a good, healthy biological environment. The child should be kept away from disease carrying germs, bacteria and viruses.
   c. *Psychosocial environment*: It includes cultural values, customs, habits, beliefs, attitudes, morals, religion, education, occupation, social and political organization, etc. Parents, members of the family, friends, classmates, neighbors, teachers, mass communication and recreation are also included in this environment. These different environmental forces have a desirable impact upon the physical, social, emotional, intellectual, moral and aesthetic development of an individual. Their influence is a continuous one which begins with the emergence of life and goes on till death.

One example of the influence of environment upon potential height is found among the first and second generations of Japanese people in the United States (US). The children are generally taller than their parents because they have had the advantages of better food and better living conditions. Another example is the children of third world countries whose growth and development have been stunted by drought and famine. As food becomes available, many of these children show marked improvement in their physical conditions.

Interaction between Heredity and Environment

Each individual enters the world with certain hereditary characteristics transmitted to him through his parents. He grows up in a certain environment with its human, social and material surroundings. Everything he does as a child or adult results from the complex interactions between heredity and environment.

- The relative influence of heredity and environment differs from one individual to another and from one human trait or condition to another.
- Heredity and environment are interdependent forces. Inheritance is an important factor in the development of artistic abilities like music. Heredity supplies the potential talent while favorable environment brings it out.
- Heredity and environment are equally important in shaping the temperament of the child. Heredity lays down the essential foundations while environment can change these foundations for better or worse.
- Heredity provides the raw material from which a person is made. How the material is molded and what he becomes depends chiefly on the environment. Good material placed in good hands results in a fine finished product. Poor material no matter how carefully fashioned can never become a first rate product.

- Our inheritance prescribes the limits beyond which it may not be possible for any individual to develop however wholesome and stimulating the environment maybe.

Today no one believes that nature or nurture alone completely determines the course of our development. Psychologists agree that development is shaped by the interaction of heredity and environment. Within this interaction our genetic endowment for many characteristics provides us with a reaction range of possible levels that we may ultimately reach depending on the quality of our experience in the environment. Heredity and environment are interdependent forces. The influence of heredity and environment is so interrelated that they are practically inseparable.

The knowledge of the mechanism of heredity and the influence of environment on the personality development is important for a nurse to understand the behavior of a patient.

BRAIN AND BEHAVIOR: NERVOUS SYSTEM, NEURONS AND SYNAPSE

- The entire behavior is effectively managed and controlled by the coordination and functioning of the nervous system.
- How we will behave in a particular situation depends upon the judgment of our brain.
- Sense impressions received through sense organs do not bear any significance unless they are given a meaning by the nervous system.
- Learning also to a great extent is controlled by the nervous system.
- Proper growth and development of nerve tissues and nervous system as a whole helps in the task of proper intellectual development.
- Any defect in the spinal cord or the brain seriously affects the intellectual growth.
- Emotional behavior is also influenced by the nervous system especially at the time of anger, fear and other emotional changes. During emotional outbursts nerve tissues alter levels of hormonal secretion by some glands consequently influencing the emotional behavior of the individual.
- The process of growth and development is also directly and indirectly controlled by the functioning of the nervous system.
- Personality of an individual is greatly influenced through the mechanism of nervous system.
- Through its receptors the nervous system keeps us in touch with our environment, both external and internal. Like other systems in the body the nervous system is composed of organs particularly the brain, spinal cord, nerves and ganglia. These in turn consist of various tissues including nerve, blood and connective tissues. Together these carry out the complex activities of the nervous system.

Human behavior involves the body-mind interaction of the various bodily factors. The most important are:

- The sense organs called receptors
- The muscles and endocrine glands called effectors
- The nervous system which is the connecting or integrating mechanism called connectors

1. Receptors (Psychology of Sensations)

Behavior in all its forms and shapes certainly has a biological or physiological base. It is based on various stimuli present both in the external environment and that lying within our body. Stimuli in the form of various sensory experiences are received by our sensory organs known as receptors.

External Receptors

External receptors are those sensory mechanisms that help us make contact with the outer world, e.g., eyes, ears, nose, tongue and skin. The specific receptor cells for receiving the external stimuli lie within these sensory organs.

Sense organs

- Our sense organs help in assimilating knowledge of the world around us. Each of our sense organs has a distinct function to perform.

- Sense organs consist of receptors which are specialized sensitive cells associated with endings of sensory nerve fibers. These receptors are stimulated by objects outside the body and also by internal conditions.
- When receptors malfunction they lead to sensory defects or disorders—visual, auditory, cutaneous, olfactory, gustatory and kinesthetic disorders.

Internal Receptors

Internal receptors are associated with internal stimuli present in our body. They are responsible for feelings of pain, hunger or nausea. Another variety of these internal receptors helps us in maintaining balance, bodily posture and equilibrium and also exercise control over the muscles.

2. Effectors (Muscular and Glandular Controls of Behavior)

Effectors are termed as organs of responses. What is received through sensory organs in the form of sensory input is responded through bodily reactions and motor activities carried out through muscles and glands particularly the hormones secreted by the ductless glands that are responsible for most of our behavior patterns. The underactivity or overactivity of these glands causes deficiency or excess of hormonal secretion. This affects the entire personality makeup of the individual.

Muscles

Our behavior and activity involves movement of different parts of our body. Muscles help the organism to carry out motor activities in order to respond to various stimuli. There are mainly three types of muscles, viz. smooth muscles, cardiac muscles and skeletal muscles.

1. **Smooth muscles** are primarily concerned with the process of digestion, excretion and blood circulation. Their contraction and relaxation produce constriction and dilation of blood vessels thus increasing or decreasing blood pressure.
2. **Cardiac muscles** function smoothly in a rythmic fashion but when one is emotionally upset their normal functioning is disturbed causing heart trouble.
3. **Skeletal or striped muscles** enable the individual to perform voluntary motor activities ranging from walking to the fine psychomotor skills like typing, etc.

Glands

Glands play an important role in human behavior. They also assist in the digestion of food, elimination of waste products, production and prolongation of emotional states and regulation of metabolism of the body. There are two types of glands: Duct glands and ductless glands.

1. **Duct glands** release their chemical secretion through little ducts or tubes into the body cavities or on the surface of the body. Some of the duct glands are:
   - Salivary glands
   - Gastric glands
   - Sweat glands
   - Lacrimal glands
   - Kidneys
   - Sex glands

   The duct glands either become overactive or underactive under the influence of emotions. There is a close and intimate connection between human behavior and secretions of duct glands.
2. **Ductless or endocrine glands** secrete chemical substances called hormones. The hormones are released into the bloodstream and are carried to all parts of the body. They play a vital role in the determination of human personality. They affect the development of the body, mind, metabolism, secondary sex characteristics and emotional behavior. The endocrine glands are:
   - Pituitary gland
   - Thyroid gland
   - Parathyroid gland
   - Adrenal glands
   - Male sex glands or gonads
   - Pancreas

   The functioning of all the endocrine or ductless glands exercises a great influence on the various aspects of growth and development of human personality. The underactivity or overactivity of these glands caused by the deficiency or excess of the hormones secreted by them affects not only the growth and development of the individual but also the entire behavior. A slight imbalance of the hormones may cause unusual restlessness, anxiety and weakness. Our physical strength, thinking and reasoning powers and decision making ability all depend upon the health of the glands **(Figure 2.5)**.

3. Connectors

Connectors or adjusters help in regulating, controlling or coordinating the activities of receptors and effectors. The ability to play a piano, drive a car or hit a tennis ball depends on muscle coordination. It is necessary for the body to provide messages to the muscles to coordinate. These messages are passed through specialized cells called 'neurons'.

Neuron

- A nerve cell with all its branches is called a neuron. These are the basic elements of the nervous system.
- A neuron has a nucleus, a cell body and a cell membrane to enclose the whole cell. There are tiny fibers extending out from the cell body called 'dendrites'.
- Their role is to receive messages through electrical impulses from the sense organs or adjacent neurons and carry them to the cell body.
- The messages from the cell body further travel the length of a nerve fiber known as the axon **(Figure 2.6)**.
- A group of axons bundled together like parallel wires in an electrical cable is referred to as the nerve.
- The axon (not all of them) is surrounded by a fatty covering called the 'myelin sheath'. It serves to increase the velocity with which the electrical impulses travel through the axons.

There are three types of neurons:

1. **Sensory neurons:** They help in the process of sensation and perception.
2. **Motor neurons:** They are responsible for physical movements and activation of glands.
3. **Interneurons or association neurons:** They carry signals in the form of memories and thoughts and add reflex or automatic activities.

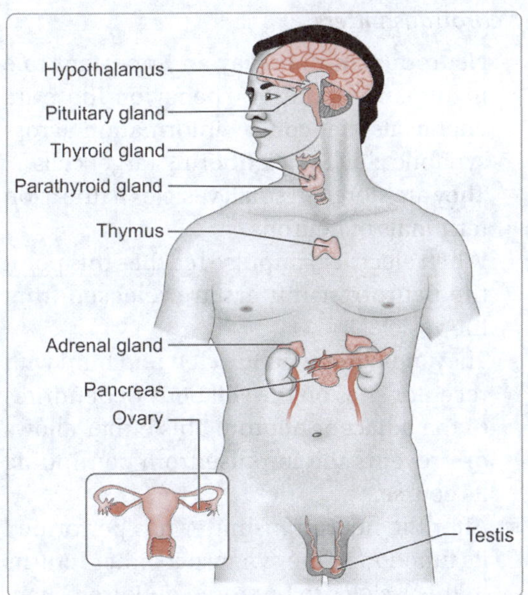

Figure 2.5: Location of major endocrine glands

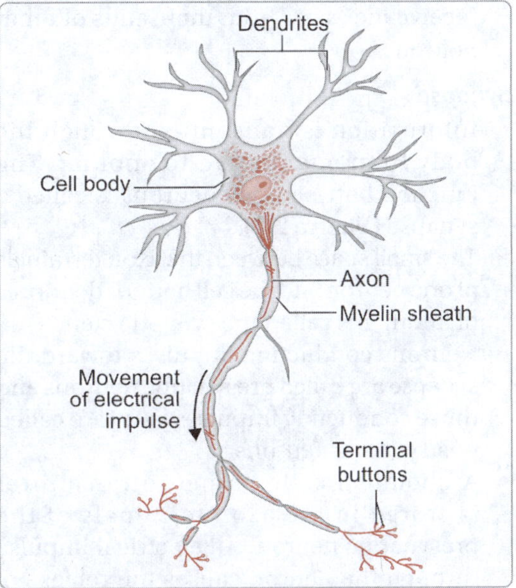

Figure 2.6: Structure of neuron

Neural Impulse

- Neurons are the receivers and transmitters of messages. These messages are always in the form of electrochemical impulses.
- A neuron in its resting position is supposed to maintain a sort of electrical equilibrium, i.e., state of polarization. This state of polarization may be disturbed on account of the effect of trigger like action of a stimulus applied to the membrane. It causes a sudden change in the electrical potentiality of the neuron resulting in depolarization and initiation of neural impulses. These impulses are carried along the neuron axons.
- There is a fluid-filled space called the synapse between the axon of the neuron and the receiving dendrite of the next neuron.
- Enlargements of the axon endings of transmitting neurons are called boutons. These contain neurotransmitter chemicals which are stored in small vesicles.
- A nerve impulse reaching these boutons causes a neurotransmitter to be released into the synapse. This enables the neurons to send messages to many other neurons.
- It makes it possible for a single neuron to receive messages from thousands of other neurons.

Synapse

- Information is transmitted through the body from one neuron to another. The junction between two neurons is called a synapse **(Figure 2.7)**.
- The small space between the axon terminals of one neuron and the cell body or dendrites of another is called the synaptic cleft.
- Neurons conducting impulses toward the synapse are called presynaptic neurons and those conducting impulses away are called postsynaptic neurons.
- A chemical called a neurotransmitter is stored in the axon terminals of the presynaptic neuron. An electrical impulse through the neuron causes the release of this neurotransmitter into the synaptic cleft.

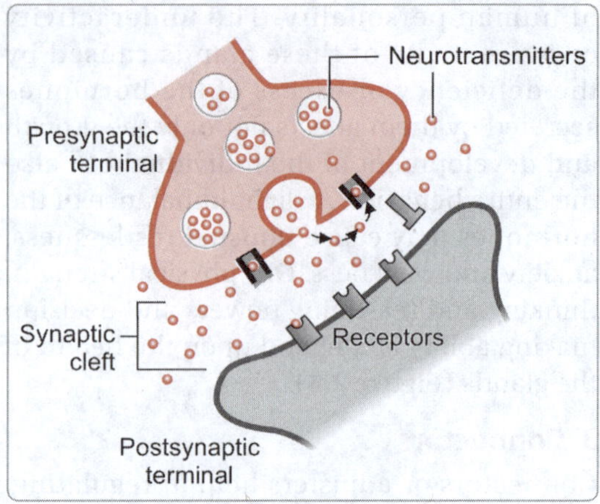

Figure 2.7: Synapse.

- The neurotransmitter then diffuses across the synaptic cleft and combines with receptor sites that are situated on the cell membrane of the postsynaptic neuron.
- The cell body or dendrite of the postsynaptic neuron also contains a chemical inactivator which is specific to the neurotransmitter released by the presynaptic neuron.
- When the synaptic transmission is complete the chemical inactivation quickly inactivates the neurotransmitter to prevent unwanted continuous impulses.

Neurotransmitters

- Neurotransmitters play an important role in human emotion and behavior. These are chemicals that convey information across synaptic cleft to neighboring target cells.
- They are stored in small vesicles in the axon terminals of neurons.
- When electrical impulse reaches this point the neurotransmitters are released from the vesicles.
- They cross the synaptic cleft and bind with receptor sites on the cell body of dendrites of the adjacent neuron. This either allows or prevents the impulse from continuing its course.
- After the neurotransmitter has performed its function in the synapse it either returns to the vesicles to be stored and used again or is inactivated and dissolved by enzymes.

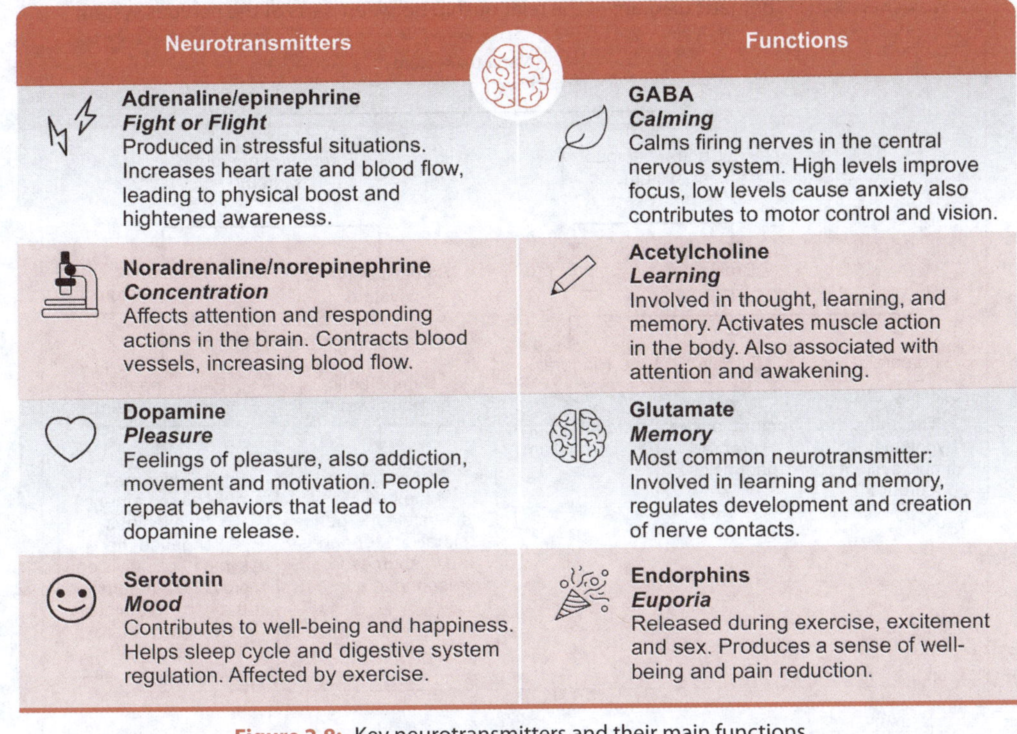

Neurotransmitters	Functions
Adrenaline/epinephrine ***Fight or Flight*** Produced in stressful situations. Increases heart rate and blood flow, leading to physical boost and hightened awareness.	**GABA** ***Calming*** Calms firing nerves in the central nervous system. High levels improve focus, low levels cause anxiety also contributes to motor control and vision.
Noradrenaline/norepinephrine ***Concentration*** Affects attention and responding actions in the brain. Contracts blood vessels, increasing blood flow.	**Acetylcholine** ***Learning*** Involved in thought, learning, and memory. Activates muscle action in the body. Also associated with attention and awakening.
Dopamine ***Pleasure*** Feelings of pleasure, also addiction, movement and motivation. People repeat behaviors that lead to dopamine release.	**Glutamate** ***Memory*** Most common neurotransmitter: Involved in learning and memory, regulates development and creation of nerve contacts.
Serotonin ***Mood*** Contributes to well-being and happiness. Helps sleep cycle and digestive system regulation. Affected by exercise.	**Endorphins** ***Euporia*** Released during exercise, excitement and sex. Produces a sense of well-being and pain reduction.

Figure 2.8: Key neurotransmitters and their main functions

- The process of being stored for reuse is called reuptake.
- Deficiency or an excess of neurotransmitters can produce severe behavioral disorders.

Some of the key neurotransmitters and their main functions are listed in **Figure 2.8**.

NERVOUS SYSTEM

Nervous system is the master controlling, communicating and the regulatory system in the body. Nervous system controls and coordinates all essential functions of the human body. It is the center of all mental activity including thought, learning and memory. Together with the endocrine system, the nervous system is responsible for regulating and maintaining homeostasis.

The human nervous system can be divided into two parts: the central nervous system (CNS) and the peripheral nervous system (PNS). While the central nervous system constitutes of the brain and the spinal cord, the peripheral nervous system constitutes of the somatic system and the autonomic system **(Flowchart 2.1)**.

Central Nervous System

Central nervous system consists of the brain and the spinal cord which act as the integrating and command centers of the nervous system. They interpret incoming sensory information and issue instructions based on past experience and current conditions. Brain is composed of three divisions: the forebrain, midbrain and hindbrain.

Forebrain

Its important structures are thalamus, hypothalamus, limbic system and the cerebrum.

Thalamus

As all sensory impulses pass through *thalamus* to the higher centers it is termed as the relay station. In addition, the thalamus exercises some control over the autonomic nervous system and also plays a role in the control of sleep and alertness.

Flowchart 2.1: Schematic diagram of the relationship between parts of the nervous system

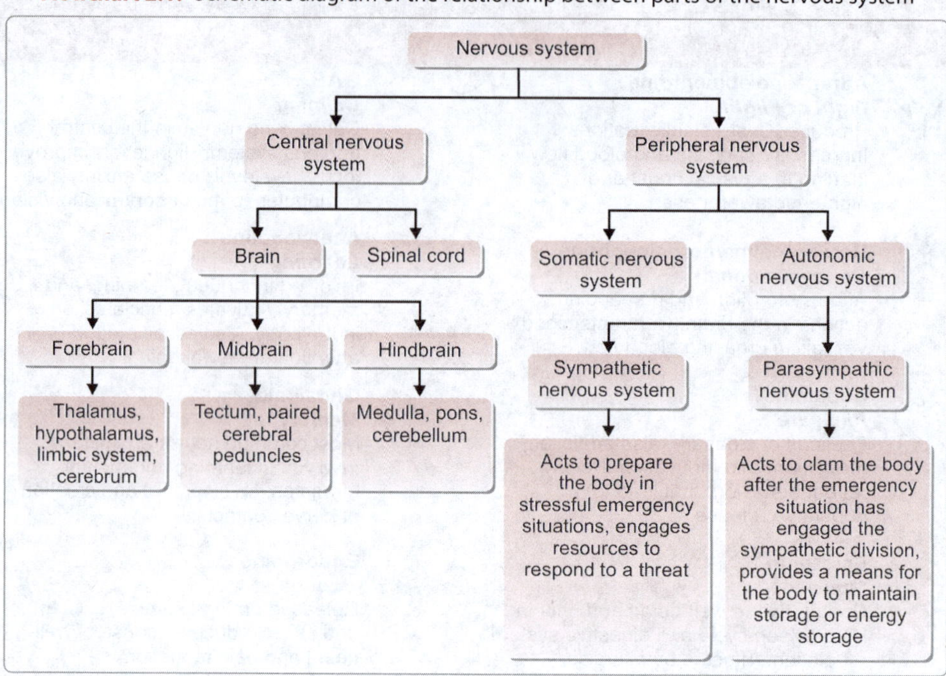

Hypothalamus

It lies below the thalamus. It exerts a key influence on all kinds of emotional as well as motivational behavior. Centers in the hypothalamus have control over important body processes like eating, drinking, sleeping, temperature control and sex. It also has control over the activities of pituitary gland.

Limbic system

It consists of structures in the thalamus, hypothalamus and cerebrum which form a ring around the lower part of the forebrain. Major structures within this system include the olfactory bulb, septal nuclei, hippocampus, amygdala and cingulate gyrus of the cerebral cortex. The limbic system often called the emotional brain functions in the emotional aspects of behavior related to survival, memory, smell, pleasure and pain, rage and aggression, affection, sexual desire, etc.

Cerebrum

It is the most complex and largest part of the brain. The cerebrum is covered by a thick layer of tightly packed neurons called the cerebral cortex. It is divided into two hemispheres—the left and right hemispheres.

Right and left hemispheres

Cerebral cortex is responsible for many higher order functions like language and information processing. The cerebral cortex is divided into sensory, motor and association areas **(Table 2.1)**.

- Sensory area receives sensory input.
- Motor area controls movement of muscles.
- Association area is involved with more complex functions such as writing.
- Each cerebral hemisphere is divided into four lobes: frontal, parietal, occipital and temporal lobes. Each part of the cerebrum is responsible for different mental functions. The visual area lying in the occipital lobe is connected with the visual organs or the eyes through the optic nerve. It is the seat of visual sensations.
- The auditory area lies in the temporal lobe and is connected with the auditory organs or the ears through the auditory nerves. It is the seat of auditory sensations and also involved in memory.

Table 2.1: Cortical areas and their functions

Cortical areas	Functions
Primary motor cortex	Initiation of voluntary movement
Primary somatosensory cortex	Receives tactile information, pain, pressure, position, movement and temperature
Motor association cortex	Coordination of complex movements
Speech center (Broca's area)	Speech production and articulation
Auditory cortex	Auditory perception and hearing
Auditory association area	Complex processing of auditory information
Sensory association area	Processing of multisensorial information
Visual association area	Primary visual perception
Wernicke's area	Comprehension of spoken language

- The parietal lobe lies in the upper rear portion of the brain and is connected with the information about special relationship and structure.
- Frontal lobes contain several parts and are concerned with organizing and planning our actions, learning new tasks, generating motivation and regulation of behavior **(Figure 2.9)**.

The cortex is divided into left and right hemispheres connected by a thick layer of cells called the corpus callosum. Specific differences between the two hemispheres are listed in **Table 2.2** and **Figure 2.10**.

Association cortex

Association cortex deals with more complex, integrative functions such as memory, emotions, reasoning, will, judgment, personality traits and intelligence. The association areas are:

- **Somatosensory association areas**: It permits the determination of exact shape and texture of an object without looking at it.
- **Visual association areas**: It relates present to the past, visual experiences with recognition and evaluation of what is seen.
- **Auditory association areas:** It determines if a sound is a speech, music or noise **(Figure 2.11)**.

Midbrain

Midbrain is concerned with the relaying of messages to the higher brain centers particularly those related to hearing and sight. One of its important structures is known as the reticular activating system (RAS). With the help

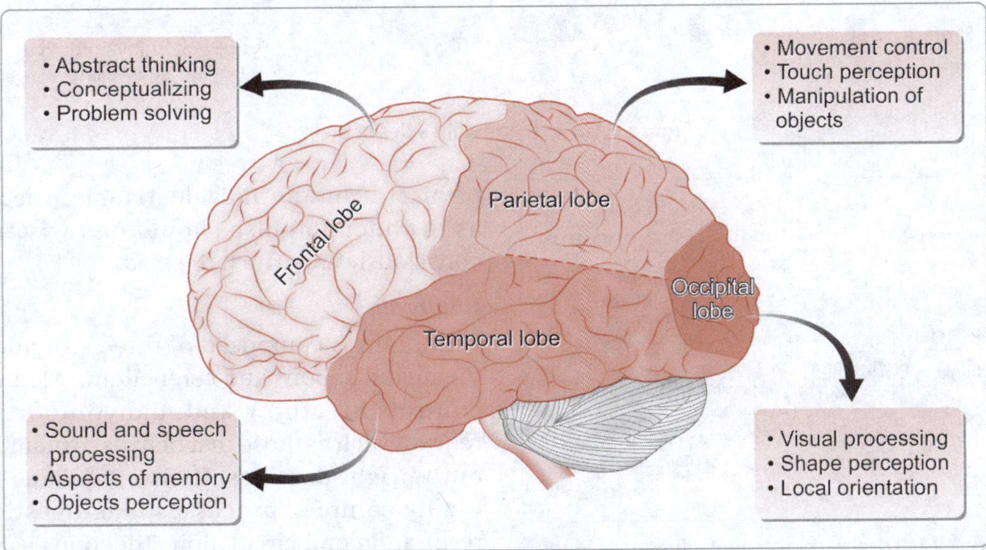

Figure 2.9: Lobes of brain and their functions

Table 2.2: Activities of right and left hemispheres

Activities	Right hemisphere	Left hemisphere
Specialties	• Copying of designs • Discrimination of shapes • Reading • Music • Holistic processing • Understanding metaphors • Expressing emotions	• Language skills • Skilled movements
Emotions	• Negative emotions	• Positive emotions
Neurotransmitters	• Higher levels of norepinephrine	• Higher levels of dopamine
Gray matter and white matter ratio	• More white matter on right	• More gray matter on the left
Shared	• Sensations on both sides of the face • Sound perceived by both ears • Pain • Hunger • Position	

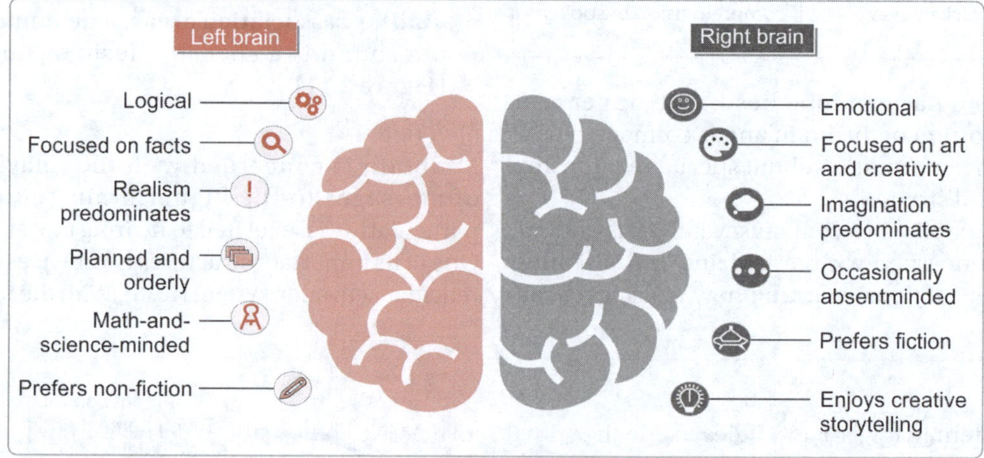

Figure 2.10: Left and right sides of brain

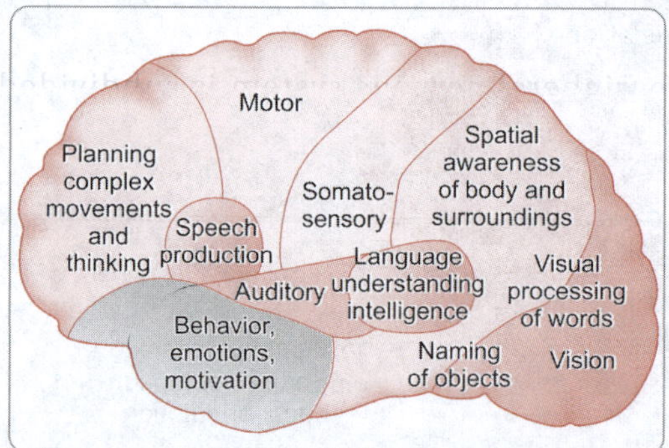

Figure 2.11: Localization of mental functions in the brain

of this structure an individual is able to decide as to which impulse should be registered consciously and which rejected.

Hindbrain

Hindbrain is composed of three structures: the medulla, pons and cerebellum. 'Medulla' controls breathing and many important reflexes such as those that help us to maintain our upright postures. It also regulates the highly complex processes like digestion, respiration and circulation. The 'pons' assist in breathing, transmitting impulses from the

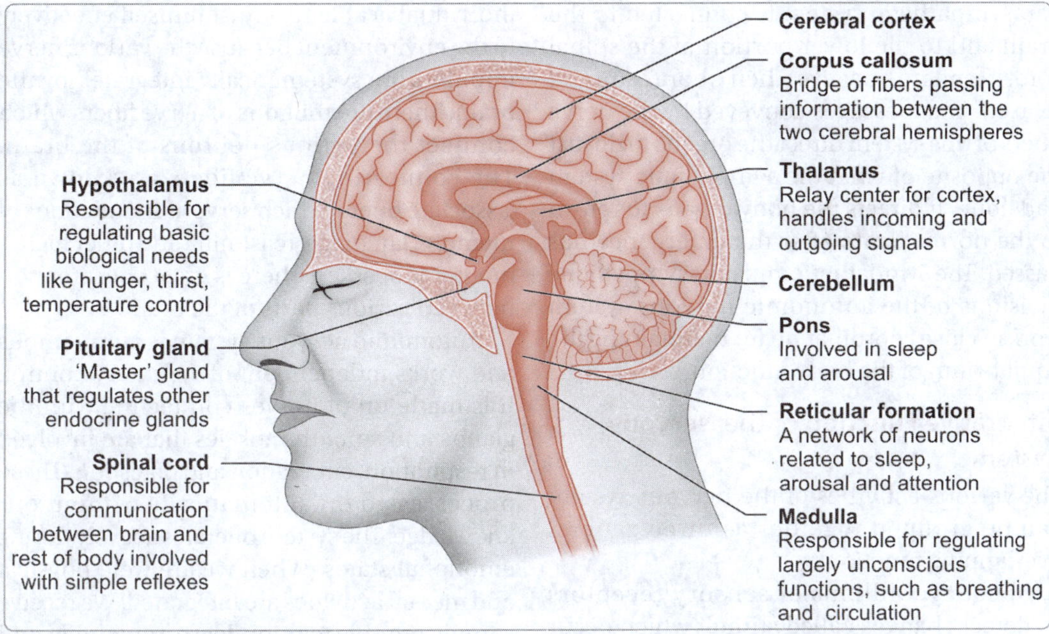

Figure 2.12: Major structures in the brain

cerebellum to the higher brain regions and in coordinating the activities of both sides of the brain. 'Cerebellum' is responsible for body balance and the coordination of body movements like dancing, typing, playing, etc. **(Figure 2.12)**.

Spinal Cord

- Spinal cord is a cylindrical structure that runs through the center of spine from brain stem to lower back. It lies inside the spinal column, which is made up of 33 bones called the vertebrae.
- Cerebrospinal fluid surrounds the spinal cord, which is shielded by three protective layers.
- This is the major conduit and reflex center between the peripheral nerves and the brain. It transmits motor information from the brain to the muscles, tissues and organs and sensory information from these areas back to the brain.
- It has 31 pairs of spinal nerves and other mixed nerves.
- At the junction it is divided into two roots: the dorsal root and the ventral root. Dorsal root contains sensory neurons while the ventral root contains motor neurons.
- It acts as an independent centre for reflex movements which are not under the conscious control of the cortex such as withdrawal of the hand when something is hot.

Peripheral Nervous System

The nerve tissues lying outside the bony case of the CNS come in the region of the peripheral nervous system. It consists of a network of nerves which helps in passing the sense impressions to the CNS as well as in conveying the orders of the CNS to the muscles. This peripheral nervous system is subdivided into two parts: the somatic system and the autonomic system.

While the somatic system is both a sensory and a motor system, the autonomic system is only a motor system consisting of two divisions: the sympathetic and the parasympathetic system. The sympathetic system is connected to the spinal cord and carries messages to the muscles and glands particularly in stress situations to prepare for an emergency. The parasympathetic system is connected to the brain and to the lower portion of the spinal cord. It tends to be active when we are calm and relaxed. The messages conveyed by the nerve fibers of this system direct the organs to do just the opposite of what the sympathetic system had done. It directs the body organs to return to the normal state after the emergency has passed. The sympathetic and parasympathetic divisions of the autonomic nervous system work in close coordination for maintaining the equilibrium of the body function.

Integrative Function of the Nervous System

The various activities of the nervous system can be grouped together as three general overlapping functions.

1. **Sensory:** Millions of sensory receptors detect changes called stimuli which occur inside and outside the body. They monitor parameters such as temperature, light and sound from the external environment. Within the body these receptors detect variations in pressure, pH, carbon dioxide concentration and levels of various electrolytes. All of this gathered information is called sensory input.
2. **Integrative:** Sensory input is converted into electrical signals called nerve impulses that are transmitted to the brain. The signals in the brain are brought together to create sensations to produce thoughts or add to the memory. Decisions are made every moment based on the sensory input. This is integration.
3. **Motor:** Based on the sensory input and integration the nervous system responds by sending signals to muscles causing them to contract or to glands causing them to produce secretions. Muscles and glands are called effectors because they cause an effect in response to detections from the nervous system. This is the motor output or motor function.

The cerebral cortex has primary areas which control the incoming sensory stimuli and the outgoing motor responses. An individual is able to adjust himself effectively to the environment because the various nerve impulses are systematically integrated by the brain. There are millions of nerve fibers which connect the various neurons of the brain. The connecting nerve fibers are known as 'associate fibers' which serve as foundations of memory, language, reasoning and other higher mental processes. There is great coordination between various parts of the brain.

Autonomic nervous system is autonomous and works independent of voluntary control. It is made up of nerves connecting with the glands and smooth muscles that are involved in respiration, circulation and digestion. These processes go on automatically without our knowledge. The system operates actively during emotional states. When we are well, physical and mental activities are integrated. We receive stimuli, are able to think, learn, remember and experience the various types of feelings. In illness, the normal healthy functioning of the body and its various organs is upset. Illness affects the threshold levels of our nervous system which may cause abnormal reactions to ordinary stimuli. It may adversely affect our co-ordination and disturb the thinking processes. Even the process of association is adversely affected resulting in funny and stray thoughts. Specific diseases and conditions have their own effects, some causing permanent damage to the nervous system and others causing only a temporary damage.

Importance of Knowledge of the Nervous System and Glands to a Nurse

- It helps the nurse to understand the physiological basis of patient behavior.
- It helps the nurse to understand how glandular secretions influence personality.
- It helps the nurse to understand the various diseases of nervous system and glands and their effect on human behavior.

PSYCHOLOGY AND SENSATION

Most of our behavior is dependent upon what our senses tell us. Vision, hearing, taste, smell and touch are the so called five senses.

The functioning of these five senses is called sensation. It is purely the result of physical stimuli operating on our nervous system.

Sensory Process

Each sensory system is a kind of a channel consisting of a sensitive element (the receptor). The nerve fibers connect these receptors to the brain or spinal cord, various relay stations and processing areas within the brain. When a sensory channel is stimulated, we experience a sensation that is characteristic of that channel. For instance, whether the eye is stimulated by light or by pressure on the eyeball, we have a visual experience. In order to know about the world around us physical energy must be converted into an activity within the nervous system. The process of converting physical energy into an activity within the nervous system is called transduction. This process occurs in the receptor cells. During the transduction process, receptor cells convert physical energy into an electric voltage or potential called the receptor potential. In some sensory systems the receptor potential itself directly triggers the nerve impulses that travel to the brain or the spinal cord. In other sensory systems the receptor potential leads to further electrical events which in turn trigger nerve impulses. This is known as the generator potential.

For any event in the environment, thousands of nerve impulses are generated and conducted to the central nervous system. Since these impulses travel along many different nerve fibers at slightly different times they form a pattern of input to the central nervous system that is the basis for our sensory experience of the event **(Flowchart 2.2)**.

Flowchart 2.2: Schematic representation of sensory experience

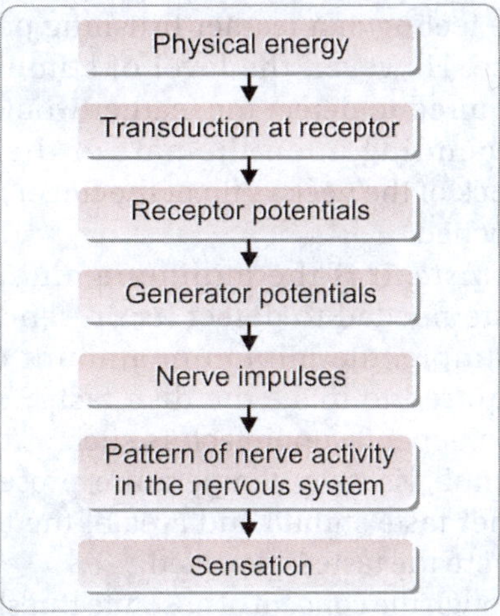

Sometimes our sensations are not accurate because our sense organs or parts of the nerve complexes which produce sensations are abnormal, sick or injured. When this happens, the information we receive is inaccurate and our responses abnormal.

General Characteristics of Sensation

- **Intensity:** Within each modality sensations vary in intensity from low to high. Thus we experience mild pain or severe pain, see faint light or bright light and so on.
- **Absolute threshold:** For any sensation to be aroused the stimulus (light, sound, smell, touch, etc.) must have a minimum intensity called the absolute threshold. The term is often applicable to any stimulus that can be detected by the human senses viz. sight, sound, smell, touch and taste.
  In hearing: It is the smallest level of tone that can be detected by normal hearing in the absence of other interfering sounds. For example, the level at which an individual can detect the ticking of a clock.
  In vision: It is the smallest level of light that an individual can detect. For example, measuring the distance at which an individual can first detect the presence of a light source in the dark. Wavelength of the light, its location and size of the stimulus are some other factors that need to be considered.
  In smell: It is the smallest concentration that an individual is able to smell. For example, the smallest amount of perfume that an individual can smell in a room. It also varies on a few other factors such as the odor, dilution, data collection methods, characteristics of the individual and environmental factors such as time of day, pressure and humidity.

In touch: It is the smallest amount of force required to detect a feeling. For example, the feeling of a feather brushing past the face. However, the level of stimulation required to detect the feather would vary depending upon the part of the body (back of the neck vs tip of the finger) being touched.

In taste: It is the minimum amount of taste needed to detect its presence. For example, the minimum amount of salt required to make the dish taste salty. It also depends upon factors such as type of stimuli, viscosity, temperature, presence of other taste stimuli and area of the tongue where the taste is detected.

Though the concept of absolute threshold is mostly explained in terms of sensation and perception, the conditions under which the observations are made play an important role in influencing it:

- *Expectations, motivations and thoughts*: One is more likely to detect a noise at a lower level if he is expecting to hear it.
- *Gender*: Women tend to have lower levels of absolute threshold for sight, smell, taste, touch and sound than men.
- *Age*: Absolute threshold varies with age. While younger people are able to detect stimulus at lower levels, a greater stimulus is required to detect the same stimuli when they grow older.
- *Time*: Absolute threshold varies for the same individual with time. For example, individual threshold for hearing the tick of a watch may be higher or lower depending upon whether he is very tired or well rested. It also differs if there are many other strong stimuli reaching the individual at the same time. For example, he will not hear a very soft sound if there are other louder sounds in the surroundings.
- *Physical condition*: Absolute threshold for the senses can be lower or higher in times of illness. A moderate sound may seem very loud, a weak light or small wrinkle in the sheet may irritate an ill person. At the same time these things may not even be felt by a partially conscious, heavily medicated or extremely fatigued patient.

- **Difference threshold:** Just as there must be a certain minimum amount of stimulation to evoke a sensory experience, there must also be a certain magnitude of difference between two stimuli before one can be distinguished from the other. The minimum amount of stimulation necessary to tell two stimuli apart is known as the difference threshold. For example, two tones must differ in intensity by a measurable amount before one can be heard as louder as the other. The difference in threshold will also vary for each person depending upon his physical condition, interest and kind of stimuli.

NORMAL AND ABNORMAL SENSATION

The nervous system is a complex system of nerve cells that send signals around the body. It receives information about the outside world through sensory inputs. The various types of sensation are: skin, smell, taste, vision, hearing, kinesthetic and vestibular.

Sensory processing disorders disrupt the processing of sensory information by the nervous system resulting in inappropriate responses, reactions or both. Individuals with sensory processing disorder cannot process certain sensory information effectively **(Figure 2.13)**.

1. Skin

The network of nerve endings and touch receptors in the skin called the somatosensory system controls the sense of touch. It is responsible for sensations such as cold, hot, smooth, rough, pressure, tickle, pain, itching, etc.

There are four categories of sensation that can be grouped under skin sensation—pain, pressure, cold and warmth. The sensitivity of the skin varies for each sensation and with the area of the body. Where there are more pain

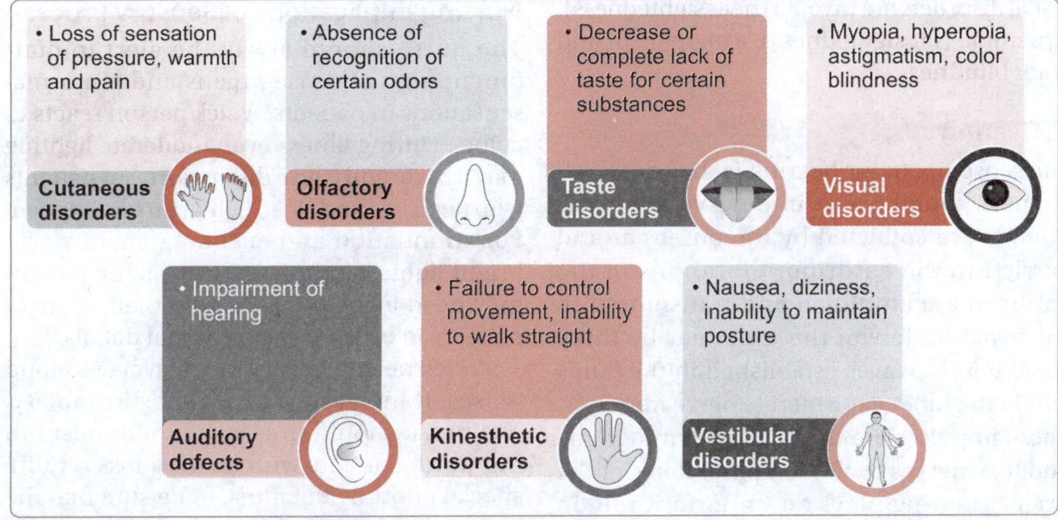

Figure 2.13: Types of sensory disorders

receptors the skin will be more sensitive and more pain will be felt.

Cutaneous disorders/factual disorders: They include loss of sensation of pressure, warmth, cold and pain.

2. Smell

Smell and taste sensations are closely related. The nerve receptors for smell are located in the lining of the upper nasal passages. When a smell is detected, the olfactory neurons generate an impulse which is passed on to the brain along the olfactory nerve. This signal is then processed by the olfactory bulb and information about the smell passed on to other areas. There are pleasant and unpleasant odors.

Olfactory disorders: These include sensitivity to odors or absence of recognition of certain odors.

3. Taste

The taste sensation occurs in the mouth when a substance reacts chemically with taste receptor cells. These are lined inside the taste buds most of which are found on the tip, sides and back of the tongue. The sensation of taste called 'gustation' gives us four basic tastes—sweet, sour, salt and bitter. The reason for difference in likes and dislikes for certain tastes is genetic. For example, a strong taste for one might seem quite bland for another. Another major reason for differences in taste is ageing during which the number of taste buds decrease with age. For example, older people are less sensitive to taste when compared to children. Similarly taste sensitivity is impaired in younger people who are heavy smokers.

Gustatory disorders: These include decrease in taste sensitivity or complete lack of taste for certain substances.

4. Vision

The retina of each eye contains receptor cells responsible for vision. There are two kinds of receptor cells in the retina—rods and cones. *Rods* respond only to varying degrees of light and dark and not to colors. They are responsible for night vision. Cones on the other hand respond both to light and dark and to colors. They are responsible for daylight vision. The *retina* is a continuation of the optic nerve. It carries the visual stimulations from retina to the occipital lobe in the brain.

Visual disorders: These may be due to deficiencies of the accessory structures of the eye such as the cornea and lens or due to inadequacies within the retina. The common visual disorders are myopia (near sightedness), hyperopia (far sightedness), astigmatism and color blindness.

5. Hearing

The sense organ for hearing is the ear which changes sound waves into nerve impulses. Sounds are collected by the outer ear and carried to the eardrum. Vibrations of the eardrum are amplified and transmitted to the oval window of the inner ear by three small bones. Waves established in the fluids within the inner ear generate nerve impulses. These impulses are then carried through the auditory nerves to the temporal lobes of the brain. Hearing plays an important role in the understanding of spoken language. It is the principal sensory modality for human communication. Sound can be loud or soft, low or high.

Auditory defects: Hearing can be impaired by injuries, fixation or disengagement of the ossicles, diseased tonsils, measles, mumps, etc.

- Varying degrees of deafness
- Deafness to certain specific tones
- A subjective ringing or roaring in the ears

6. Kinesthetic Sense

Kinesthetic senses perform the very important function of providing cues to our movements and maintain smooth and continuous action.

Kinesthetic disorders: These refer to a failure to control movements and inability to walk straight, etc.

7. Vestibular Senses

The vestibular senses monitor equilibrium and awareness of body position and movement. The receptors for these are the vestibules in the inner part of the ear.

Vestibular disorders: Nausea and dizziness, inability to maintain equilibrium and posture.

Nursing Implications of Sensory Process

The nurse should always be alert to malfunctioning of sense organs and abnormal sensations in patients. A sick person reacts to colors. During illness even moderate lighting may irritate and cause discomfort. For patients who need rest and sleep lights can be subdued. For stimulation and encouragement warm bright lights can be used. An ageing patient may need a great deal of help than younger patients in order to see the visual details.

A sick person is very much averse to loud noises. It increases the patient's irritability. The nurse should thus avoid loud noises in the ward. Patients with hearing loss require special effort by the nurse to be sure that the instructions are given clearly and questions are answered and understood.

Patients with loss of skin sensation require special attention to prevent further injuries to the skin while treating or using treatments or applications of any kind. Bandages, adhesive tapes, plaster casts, heat or cold, even wrinkled linens may be very irritating to a patient. Gentle skin care is necessary to prevent irritation. Patients should always be handled smoothly and gently to avoid pain and discomfort.

In healthcare environment the possible sources for bad odor are: body eliminations, treatment procedures, dressings, drainages and medications. These must be controlled to the maximum extent possible by proper ventilation and prompt disposal of waste.

A sick person may not relish his food. Taste can be improved with good mouth care and well prepared, clean and fresh food served in an appetizing way. Those experiencing dizziness may need help in walking and protection from accidents and injury. Rough, fast or jerky movements may cause discomfort and irritation to the patient.

The nurse can use her knowledge of sense organs for training her own senses. This will train her sense organs to observe her own functions.

SYPNOSIS

- Psychology studies human behavior, involves both body and mind.
- Body and mind are two aspects of the living, dynamic and adjusting personality.
- Heredity and environment are equally important initiating the temperament of the child.
- The entire behavior is effectively managed and controlled by the co-ordination and functioning of the nervous system.
- Nervous system controls and co-ordinates all essential functions of the human body.
- The various activities of the nervous system can be sensory, integrated and motor activities.
- Most of our behavior is dependent on the functioning of our senses.
- The nurse should always be alert to malfunctioning of sense organs and abnormal sensations in patients.

Review Questions

Long Essays

1. Explain physiological basis of behavior.
2. Describe endocrine system and its influence on development of behavior.
3. Define perception. Explain organization of perception.
4. What are the factors influencing perception? Explain the relationship between sensation and perception.
5. Describe sensory disorders. Explain nursing implications for sensory abnormalities.

Short Essays

1. Role of environment in behavioral change.
2. Write a short note on sense organs.
3. What is the role of heredity and environment in shaping behavior?
4. Genetics and behavior.
5. Heredity and environment.
6. Level of functioning.
7. Explain sensory process.
8. Discuss the salient features of sensation and perception.

Short Notes

1. Principles of heredity
2. Genes
3. Integrated responses
4. Heredity
5. Chromosomes
6. Environment
7. Identical and fraternal twins
8. Name any four endocrine glands
9. What are 'endocrine glands'?
10. Principles of heredity
11. Glands
12. Parts of a neuron
13. Levels of consciousness
14. Meiosis
15. Sensation

Multiple Choice Questions

1. Which among the following is the basic unit of nervous system?
   a. Brain
   b. Neuron
   c. Spinal cord
   d. Axon

2. Which among the following is a part of the neuron that receives messages from other neurons?
   a. Axons
   b. Terminal buttons
   c. Dendrites
   d. Cell bodies

3. A narrow gap that separates the neurons is called:
   a. Axon tip
   b. Cell body

c. Synaptic cleft
d. None of the above

4. Information is passed from one neuron to another at synapse by:
a. Cell membrane
b. Neurotransmitters
c. Nerve impulses
d. None of the above

5. Part of the brain that regulates higher levels of cognitive and emotional functions is the:
a. Cerebellum
b. Cerebrum
c. Limbic system
d. None of the above

6. The brain structure located in the center of the brain which has a role in emotions is:
a. Cerebellum
b. Limbic system
c. Pituitary
d. Caudate nucleus

7. The following plays an important role in long-term storage of information:
a. Hypothalamus b. Thalamus
c. Hippocampus d. Amygdala

8. The cerebrum controls:
a. Cognitive functions
b. Motor functions
c. Coordination
d. All of the above

9. What controls feeding, drinking, temperature regulation, sexual behavior, fighting or activity level?
a. Basal ganglia
b. Hypothalamus
c. Thalamus
d. Pituitary gland

10. The goal of physiological psychology is to understand the function of the brain and its relation to:
a. Communication
b. Behavior
c. Biology
d. Neurotransmitters

11. Which of the following areas of the brain deals with psychological processes like reasoning and memory?
a. Motor area
b. Premotor area
c. Association area
d. Sensory area

12. Two parts of the autonomic nervous system are:
a. Brain and spinal cord
b. Somatic and parasomatic
c. Anterior and posterior
d. Sympathetic and parasympathetic

13. Which of the following experiences do not easily reach to awareness?
a. Conscious
b. Preconscious
c. Unconscious
d. Semiconscious

14. The study of inheritance of physical and psychological characteristics from ancestors is referred to as:
a. Biopsychology
b. Genetics
c. Chromosomes
d. Anthropology

15. Another way of stating the nature versus nurture issue is:
a. Heredity versus environment
b. Education versus nutrition
c. Physical versus mental activity
d. Learned versus unlearned behavior

16. After a successful job interview Mr Rajan felt relaxed and calm. He stopped sweating and felt hungry. Which part of his nervous system was activated?
a. Sympathetic b. Somatic
c. Parasympathetic d. Central

17. How many chromosomes does a zygote contain?
a. 2 b. 23
c. 46 d. 92

18. Which of the following factors supports the nurture argument?
   a. Hereditary factors
   b. Maturation
   c. Genetic makeup
   d. Environmental factors

19. The central nervous system is composed of the ______ and ______.

20. Each hemisphere controls the _____ side of the body.

21. Non-verbal realms such as emotions and music are controlled primarily by the ____ hemisphere of the brain, whereas the ___ hemisphere is more responsible for speaking and reading.

22. The left hemisphere tends to consider information______, whereas the right hemisphere tends to process information_____.

23. Stimulus operating on our nervous system is termed as:
   a. Sensation
   b. Observation
   c. Attention
   d. Perception

ANSWER KEY

1. b	2. c	3. c	4. b	5. b	6. b
7. c	8. d	9. b	10. b	11. c	12. d
13. c	14. b	15. a	16. c	17. c	18. d
19. Brain, spinal cord	20. Opposite	21. Right, left	22. Sequentially, globally	23. a	

CHAPTER

3 Mental Health and Mental Hygiene

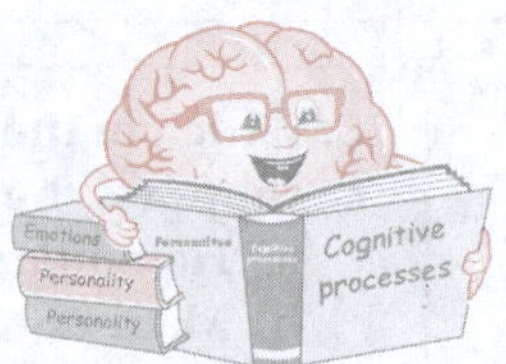

CHAPTER OUTLINE

- Concepts of mental health—mental health and mental hygiene
- Characteristics of a mentally healthy person
- Warning signs of poor mental health
- Promotive and preventive mental health services
- Ego defense mechanisms and their implications
- Frustration and conflict
- Role of a nurse in reducing frustration and conflict

MENTAL HEALTH

Mental health is a state of balance between the individual and the surrounding world, a state of harmony between oneself and others, a co-existence between the realities of the self and other people and the environment.

Definitions

- An adjustment of human beings to the world and to each other with maximum effectiveness and happiness.

  —Karl Menninger (1947)

- Simultaneous success at working, loving and creating with the capacity for mature and flexible resolution of conflicts between instincts, conscience, important other people and reality.

  —The American Psychiatric Association (APA) (1980)

Thus, mental health would include not only the absence of diagnostic labels such as schizophrenia and obsessive-compulsive disorder but also the ability to cope with the stressors of daily living, freedom from anxieties and generally a positive outlook towards change in fortunes and to cope with those.

CONCEPTS OF MENTAL HEALTH—JAHODA (1958)

Jahoda described six concepts of mental health in her book titled 'Current concepts of positive mental health' **(Figure 3.1)**.

Positive Attitude towards Self

A positive attitude towards self includes an objective view of self together with the knowledge and acceptance of strengths and limitations. The individual feels a strong sense of personal identity and security within the environment.

Achievement of Tasks

It is the ability of the individual to successfully achieve the tasks associated with each level of development.

Integration

Integration includes the ability to adaptively respond to the environment and the development of a philosophy of life both of which help the individual maintain anxiety at a manageable level in response to stressful situations.

Autonomy

Autonomy refers to the individual's ability to perform in an independent self-directed

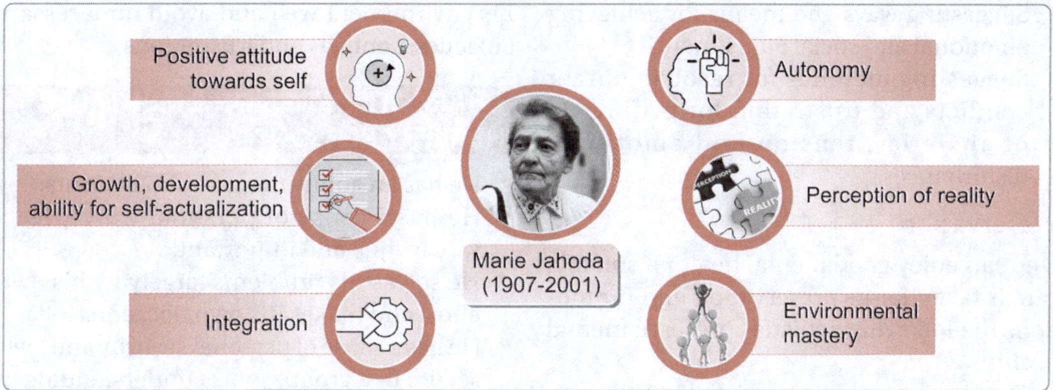

Figure 3.1: Concepts of mental health

manner, making choices and accepting responsibility for the outcomes.

Perception of Reality

Perception of reality includes perception of the environment without distortion, as well as the capacity for empathy and social sensitivity—a respect and concern for the wants and needs of others.

Environmental Mastery

Environmental mastery indicator suggests that the individual has achieved a satisfactory role within the group, society or environment. He is able to love and accept the love of others.

MENTAL HYGIENE

Mental hygiene is the science which studies laws and means of curing and preventing mental diseases, personality disorders and other abnormalities for balancing adjustment and healthy development of personality.

Definition

Mental hygiene consists of measures to reduce the incidence of mental illness through prevention and early treatment and promote mental health. —**Singh and Tiwari (1971)**

CONCEPTS OF MENTAL HYGIENE

Mental hygiene is the application of body of hygienic information for the purpose of improvement of mental health. The concepts in mental hygiene are depicted in **Figure 3.2**.

Prevention

Measures to prevent mental illness are:

- Identifying the causes leading to maladjustment, whether personal or social and taking suitable precautions to eliminate the same.

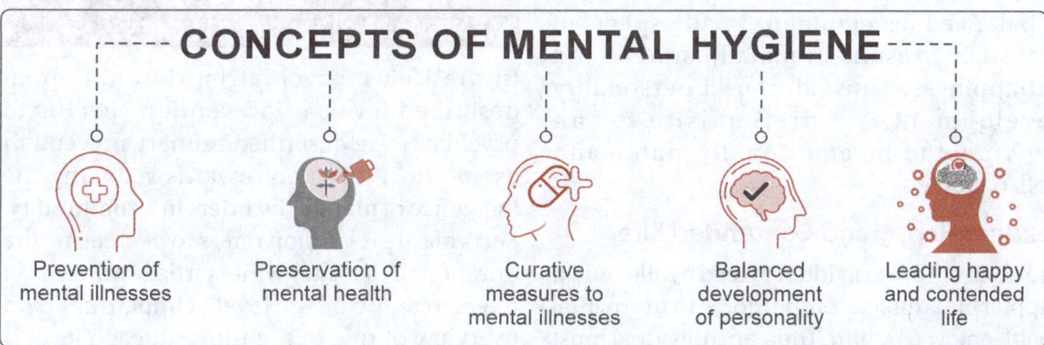

Figure 3.2: Concepts of mental hygiene

- Suggesting ways and means for achieving emotional and social adjustment.
- Suggesting methods for resolving inner conflicts and frustration for getting rid of anxieties, tension and emotional disturbances.

Preservation

One can enjoy good mental health if suitable care is taken for its preservation and promotion. The following activities preserve mental health:

- Developing an inner potential.
- Attaining emotional maturity and stability.
- Achieving personal and social security and adequacy.
- Promoting healthy human relationships and group interaction.

Curative Measures

An individual can enjoy good mental health to the extent one is cured as early as possible of mental illnesses and diseases he is suffering from. The following are some curative measures:

- Adequately equip with the knowledge regarding types of mental illnesses and disorders.
- Suggest various therapies for treatment and curing mental illnesses and disorders.
- Suggest methods for rehabilitation and readjustment of mentally ill persons.

Balanced Development of Personality

Balanced development of personality holds the key for an individual's adjustment with one's own self and the environment. Lack of balanced development in all aspects of personality results in maladjustment and unhappiness. Thus, all round personality development is a prerequisite for an individual to be emotionally stable and well-balanced.

Leading Happy and Contended Life

The ability of an individual to lead a fuller and a happier life is directly proportional to the mental health enjoyed by him. Thus, an individual must always strive to get along with himself and his environment well and avoid unnecessary anxieties, conflicts and frustrations.

CHARACTERISTICS OF A MENTALLY HEALTHY PERSON

- He has an ability to make adjustments.
- He has a sense of personal worth, feels worthwhile and important.
- He solves his problems largely by his own effort and makes his own decisions.
- He has a sense of personal security and feels secure in a group, shows understanding of other people's problems and motives.
- He has a sense of responsibility.
- He can give and accept love.
- He lives in a world of reality rather than fantasy.
- He shows emotional maturity in his behavior, and develops a capacity to tolerate frustration and disappointments in his daily life.
- He has developed a philosophy of life that gives meaning and purpose to his daily activities.
- He has a variety of interests and generally lives a well-balanced life of work, rest and recreation.

WARNING SIGNS OF POOR MENTAL HEALTH

Symptoms of mental disorders vary depending upon the type and severity of the condition. Warning signs of poor mental health among children, adolescents and adults are presented in **Figure 3.3**.

PROMOTIVE AND PREVENTIVE MENTAL HEALTH STRATEGIES

In the 1960s, psychiatrist Gerald Caplan described levels of prevention specific to psychiatry. He described primary prevention as an effort directed towards reducing the incidence of mental disorders in a community. Secondary prevention refers to decreasing the duration of disorder while tertiary prevention refers to reducing the level of impairment. An overview of role of the nurse in each level is presented in **Table 3.1.**

Younger Children

- Changes in school performance
- Poor grades despite strong efforts
- Excessive worrying or anxiety

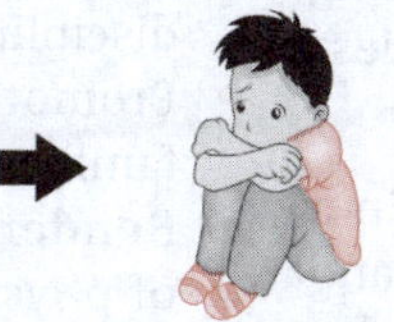

- Hyperactivity
- Persistent nightmares
- Persistent disobedience and/or aggressive behavior
- Frequent temper tantrums

Adolescents

- Abuse of drugs and/or alcohol
- Inability to cope with daily problems and activities
- Changes in sleeping and/or eating habits
- Long-lasting negative mood, often along with poor appetite and thoughts of death

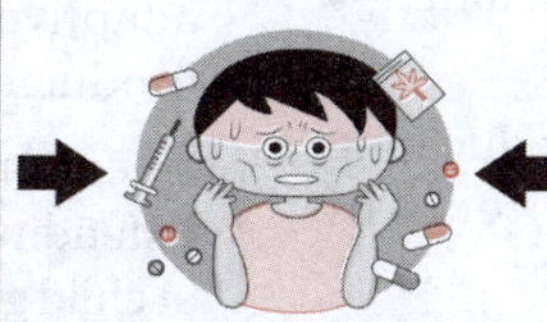

- Defying authority, skipping school, stealing or damaging property
- Intense fear of gaining weight
- Frequent outbursts of anger
- Excessive complaints relating to physical problems

Adults

- Confused thinking
- Long-lasting sadness or irritability
- Extreme highs and lows in mood
- Excessive fear, worrying or anxiety
- Social withdrawal
- Abuse of drugs and/or alcohol
- Thoughts of suicide
- Strong feelings of anger

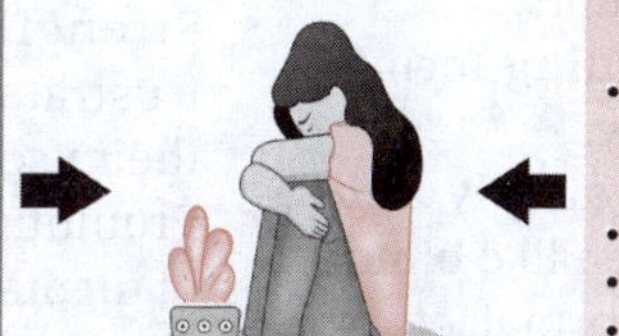

- Delusions or hallucinations (seeing or hearing things that are not really there)
- Increasing inability to cope with daily problems and activities
- Denial of obvious problems
- Unexplained physical problems
- Dramatic changes in eating or sleeping habits

Figure 3.3: Warning signs of poor mental health

Table 3.1: Promotive and preventive mental health strategies: Role of a nurse

Primary prevention strategies	Secondary prevention strategies	Tertiary prevention strategies
• Individual centered interventions • Child oriented interventions at school • Family centered interventions • Crisis intervention strategies • Mental health education • Society centered preventive measures	• Early diagnosis and case finding • Training of health professionals • Screening programs • Early reference • Prompt treatment • Consultation services • Crisis intervention	• Family involvement • Community-based programs • Collaboration • Training in community living • Dealing with stigma • Foster healthy attitude towards the mentally ill member

Primary Prevention

Primary prevention seeks to prevent the occurrence of mental disorders by strengthening individual, family and group coping abilities.

Role of a Nurse in Primary Prevention

Community mental health nurses are in a key position to identify individual, family and group needs, conflicts and stressors. They play a major role in identifying high risk groups and preventing the occurrence of mental illnesses among them. Some interventions include:

Individual centered interventions

- Antenatal care to the mother and educating her regarding the adverse effects of irradiation, drugs and prematurity.
- Ensuring timely and efficient obstetrical assistance to guard against the ill effects of anoxia and injury to the newborn at birth.
- Dietary corrections to those infants suffering from metabolic disorders.
- Correction of endocrine disorders.
- Liberalization of laws regarding termination of unwanted pregnancy.
- Training programs for physically and mentally handicapped children like blind, deaf, mute and mentally subnormal, etc.
- Counseling the parents of physically and mentally handicapped children with particular reference to the nature of defects. Parents need to accept and support the child emotionally, and be satisfied with achievement of limited goals in various fields.
- Fostering bonding behaviors, explaining importance of warm, accepting, intimate relationship and avoiding the prolonged separation of mother and child are essential.

Child oriented interventions at school

- Sensitizing parents and teachers on concepts of growth and development.
- Identifying problems related to scholastic performance and emotional disturbances among school children and providing timely intervention. School teachers can be taught to recognize the beginning symptoms of problems and refer it to appropriate agencies.

Family-centered interventions to ensure harmonious relationship

- Consulting parents about appropriate disciplinary measures.
- Promoting open health communication in families.
- Rendering crisis counseling to parents of physically and mentally handicapped children.
- Ensuring harmonious relationship among members of the family and teaching healthy adaptive techniques at the time of stress producing events.

Interventions oriented to keep families intact

- Extending mental health education services at child guidance clinics regarding child rearing practices; at parent teacher associations regarding the triad relationship between teacher, child and parent and at various extramural health agencies regarding integration of mental health into general health practice.
- Strengthening social support for the frustrated aged and helping them retain their usefulness.
- Promoting educational services in the field of mental health and mental hygiene.
- Developing parent-teacher associations.
- Rendering home-maker services—in the event of mother's prolonged absence from home due to illness or other reasons, a public health nurse can be arranged for providing basic services.
- Providing counseling for those with marital problems.

Interventions for families in crisis

In developmental crisis situations such as the child passing through adolescence, birth of a new baby, retirement or menopause, death of a wage earner in the family, desertion by the spouse, etc., crisis intervention can be given at:

- Mental hygiene clinics
- Psychiatric first-aid centers
- Walk-in clinics

Mental health education

- Conduct mass health education programs on prevention of mental illnesses and promotion of mental health in the community using film shows, flashcards and appropriate audio-visual aids.

- Educate health workers on prevention of mental illness so that they can function effectively in all the areas of prevention.

Society-centered preventive measures

- Community development.
- Culturally deprived families need biological and psychosocial supplies to avoid incidents of psychopathy, alcoholism, drug addiction, crime and mental illness. They require better hygienic living conditions, proper food, education, health facilities and recreational facilities.
- Collection and evaluation of epidemiological, biostatistical data.

Secondary Prevention

Secondary prevention targets those people who show early symptoms of mental health disruption but are able to regain premorbid level of functioning through aggressive treatment.

Role of a Nurse in Secondary Prevention

At secondary prevention level the mental health nurse should focus on detecting mental disorders early so as to ensure prompt intervention. Some of the interventions are as follows:

- **Early diagnosis and case finding:** This can be achieved by educating the public, community leaders, industrialists, *mahilamandals, balwadis*, etc., on how to recognize early symptoms of mental illness. Case finding can be done through screening and periodic examination of population at risk, monitoring of patients, etc. Community mental health nurses should detect early signs of increased anxiety levels, decreased ability to cope with stress, failure to perceive self, environment and/or reality accurately in clinics, schools, home, health care and workplace and provide direct services as appropriate.
- **Training of health personnel:** Orientation courses should be provided to health workers to detect cases in the course of their routine work.
- **Screening programs:** Simple questionnaires should be developed to identify the symptoms of mental illness and the same administered in the community for early identification of cases. These questionnaires can be translated into local languages for wide use in colleges, schools, industries, etc.
- **Early reference:** Public should be educated to refer such cases to hospitals as soon as the early symptoms of mental illness are recognized.
- **Prompt treatment:** Early and effective treatment for patient and counseling services to care givers of mentally ill patients should be provided.
- **Consultation services:** Nurses working in general hospitals may come across patients suffering from puerperal psychosis, anxiety states, peptic ulcer, ulcerative colitis, bronchial asthma, etc. These basic care providers need guidance and consultation to deal with such conditions in an effective manner.
- **Crisis intervention:** If the crisis is not tackled in time it may lead to mental disorders or even suicide. Anticipating the crisis situation and guiding the individual can help him cope with the crisis situation in a better way.

Tertiary Prevention

Tertiary prevention targets those with mental illness and helps to reduce the severity, discomfort and disability associated with it. This stage encompasses methods of minimizing negative effects and preventing future complications.

Role of a Nurse in Tertiary Prevention

In this form of prevention community mental health nurses play a vital role in monitoring the progress of discharged patients in halfway homes, houses, etc., especially with regard to their medication regimen and co-ordination of care. Some of the interventions are as follows:

- **Family involvement:** Family members should be actively involved in the treatment program to ensure effective follow up. Occupational and recreational activities should be organized in the hospital to prevent idling.

- **Community-based programs:** These programs can be launched by meeting the family members during which the need for discharge from the hospital should be emphasized. These programs can be implemented through day hospitals, night hospitals, aftercare clinics, halfway homes, ex-patient hostels, foster care homes, etc. Follow-up care can be handed over to community health nurses.
- **Collaboration:** There should be constant communication between community health nurses and the mental health institution regarding follow-up of the discharged patient as ultimate aim of the hospital and community-based programs is to resocialize and remotivate the patient for a functional role in the community consistent with its resources. There are a wide range of services that need to be provided to patients as a part of the tertiary prevention program. Nurses need to be familiar with the community agencies that render these services. Collaborative relationships between mental healthcare providers and community agencies are absolutely essential if rehabilitation is to succeed.
- **Training in community living:** An important intervention in the maintenance of patients at their own homes in the community is the training in community living (TCL) program designed by 'Stein and Test.' In this model, when a patient is referred for hospital admission, the staff goes to the community and stays with the patient rather than the patient going to the hospital and being with the staff. This real world experience with the patient enables the nurse to accurately assess the skills that the person needs to develop and mutually agree on realistic goals.
- **Dealing with stigma:** Another aspect of community life that is more difficult to assess accurately and deal with effectively is the stigma attached to mental illness. Many patients and their families try to avoid stigma by keeping the nature of the person's illness a secret. The need for secrecy places additional stress on the family system as there is always the fear of truth being revealed. Nurses in the community are in a key position to monitor community attitudes and help foster a realistic attitude towards the mentally ill.
- **Foster healthy attitude towards the mentally ill member:** For some patients the emotional climate of the family to which they return can have a significant effect on their adjustment and eventual recovery from the debilitating effects of chronic mental illness. Families sometimes view mental illness as a weakness of character that can be overcome by exertion of moral effort. This type of familial attitude may result in guilt on the part of the patient who believes that he has disappointed his significant others. Guilt leads to increased anxiety and decreased self-esteem. These conditions interfere with a high level of functioning. Therefore, nurses working with families need to foster healthy attitudes towards the mentally ill member.

MENTAL HEALTH SERVICES

Mental health services are devoted to the treatment of mental illnesses and improvement of mental health in general population. The various institutions involved in providing such services in India are listed in **Figure 3.4.**

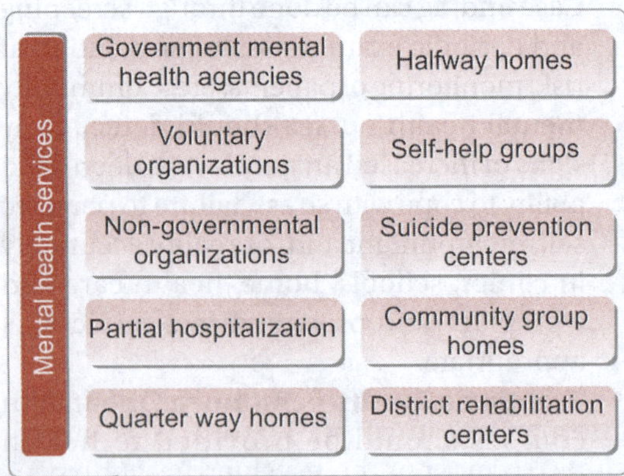

Figure 3.4: Mental health services

Mental Health Agencies—Government at National Level

Lancet Psychiatry 2020 study states that in 2017 there were 197.3 million people with mental disorders in India, comprising 14.3% of the total population of the country. There are 43 mental hospitals in the country that cater mental health services to people with common mental disorders.

Voluntary Organizations

Voluntary organizations are a valuable community resource for mental health. They are more often sensitive to the local realities than centrally driven programs and strongly committed to innovation and change. They often play an extremely important role in the absence of a formal or well-functioning mental health system thus filling the gap between community needs and available community services and strategies.

Voluntary organizations can also play an important role in developing suicide prevention and crisis support for individuals through formation of self-help groups, organizing community-based housing facilities for short-term and long-term care of persons with chronic illnesses, setting up of day-care centers, sheltered employment facilities, life skills programs for school drop-out children and public mental health education.

Non-governmental Organizations

Non-governmental organizations (NGOs) are recognized by Governments as non-profit or welfare oriented organizations that play a key role as advocates, service providers, activists and researchers on a range of issues pertaining to human and social development. Mental health non-governmental organizations (MHNGOs) are located throughout India. While many are formed in urban areas they have begun to extend services in rural areas too.

Partial Hospitalization

Partial hospitalization is an innovative alternative to hospitalization. It is ideally suited to most of the psychiatric syndromes particularly chronic psychotic disorders, neurotic conditions, personality disorders, drug and alcohol dependence and mental retardation. Day-care centers, day hospitals and day treatment programs fall under partial hospitalization. It has the advantage of lesser separation from families, greater involvement in the treatment program and a lessening of patient's preoccupation with the illness which may otherwise be intensified by full hospitalization.

Quarterway Homes

Quarter way home is a place usually located within the hospital campus itself with no regular hospital services. While routine nursing staff or routine rounds may not be available, most of the activities at the home are taken care of by the patients themselves.

Halfway Homes

A halfway home is a transitory residential center for mentally ill-patients who no longer need the full services of a hospital but are not yet ready for a completely independent living. It attempts to maintain a climate of health rather than that of illness and develop and strengthen individual capacities. Simultaneously, it enables the recognition of problems that require medical attention and permits the discovery of conditions in the community that are acting adversely on the individual. Thus, halfway homes play a major role in the rehabilitation of mentally ill individuals.

Self-help Groups

- Self-help groups (SHGs) are informal associations of people with similar socio-economic background and a desire to cope with a specific problem or life crisis. These groups improve the emotional health and wellbeing of its members. Usually, organized with a particular task in mind such groups do not attempt to explore individual psychodynamics in great depth or change personality functioning significantly.
- A distinguishing characteristic of self-help groups is their homogeneity. Its members have similar disorders and share their

experiences good or bad, successful or unsuccessful with one another. They work together using their strengths to gain control over their lives. By doing so they educate each other, provide mutual support and alleviate the sense of alienation usually felt by people drawn to this kind of a group. In other words, self-help groups are based on the premise that people who have experienced a particular problem are better positioned to help others experiencing similar problems.

Suicide Prevention Centers

There are many suicide prevention centers in India in the voluntary sector doing good work and helping those in need. Some of them are:

- Helping Hands and Medico-Pastoral Association (MPA) in Bengaluru
- Sneha in Chennai
- Sahara in Mumbai
- Sanjivini and Sumaitri in New Delhi

Other Mental Health Services

- Community group homes
- Large homes for long-term care
- Hostels
- Home care programs
- District rehabilitation centers

DEFENSE MECHANISM AND ITS IMPLICATIONS

When aspirations are not realized or goals not met they lead to frustration. These failures and frustrations hurt our ego leading to anxiety, stress and a feeling of guilt. Under such circumstances individuals attempt to handle the negative emotions and maintain harmony with the environment by resorting to either direct and indirect methods.

Direct Methods

Direct methods are employed by an individual at the conscious level. These include:

- **Increasing trials or improving efforts:** When one comes across obstacles or finds it difficult to solve a problem, he can improve his efforts and behavioral process and attempt with a new zeal to cope with the environment.
- **Adopting compromising means:** For maintaining harmony between himself and the environment the individual may adopt the following compromising postures:
  - He may altogether change his direction of efforts by changing the original goals, i.e., an aspirant for Indian Administrative Service (IAS) may direct his energies to become an officer in a nationalized bank.
  - He may seek partial substitution of the goal by opting for selection to provincial civil services instead of the IAS.
- **Withdrawal and submissiveness**: One may learn to cope with one's environment by simply accepting defeat and surrendering oneself to the powerful forces of environment and circumstances.

Indirect Methods

Indirect methods are those by which a person tries to seek temporary adjustment to protect himself for the time being against a psychological danger. These are purely psychic or mental devices or ways of perceiving situations as he would want to see himself in and imagining that things would happen according to his wishes.

The ego usually copes with anxiety through rational means. When anxiety is too painful the individual protects his ego and reduces the anxiety using defense coping mechanisms. Such mechanisms are called mental mechanisms or ego defense mechanisms.

Ego Defense Mechanisms

Ego defense mechanisms are methods to protect self and cope with basic drives or emotionally painful thoughts, feelings or events. Though originally conceived by Sigmund Freud much of the development of defense mechanisms was done by his daughter Anna Freud. Also referred to as defense mechanisms these are considered as protective barriers to manage instinct and affect in stressful situations (Freud, 1946).

Defense mechanisms (or coping styles) are automatic psychological processes that protect the individual against anxiety and from the awareness of internal or external dangers or stressors. Individuals are often unaware of these processes as they operate. Defense mechanisms mediate the individual's reaction to emotional conflicts and to internal and external stressors.

Purpose of Defense Mechanism

Defense mechanisms are conscious or unconscious psychological processes that individuals can use to protect themselves from anxious, inconvenient or unpleasant feelings and thoughts. Some of the purposes are:

- To reduce or eliminate anxiety
- To resolve mental conflict
- To protect one's self-esteem
- To maintain a sense of security
- To decrease conflict between the superego and the id
- To contribute to mental homeostasis

They can be helpful when used in very small doses and if overused become ineffective leading to breakdown of the personality. Most defense mechanisms operate at the unconscious level of awareness.

Types of Defense Mechanisms

Defense mechanisms are classified into either primitive defenses or mature defenses or higher-level defense mechanisms. Other classification includes adaptive or maladaptive depending on how much they help or harm an individual or the people in their lives.

- Primitive defense mechanisms are the first to occur developmentally. These include regression, repression, conversion, denial, projection, fantasy, identification, rationalization, reaction formation, acting out, etc.
- Mature defense mechanisms involve accepting reality even if it is disliked. Uncomfortable thoughts, feelings and situations are interpreted and addressed in less threatening forms instead of being denied. They are helpful for the psychological development of an individual as well as improving mental hygiene. These include sublimation, displacement, compensation, humor and suppression, etc. People can practice choosing to use mature defense mechanisms. This often requires intension, practice and effort. The commonly used defense mechanisms are presented in **Table 3.2.**

Table 3.2: Commonly used defense mechanisms

Defense mechanism and description	Example	Overuse may lead to
Repression: Unconscious and involuntary forgetting of painful ideas, events and conflicts	Forgetting a loved one's birthday after a fight	Conscious perception of instincts and blockage of feelings
Denial: Unconscious refusal to admit an unacceptable idea or behavior	Mother of a child who is fatally ill though fully informed of the diagnosis and the expected outcome refuses to admit it. It is because she cannot tolerate the pain that acknowledging the reality would cause	Repression, dissociative disorders
Displacement: Unconscious discharging of pent-up feelings to a less threatening object	A husband yells at his wife after a bad day at work	Loss of friends and relationships, confusion in communication
Reaction formation: Replacement of unacceptable feelings with their exact opposites	A boy who is jealous and hates his elder brother shows him exaggerated respect and affection	Failure in resolving internal conflict

Contd...

Contd...

Defense mechanism and description	Example	Overuse may lead to
Rationalization: Justification of failures and offering socially approved reasons for socially unacceptable behavior	A student complains about the unfavorable hostel atmosphere for his failure in the examination	Self-deception
Sublimation: Conscious or unconscious channeling of instinctual drives into acceptable activities	Aggressiveness being transformed to competitiveness in business or sports	Channeling of instincts rather than being blocked or diverted
Compensation: Conscious covering up for a weakness by over emphasizing or making up a desirable trait	A student who fails in his studies compensates for it by becoming the college champion in athletics	Modest instinctual satisfaction
Projection: Unconscious (or conscious) blaming of someone else for one's difficulties.	A surgeon blames the theater nurse for an unsuccessful operation. Here the surgeon blames the theater nurse for his own mistake using the projection mechanism	Failure in taking personal responsibility; building up of delusional tendencies
Intellectualization: Undue emphasis on the inanimate to avoid intimacy with people; increased attention on external reality to avoid expression of inner feelings; excessive stress on irrelevant details to avoid perceiving the whole.	Person shows no emotional expression when discussing a serious car accident	Limiting of affective expression on experience
Undoing: Reversing or undoing a thought or feeling by performing an action that signifies an opposite feeling than original thought or feeling	Buying a gift for someone for whom there is a feeling of dislike	Sending a double message
Regression: Reverting to an older, less mature way of handling stresses and feelings	An adult throwing a temper tantrum when he does not get his own way	Interference with progression and development of personality
Dissociation: Unconscious separation of painful feelings and emotions from an unacceptable idea, situation or object	Amnesia preventing recall of previous days auto accident. Adult remembering nothing of childhood sexual abuse	Dissociative disorders
Conversion: Unconscious expression of intrapsychic conflict symbolically through physical symptoms	Student awakening with a migraine headache in the morning of a final examination and feeling too ill to take the exam	Inability in dealing with anxiety which may lead to actual physical disorders such as gastric ulcers
Suppression: Voluntary rejection of unacceptable thoughts or feelings from conscious awareness	Student failing in an examination not forthcoming about his marks	Acknowledging the discomfort though not willingly

Contd...

Contd...

Defense mechanism and description	Example	Overuse may lead to
Substitution: Unconscious replacement of unacceptable impulses, attitudes, needs or emotions with those that are more acceptable	Student nurse taking up teaching as she is unable to master clinical competencies	Acknowledging the discomfort though not willingly
Isolation: Attempt to avoid a painful thought or feeling by objectifying and emotionally detaching oneself from the feeling	Acting aloof and indifferent towards someone who is disliked	Loss of ability in dealing with true feelings and increased stress

Implications

- Defense mechanisms enable a person to resolve conflicts. They are essential to the maintenance of normal equilibrium.
- Difficulties arise only if the defense mechanisms are inadequate to deal with anxiety or inappropriate to the situation in which they are used.
- Most mental mechanisms are a means for compromising with forbidden desires, feeling of guilt, etc.
- Mental mechanisms when used moderately are harmless, protect the ego and help face the conflicts and frustrations easily. They also help to relieve tensions and make the person feel comfortable.
- Excessive and persistent use of these defense mechanisms is harmful. They do not solve the problems but only relieve the related anxiety. Too much dependence makes us incapable of facing problems. For example, if a student is unable to face the examination and withdraws from taking it, he may experience greater difficulty in the next attempt. Hence, it is better to face the problems than resorting to such mechanisms.
- Many a times more than one mechanism may operate in the process of adjusting to the situation.
- If defense mechanisms are identified during adolescent period, it can help to predict personality disorders.
- Hence early identification of defense mechanisms can have great clinical significance.

Relevance to Nursing Practice

The nurse must recognize and understand maladaptive defense mechanisms used by the patients. While carefully pointing out these mechanisms and discouraging them she should work with the patients to encourage adaptive behavior.

FRUSTRATION

Every action arises in response to a need and is directed towards a goal. The blocking of activity directed towards a goal results in frustration. It always produces unpleasant feelings like anger, despair, irritation, anxiety, etc. This produces mental tension. For example, over restrictive parents would be a source of frustration to an adolescent girl wanting to attend a party or lack of water would be a source of frustration to a man lost in the desert.

Definition

The word frustration has been derived from the Latin word 'Frustra' meaning 'obstruct'. Frustration refers to the blocking of behavior directed towards the goal. Frustration means emotional tension resulting from the blocking of a desire or need.

—Good, Carter V

Characteristics of Frustration

- Frustration produces an unpleasant emotional state. The tension or stress created varies from simple annoyance to heated anger adversely affecting the vital balance.
- Frustration is a stage or condition in which failure dominates the attempts.

- In this state one experiences a major obstacle in the satisfaction of basic needs or goals.
- Significance of the goal and strength of the blockade increases the degree of frustration.
- The cause of frustration lies both in the individual himself and his environment.

Causes or Source of Frustration

There are two kinds of frustration: external and personal. External frustration is caused by conditions outside of oneself. Personal frustration is caused by conditions within oneself. These conditions can be categorized into external and internal factors.

External Factors (Environmental Factors)

- **Physical factors:** Natural calamities, obstacles in environment to reach a goal, environmental situations or conditions beyond our control. For example, a contagious disease, death of a friend or a beloved relative.
- **Social factors:** Conflicts with other people, customs, traditions, restrictions, taboos, laws, codes, etc.
- **Economic factors:** Financial problems.

Internal Factors

- Physical abnormalities or defects
- Conflict of motives within the individual
- Individual's morality and high ideals
- High levels of aspiration
- Lack of persistence and sincerity in efforts

Reactions to Frustration

Important reactions to frustration are as follows **(Figure 3.5)**:

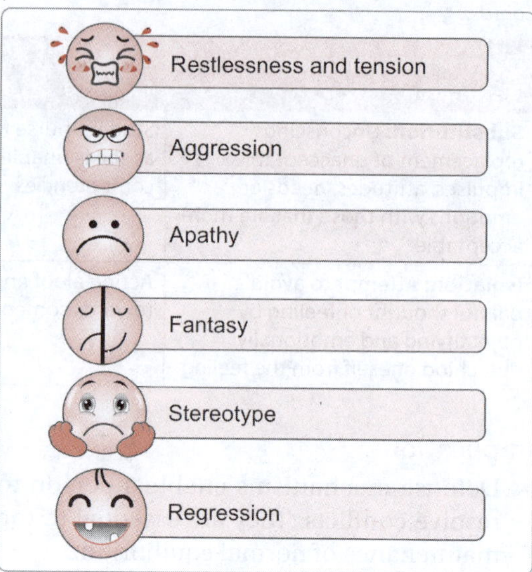

Figure 3.5: Reactions to frustration

Restlessness and Tension

When increased effort and variation in attack fail and substitute goals are unavailable and unacceptable the person exhibits restlessness and tension behavior.

Aggression

- **Direct aggression:** Aggression is at times expressed directly against an individual or object which is the source of frustration.
- **Displaced aggression:** When circumstances block direct attack on the cause of frustration, aggression may be 'displaced'. Displaced aggression is an aggressive action against an innocent person or object rather than against the actual cause of the frustration.

Apathy

Those who realize that they have no power to satisfy personal needs by means of own actions, whose aggressive outbursts are never successful may well resort to apathy and withdrawal when confronted with a frustrating situation.

Fantasy

When problems become too much for an individual to handle, he sometimes seeks the solution of escape into a dream world, a solution based on fantasy rather than reality.

Stereotype

Stereotype is a repetitive, fixed behavior. When repeated frustration baffles a person, some flexibility appears to be lost and the person stupidly makes the same effort again and again though experience has shown its futility.

Regression

Regression is defined as a return to more primitive modes of behavior, i.e., to modes of behavior characterizing a younger age.

Individuals show considerable variability in behavior when their goal-seeking behavior is blocked.

Approaches to Resolve Frustration

- Increasing trials or improving efforts
- Changing goals to more attainable ones
- Adopting compromising ways and methods

CONFLICT

Conflict in life is one cause of stress. It is a painful state or condition of an individual during which the person experiences an intense emotional tension. Conflict occurs when one has to choose between equally desirable or equally undesirable goals. These desires are contradictory in nature and therefore cannot be satisfied simultaneously. Thus, becoming a victim of the two opposing desires he suffers from an inner conflict to either satisfy or not satisfy one or the other desire.

Definition

Conflict means a painful emotional state which results from a tension between opposed and contradictory wishes.

—**Douglas and Holland**

Types of Conflict

Approach-Approach Conflict

Approach-approach conflict occurs when a person is forced with two attractive alternatives while only one of them can be selected. For example, two interesting classes a student always wanted to attend are scheduled at the same time. Approach-approach conflicts are usually easy to resolve but become serious if the choice of one alternative means the loss of an extremely attractive alternative **(Figure 3.6)**.

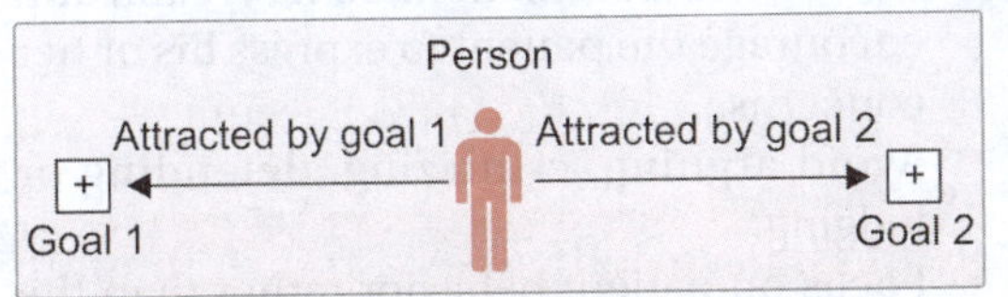

Figure 3.6: Approach-approach conflict

Avoidance-Avoidance Conflict

Avoidance-avoidance conflict arises when a person faces two undesirable situations and avoidance of one forces exposure to the other. These types of conflicts are very difficult to resolve and create intense emotions. For example, a woman trying to choose between continuing an unwanted pregnancy and getting an abortion done (she may morally be opposed to abortion) **(Figure 3.7)**.

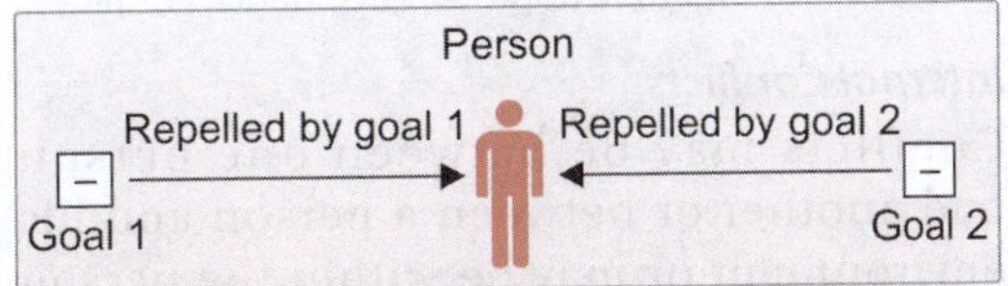

Figure 3.7: Avoidance-avoidance conflict

Approach-Avoidance Conflict

Approach-avoidance type of conflict exists when one event or activity has both attractive and unattractive features. The result is continuing oscillation between approach and avoidance creating a great deal of emotional conflict and stress. For example, to marry or not to marry **(Figure 3.8)**.

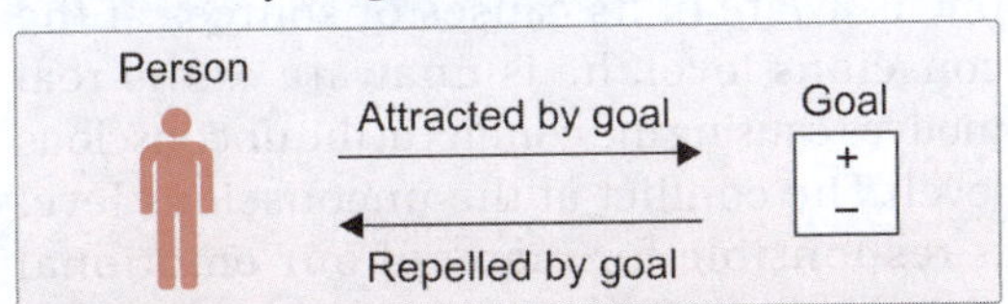

Figure 3.8: Approach-avoidance conflict

Multiple Approach-Avoidance Conflict

Multiple approach-avoidance conflict exists when a choice must be made between two or more alternatives each of which has both positive and negative features. Such conflicts are the most difficult to resolve and to make the right decision the individual must analyze the expected values of each course of action.

For example, a person may have the alternative of accepting any of the two jobs of which one may be boring but with a very good pay while the other may be interesting but with a very poor pay. Either choice has a positive and a negative quality, so which one does he choose? The choice will depend on the person involved and his feelings about the pay or work involved.

When it is difficult to decide in a double approach-avoidance conflict people usually vacillate and go back and forth between the two choices **(Figure 3.9)**.

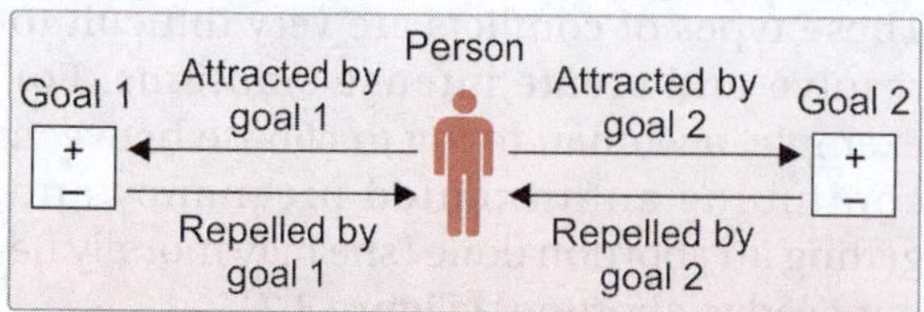

Figure 3.9: Multiple approach-avoidance conflict

Internal Conflicts

Conflicts may be between one person and another or between a person and his environment or may be within the person himself. The most dangerous and serious conflict is the one within a person. This is called internal conflict, the conflict between one's motives, desires, sentiments and attitudes. Freud describes it as a conflict between the three dynamic aspects of one's personality: id, ego and superego.

Our internal conflicts may either be conscious or unconscious in nature. While one is aware of its causes or sources at the conscious level, he is unaware of the real motives causing the conflict at the unconscious level. The conflict at the unconscious level is responsible for many of our emotional disorders and mental illnesses.

Measures to Overcome Frustration and Conflict

Frustration and conflict lead to stress and anxiety causing harm to the body. Some methods of relieving frustration are:

- Identify the source of frustration and make an attempt to change or control it. If not, learn to accept it.
- Decide upon important things carefully and double check everything before taking the final decision.
- Review the situation again.
- Change the goals or modify the desires.
- Substitute goals with those that are equally satisfying but different and obtainable.
- Seek advice from friends, relatives and experts.
- Encourage full expression of positive and negative feelings within an accepting atmosphere.
- Avoid indecision. Stick with decisions taken and forget other choices.

ROLE OF NURSE IN REDUCING FRUSTRATION AND CONFLICT AND ENHANCING COPING

Conflict is an inevitable part of life whether at home or at work, with patients or with colleagues. Since conflict and frustration have direct implications for patients, their positive resolution is essential to promote safe and effective delivery of care.

To resolve conflict and frustration the nurse should first identify or recognize the key factors or situations that are associated with escalation of conflict in patients and their families. Some of the adaptive mechanisms that patients need to be taught for resolving conflict are as follows:

- Encourage the patient to accept reality, prioritize the goals, change or reset them if not achieve them.
- Help the patient to set achievable goals thus resolving the conflict situation.
- Teach the patient problem solving techniques and help him analyze the pros and cons of each alternative solution. This will enable him to choose the best possible solution for the problem.
- Having an open mind can help solve one's problems easily.

A nurse can implement many different strategies to resolve conflict in patients. Conflict management strategies should be tailored to suit each patient situation. The nurse should decide the most appropriate strategy for each patient. Some such strategies to be adopted by a nurse are:

- During conflict situation, remain calm and encourage the patient to express his or her concerns.
- Avoid arguing, criticizing, defending or judging.
- Focus on patient behavior rather than the personality.

- Involve the patient, his family and health care team members in developing strategies to prevent or manage conflict situations.
- Employ patient-centered strategies to prevent behaviors that contribute to escalation of conflict.
- Try to understand patient health care needs and acknowledge feelings that stimulate patient behavior.
- Ask open-ended questions to collect more information.
- Engage in active listening—use verbal and non-verbal cues to acknowledge what is being said.
- Use calm, respectful and attentive attitude, respect client's wishes, concerns, values and priorities from the patient point of view.
- Anticipate situations which have earlier resulted in conflict and create a care plan to prevent its occurrence or escalation.
- As a member of the health care team be ready to work in collaboration with other healthcare members to deliver safe and effective patient care.
- Promote a respectful work environment by modeling professional behavior, reflect on personal attitudes, motives, values and beliefs that affect relationships with colleagues.
- Take adequate steps to manage personal stress as it may affect professional relationships.

SYNOPSIS

- Mental health is a state of balance between the individual and the surrounding world.
- Mental hygiene consists of measures to reduce the incidence of mental illness. It includes prevention, preservation and curative measures.
- Symptoms of mental disorders vary depending upon the type and severity of the condition.
- Primary prevention directed towards reducing the incidence of mental disorders in a community.
- Secondary prevention decreases the duration of disorder.
- Tertiary prevention reduces the level of impairment.
- Mental health services include Government mental health services, voluntary organizations, non-governmental organization (NGO), quarterway homes, halfway homes, self-help groups and suicide prevention centers.
- Ego defense mechanisms are methods of protect self and cope with basic drives or emotionally painful thoughts, feelings or events.
- The purpose of defense mechanisms is to reduce anxiety, resolve mental conflict and maintain a sense of security.
- Frustration refers to the blocking of behavior directed towards the goal.
- Conflict is a painful state of an individual during which the person experiences an intense emotional tension.
- The nurse should identify and recognize the key factors associated with conflict in patients and their families.

Review Questions

Long Essays

1. Define defense mechanisms. Explain any two with examples.
2. Define mental health. Discuss the characteristics of a mentally healthy person.
3. Discuss the role of a nurse in promotion of mental health.
4. Explain the different measures that can be taken in prevention of emotional and mental disturbances.
5. Define frustration and conflict. Explain sources of frustration.
6. What are conflicts? Explain different types of conflicts with examples.

Short Essays

1. Strategies of promotive and preventive mental health.
2. Briefly explain the preventive strategies in mental health.
3. Characteristics of a mentally healthy person.
4. Concepts of mental hygiene and mental health.
5. Explain the steps in prevention of mental and emotional disturbances.
6. Role of a nurse in preventing mental disturbances.
7. Community organization for care and rehabilitation of mentally retarded.

Short Notes

1. Rationalization
2. Ego defense mechanism
3. Adjustment
4. Mental health
5. Sublimation
6. Conflict
7. Frustration
8. Types of conflict
9. Conflict resolution
10. Conflict in motives
11. Approach-avoidance conflict

Multiple Choice Questions

Mental Hygiene

1. Mental hygiene is:
   a. A general set of principles that promotes healthy personality
   b. A general set of principles that promotes healthy learning
   c. A general set of principles that promotes positive emotions
   d. A general set of principles that promotes good intellectual capacity

2. Which of the following is a predisposing factor for mental illness?
   a. Genetic makeup
   b. Brain damage
   c. Psychological stress
   d. All of the above

3. Basics for a child's good mental health include:
   a. Unconditional love
   b. Minor illness
   c. Immunization
   d. Weaning

4. One of the characteristics of a mentally healthy individual is:
   a. Ability to make adjustments
   b. Ability to control anger
   c. Ability to be courageous
   d. Genuine concern towards others

5. Which of the following is a sign of poor mental health during adolescent period?
   a. Frequent temper tantrums
   b. Hyperactivity
   c. Abuse of drugs or alcohol
   d. Poor grades in school

6. The aim of primary prevention is:
   a. Decreasing the duration of disorder
   b. Reducing the incidence of mental illness

c. Reducing the impairment of mental illness
d. Reducing complications of mental illness.

7. ______________ **described levels of prevention specific to psychiatry.**

8. **In the process of development the individual strives to maintain, protect and enhance integrity of the self. This is normally accomplished through the use of:**
a. Affective reactions
b. Withdrawal patterns
c. Defense mechanisms
d. Strong emotional forces

9. **A male college student who is smaller than average and unable to participate in sports becomes the life of a party and a stylish dresser. This is an example of which type of mechanism?**
a. Rationalization
b. Sublimation
c. Compensation
d. Reaction formation

10. **After a horrible day at work, a father comes home and yells at his children for a minor mess. This is an example of:**
a. Repression
b. Rationalization
c. Projection
d. Displacement

11. **Sublimation is a defense mechanism that helps the individual to:**
a. Act out in reverse to something already done or thought
b. Return to an earlier, less mature stage of development
c. Exclude from the conscious things that are psychologically disturbing
d. Channel unacceptable sexual desires into socially approved behavior

12. **An example of displacement is:**
a. Imaginative activity to escape reality
b. Ignoring unpleasant aspects of reality
c. Resisting any demands made by other
d. Pent up emotions directed to other than the primary source

ANSWER KEY

1. a	2. d	3. a	4. a	5. c	6. b
7. Gerald Caplan	8. c	9. c	10. d	11. d	12. d

CHAPTER

4 Developmental Psychology

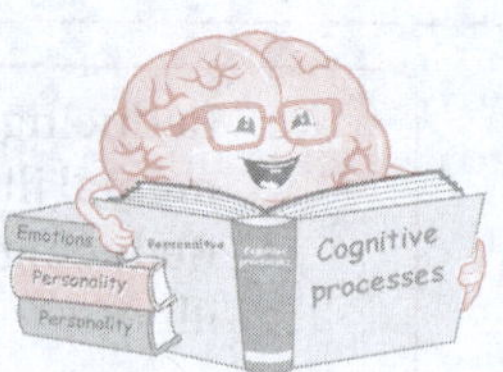

CHAPTER OUTLINE

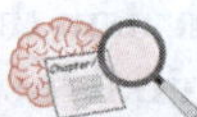

- Physical, psychosocial and cognitive development across lifespan
- Role of nurse in supporting normal growth and development across the lifespan
- Psychological needs of various groups in health and sickness—role of a nurse
- Introduction to child psychology and role of nurse in meeting the psychological needs of children
- Psychology of vulnerable individuals—role of a nurse

Growth is a process of physical maturation resulting in an increase in body size and organs. It occurs by multiplication of cells and an increase in intracellular substance. Quantitative change in the body is a measurable and progressive phenomena which can be measured in inches/centimeters/kilograms, etc.

Development is the process of physiological maturation of the individual. It also includes the progressive increase in skill and capacity of function along with psychological, emotional and social changes. It is a qualitative aspect of maturation which is difficult to measure.

Developmental psychology examines how people grow and change from the moment of conception through death. It is important for a nurse to know the basic principles of normal growth and development, to understand what can be expected from the child and to know the reason for particular conditions and illnesses that occur in various age groups. This knowledge forms the basis for teaching the patients.

Meaning of Developmental Psychology

Developmental psychology describes the processes and factors that influence the growth and development of an individual in relation to his behavior from birth to old age. It focuses on how people grow and change over the course of a lifetime. It is further subdivided into branches like child, adolescent, adult and old-age psychology.

PHYSICAL, PSYCHOSOCIAL AND COGNITIVE DEVELOPMENT ACROSS LIFESPAN

Development is a continuous lifelong process that proceeds from prenatal through early childhood, middle to late childhood through adolescence, early and mid-adulthood to late adulthood. It can be studied scientifically across three developmental domains—physical, psychosocial and cognitive.

Physical development is a continuous process from neonatal to adulthood. Though growth ceases after adolescence, it is not the end of development. Each development stage has a new set of challenges and opportunities. It involves growth and change in the body and brain, senses, motor skills, health and wellness. It also includes puberty, sexual health, fertility, menopause, changes in sense organs, etc.

Psychosocial development refers to how individual's needs interact with needs or demands of the society. It involves changes in behavior and social cognition. It includes emotions, personality, self-esteem and social relationships. Erik Erikson is the founder of psychosocial theory who described psychosocial development across the lifespan.

Cognitive development refers to how individuals organize their ideas and make sense of the world they live in. The five important aspects in cognitive development are—language development, problem solving, memory, moral development, and abstract thinking. It involves learning, attention, memory, language, thinking, reasoning and creativity. As the individual progresses through various developmental stages, his intellectual and cognitive ability increases. Jean Piaget developed the cognitive development theory. According to him, cognitive development occurs in a series of stages through the interaction of innate capabilities and environmental events through which all the children pass. The process of physical, psychosocial and cognitive development is detailed in **Tables 4.1 to 4.3**.

Table 4.1: Physical development across the lifespan

Developmental stages	Description
Prenatal ◆ Starts at conception, continues through implantation in the uterine wall by the embryo and ends at birth.	◆ It occurs in three stages—Zygote: Conception to 2 weeks, Embryo: 2 to 8 weeks and Fetus: 8 weeks to birth. All major structures of the body are formed during this period.
Infancy and toddler ◆ Starts at birth and continues up to two years of age.	◆ The infant is called a neonate for the first 4 weeks after birth. During the first 12 months, the infant shows very rapid motor development and learns to sit, stand and begins to walk. Infant weight triples from birth weight by 1 year. Length increases by almost 50% from birth. Infants grow rapidly reaching approximately half of their adult height by the time they are two years old. At around one year of age, infants begin to walk and by two years of age they begin to run. Physical growth during the first year is marked by a quick gain in body height and weight. ◆ Two aspects of physical development during this period are gross motor skills and fine motor skills. Gross motor skills are essential for walking, running, ball throwing, etc. Fine motor skills are actions that require the use of smaller muscles of the hands, fingers and toes. These are essential for dressing, scribbling, picking objects and stacking toys, etc. During this period, the child learns to control its body and movements.
Early childhood ◆ Starts at two years of age and continues until six years of age.	◆ Children continue to grow at a steady pace and develop strength and co-ordination. The average child becomes two and one-half inches taller and 5 to 7 pounds heavier during each year of early childhood. During this period, the child learns to walk, run, climb, jump and balance; develops fine motor skills and muscular co-ordination. ◆ Major development during this period is the development of fine motor skills and gaining good control over their smaller muscles. ◆ The child also develops sensory perception of size, learns to speak, dress and care. Other important achievements during this period are learning, how to use writing tools, identifying letters, numbers and sounds.

Contd...

Contd...

Developmental stages	Description
Middle and late childhood ◆ Starts at six years of age and continues until the onset of puberty.	◆ During this period physical growth is slow and gradual. The average child grows 2 to 3 inches in height and gains about 3 to 5 pounds of weight in a year. The child achieves good strength and control over body movement and develops better balance. Increased muscular development and resistance to fatigue makes new skills and activities possible. ◆ Children develop much smoother and well co-ordinated muscle movements during this age. They become capable of many muscular activities such as running, swimming, riding a bicycle and throwing or catching a ball. Writing or reading and the ability to handle language are two important achievements during this age. The child is now able to make the finer movements necessary for writing.
Adolescence ◆ Starts at the onset of puberty and continues until 18 years.	◆ Adolescence is a period of rapid physical, intellectual, emotional and social growth. Physically, the boy or girl becomes an adult; sex organs mature. Adolescence begins with very rapid changes in the body. Changes can be seen in height and weight, shape of the body, sound of the voice, presence of pubic and facial hair and other external sex characteristics. The initial spurt in growth usually begins about 2 years earlier in girls than in boys. Puberty in girls often starts between the ages of 11 and 13. In boys, puberty generally starts later often between 13 and 15 years of age. ◆ Puberty is the most important physical change during adolescence. The adolescent becomes mature and is capable of sexual reproduction. Endocrine glands regulate puberty through secretion of hormones. Adolescent girls and boys become very interested in sexual development and relationships with members of the opposite sex.
Early adulthood ◆ Starts at 19 years and continues until 40 years.	◆ Young adults reach the peak of their physical fitness between the ages of 19 and 28. By this age, young adults have reached their full height and strength. A number of sensory and neural functions are also at optimal levels during this period. For women, reproductive capacity is at its peak during young adulthood.
Middle adulthood ◆ Starts at 40 years and continues until 65 years.	◆ Middle adulthood commonly called the midlife brings with it dramatic changes in physical development. Adults may gradually lose some strength and speed. The slow decline of physical development which begins during the late years of early adulthood appears to speed up and is much more visible as a person steps into late 40. ◆ In middle age, adults put on weight, skin loses some of its elasticity, hair begins to thin out and often turns grey or white. Muscular strength declines slowly and steadily young adulthood onwards. A major physical change occurs in the cardiovascular system of the person during middle adulthood. The older heart cannot pump as much blood as the younger heart. Blood pressure usually rises during middle adulthood. ◆ During middle adulthood, men and women undergo a number of changes in their reproductive and sexual organs, a process that generally is referred to as the climacteric. These changes are linked to decrease in the production of sex hormones, specifically estrogen and testosterone. ◆ For women in mid-40 cessation of menstruation occurs which is termed as menopause. A number of unpleasant symptoms have been correlated with menopause which include profuse sweating, hot flashes, dizziness, headache, irritability, depression, insomnia and weight gain. The male climacteric occurs at about fifty years of age during which men experience a gradual decline in testosterone.

Contd...

Contd...

Developmental stages	Description
Late adulthood ◆ Starts from 65 years onwards.	◆ It is the period of retirement from active work. In later adulthood there are many changes associated with the aging process. By the age of 80, individuals may have lost as much as 5 cm in height. This is caused by change in posture and compression of the spinal discs and joints. ◆ The aging process also continues with further loss of mobility, strength and muscle loss, as well as a reduction in stamina. Mobility and dexterity become more difficult. Deterioration of body systems and senses causes visual and hearing problems. The resistance to disease and injury diminishes. All these interfere with daily life. ◆ Of all physical changes, a loss in the efficiency of cardiovascular system has the maximum impact upon a person in late adulthood. Changes in appearance, skin wrinkles, gray hair, poor balance, risk of falling, other chronic diseases such as cancer, arthritis, loss of hearing and vision are the common problems during old age.

Table 4.2: Psychosocial development across the lifespan

Developmental stages	Erikson's psychosocial stages of development	Description
Infancy	**Trust vs. Mistrust** (0–1 year) ◆ Develop trust when basic needs such as food and affection will be met	◆ Infants need to develop a sense of security. Become depressed or frustrated when being separated from parents or caregivers if they lack the sense of security. Develop attachment with family members/caregivers.
Childhood	**Autonomy vs. Shame/doubt** (1–3 years) ◆ Develop a sense of independence in many tasks	◆ Do not know how to explain their own feelings and emotions. The most common development in early childhood is to establish self-identity. Feeling of being valuable to friends and family is important. ◆ During this period, children join same sex relationship groups. Friendship groups influence values, beliefs and behavior.
	Initiative vs. Guilt (3–6 years) ◆ Take initiative in some activities, may develop guilt when unsuccessful	◆ The child experiences emotions of love and hate, jealousy and anxiety, learns to tolerate a certain degree of frustration and disappointment and deal with own difficulties independently.
	Industry vs. Inferiority (7–11 years) ◆ Develop self-confidence in abilities when competent or sense of inferiority when not	◆ The child requires protective environment, encouragement, discipline, provision for self-expression, guidance and direction to understand what behavior is expected.
Adolescence	**Identity vs. Confusion** (12–18 years) ◆ Experiment and develop identity and roles	◆ An adolescent needs to develop and secure self-concept. Acceptance of a new body and separation from home and establishing oneself as an independent adult in society are the significant challenges in puberty. ◆ Adolescents are more independent. They have high emotional tension due to hormonal changes, become emotionally unstable and are easily aroused by self-consciousness. They try to build intimate relationships. Peers become more important than family members as they explore new roles and form own identity.

Contd...

Contd...

Developmental stages	Erikson's psychosocial stages of development	Description
		◆ An adolescent has many fluctuations in mood and experiences variations between excessive bursts of energy and periods of laziness. They include extreme sensitiveness, self-consciousness, and a desire to be intellectually and emotionally independent.
Adulthood	**Intimacy vs. Isolation** (19–29 years) ◆ Establish intimacy and relationships with others	◆ Adulthood is a transitional time between the end of adolescence and before individuals acquire all the standards of adulthood. ◆ Adults demonstrate full independence from parents and establish own social networks. They adapt to different roles and relationships such as being a partner, parent and an employee. ◆ During this period, developing intimate relationships, establishing families and work are primary concerns. They search for intimate and secure relationships. Separation in intimate relationship or marriage creates severe emotional problems. ◆ Psychosocial development continues across adulthood with similar developmental issues of family, friends, parenting, romance, divorce, remarriage, blended families and caregiving for elders.
	Generativity vs. Stagnation (30–64 years) ◆ Contribute to society and be part of family	◆ Young women have additional psychological differences related to body changes. About 75% of all women in young adulthood experience mood swings with the cycle of menstruation. These are believed to be caused by hormonal changes in the body. ◆ Choosing a career and life partner are top priorities during this period. Child rearing is usually an important part of young adulthood. ◆ During this period behavior is governed more by intelligence than emotions. Adults adapt easily to social situations, face reality objectively, have normal drive to work or play and act according to one's own age. Adults are vocationally adjusted and are able to think and decide things on their own.
Elderly	**Integrity vs. Despair** (65 and above age) ◆ Make sense of life and meaning of contributions	◆ Older people need a secure sense of self to enable them cope with the physical changes associated with aging and death. During this period retirement, coping with losses and death are primary concerns. ◆ Erikson said that elderly reflect on their lives and feel either a sense of satisfaction or a sense of failure. People who feel proud of their accomplishments feel a sense of integrity and are able to look back on their lives with few regrets. People who are not successful at this stage may have feelings of bitterness, depression and despair.

Table 4.3: Cognitive development across the lifespan

Developmental stages	Piaget's stages of cognitive development	Description
Infancy	Sensorimotor (Birth–2 years)	Infancy and early childhood stages have rapid intellectual development. They understand the world through sense and motor actions.
Early childhood	Preoperational stage (2–7 years)	During this stage, children use symbols to represent their earlier sensorimotor discoveries. They use language to communicate. Piaget believes that children at this stage cannot properly understand how ideas like numbers, mass and volume really work. Questioning skills develop during this period. They also start to see the world from other people's perspective.
Middle and later childhood	Concrete operational (7–11 years)	During this period children have the ability to use language, think logically about the concrete world around them, understand simple logical principles, are capable of solving problems, learn new skills and abilities. However, these abilities are confined to things that he/she could see in daily life. They are unable to imagine things which they have not encountered before.
Adolescence	Formal operational (11–16 years)	Adolescents develop an ability to think logically about the abstract world, reason abstract concepts systematically and understand ethics and scientific reasoning. They are able to manipulate ideas and think hypothetically the possible outcomes of a problem. Abstract thinking enables individuals to think through complicated ideas in their heads without having to see the concrete image.
Adulthood		Adults can think through problems and make sound judgments using life experiences. Memory abilities and different forms of intelligence tend to change with age.
Elderly		Changes in the brain can cause short-term memory decline and slower thought processes and reactions.

ROLE OF NURSE IN SUPPORTING NORMAL GROWTH AND DEVELOPMENT ACROSS THE LIFESPAN

Nurses play an important role in identifying individual, family and group needs across the lifespan. They serve as educators, advocates, counselors and carers in matters related to people's health. They also play a key role in identifying risk groups and preventing the occurrences of health issues among all age groups. Nurses should utilize holistic approach in assessing and identifying health care problems of individuals and provide appropriate and timely interventions.

During childhood: The first five years of life are the most crucial in the emotional and psychological development of children. The earlier a developmental problem is identified, the faster it can be corrected. Nurse plays an important role in children's growth monitoring and promoting developmental process. She should be aware of the five factors contributing to growth and development at early childhood—nutrition, parent's behaviors, parenting, social and cultural practices and environment. If children do not receive appropriate care, it may lead to malnutrition thereby affecting their health adversely. Some of the nursing interventions that support normal growth and development during childhood are:

- Ensuring adequate antenatal care to the mother, educating her regarding the adverse effects of irradiation, drugs and prematurity.

- Ensuring timely and efficient obstetrical assistance to guard against the ill-effects of anoxia and injury to the newborn at birth.
- Ensuring that the mother has support from her family/community in seeking care at time of delivery/postnatal/lactation period.
- Imparting prenatal education about child's growth and development, motor, personal-social and language skills. Videos and videotaping may be used as a strategy.
- Teaching mothers and family members on how to identify clinical signs and seek health centers in case of any deviations from normal.
- Assessing and monitoring child growth and development.
- Promoting exclusive breastfeeding, immunization, timely care during illness all contribute to child's healthy growth and development.
- Ensuring clean air, water and sanitation and safe places for play and recreation. These are important for younger children to explore and learn.
- Ensuring adequate nutrition and good health in addition to making the child feel safe and secure and have opportunities for learning.
- Monitoring for malnutrition in children.
- Guiding parents to stimulate children through touching, speaking and playing.
- Identifying temperament traits and managing them with quality time and rewards.
- Promoting parent-child interaction.
- Ensuring that children are not only receiving adequate amount of micronutrients but also consuming iodized salt at the household level.
- Promoting mental and social development through talking, playing and providing a stimulating environment.
- Implementing interventions to prevent diseases which include immunization, safe waste disposal, appropriate handwashing, appropriate home treatment for infections, appropriate actions to prevent and manage child injuries and accidents.
- Preventing child abuse and neglect and taking appropriate action at the time of occurrence.
- Early identification of scholastic problems and emotional disturbances among school children and providing timely intervention.
- School teachers can be taught to recognize the beginning symptoms of physical health and emotional problems and referring to appropriate agencies.
- Ensuring active participation of men in providing child care in addition to family healthcare responsibilities.

During adolescent period: Adolescence is a period of rapid physical, intellectual, emotional and social growth. Puberty is the most important physical change during this period. To ensure optimal growth and development among adolescents, nurses are expected to identify their unique needs and ensure timely interventions. These include:

- Guiding the parents of adolescents' to not only appreciate the fact that every child is unique but also desist from unhealthy comparison which can lead to adolescent stress and subsequent behavioral problems.
- Reaching out to the adolescents in the community, at home, school and religious gatherings so as to provide intense education on developmental processes of adolescents, sexual and reproductive health as well as societal expectation during this period.
- Providing information on personal hygiene, menstrual hygiene, adequate nutrition, exercise and ill effects of illicit use of drugs, matters related to puberty and sexuality.
- Liaisoning with the schools to provide a safe and conducive physical, emotional and social environment for adolescents.

During adulthood period: Adulthood is a critical period of development with long-lasting implications for a person's economic security, health and well-being. Adults are key contributors to the nation's workforce. Common health issues among adults are motor vehicle accidents, homicides, mental health problems, sexually transmitted infections, substance abuse, obesity problems, etc. Behaviors associated with mortality and morbidity across the lifespan tend to emerge or peak during young adulthood. For example, use of tobacco, and low level of fitness and poor nutrition increase the probability of developing cardiovascular and pulmonary diseases and cancers later on in life. Some of the specific nursing interventions suitable for this period are:

- Encouraging positive health behaviors such as wearing seat belt to prevent vehicle injuries, immunization for preventable diseases such as COVID vaccine, tetanus vaccine, etc., regular exercise program, healthy diet, dietary modifications, stress management, weight management, smoking and drinking cessation, disease control for existing diseases, regular screening for chronic diseases, etc.
- Educating on special programs related to substance use, sexually transmitted infection, educational and vocational skills, suicide prevention and mental health.
- Identifying individuals with high disease risk factors through screenings and regular care.
- Conducting outreach programs to screen for various chronic illnesses.

During old age: Nurses act as a support function to motivate and empower the elderly, utilize their expertise in age-related issues to promote independence and functional abilities. Some of the nursing interventions specific to the elderly are:

- Assessing functional, mental and emotional status of the elderly.
- Early identification of complex comorbid physical and mental conditions.
- Assisting and training the elderly for daily living activities such as hygiene, toileting, medication management and nutritional needs.
- Preventing prevent risk of falls, malnutrition and other health problems.
- Encouraging physical exercises, yoga and other brain stimulating activities such as crossword puzzles or Sudoku.
- Facilitating connections with family members and loved ones who may be living in other parts of the country or abroad through video calls or messaging apps.
- Encouraging participation in traditional social events and cultural activities such as festivals or religious ceremonies.
- Enabling them to access technology.
- Promoting healthy lifestyle that can prevent or delay the onset of chronic diseases.
- Providing training and motivation to patients and caregivers to handle age-related conditions.
- Counseling on recommended self-care practices.
- Guiding older adults on their wellness journey.

Nurses help individuals across the health continuum to lead healthier and more fulfilling lives. They educate, inform and support individuals.

PSYCHOLOGICAL NEEDS OF VARIOUS GROUPS IN HEALTH AND SICKNESS—ROLE OF A NURSE

Psychological needs are essential nutrients that we all need to fulfill our natural tendencies for growth, development and wellbeing. Just like our body needs proper nutrition, our mind also needs proper psychological nutrients for optimal and healthy functioning.

1. Psychological Needs of an Infant

It includes need for security, love, affection, warmth, comfort, acceptance, nourishment, understanding and physical contact. The infant needs to be cuddled and fondled frequently and recognized consistently.

Children in Hospital

Small children cannot bear to be separated from parents for long. Bowlby (1951) argued strongly that disturbances in mental health and personality development resulted from maternal deprivation. There is strong evidence that very small children suffer from a sense of loss, mourning and grief when away from their mothers (Robertson, 1970; Hawthorn, 1974). At first the child may be fearful or angry;

later there is a stage of resignation with lack of interest and an apparent inability to accept love or return affection. How much this affects the child's development and its ability to form relationships with other people later on in life depends to some extent on the nature and duration of the separation from its mother and on the mother-child relationship before separation (Clarke and Clarke, 1976). Rutter (1981) argues that the concept of 'maternal deprivation' has been used to cover a wide range of different childhood experiences which have different effects on development.

On admission to hospital, children experience many distressing events such as the fact of being ill, strange medical and surgical procedures, different daily routines and a variety of unknown people. Nearly always, the child's rate of progress is affected both physically and mentally when separation from its mother is lengthy or repeated. On returning home, the child may refuse to recognize its mother and remain detached and unresponsive for some time. Bowel or bladder control achieved earlier might be lost. There may be excessive clinging, nightmares and other emotional disturbances.

Role of a Nurse

- The growth and development of an infant is all round—physical, mental, social and emotional. The nurse in charge of infant care must realize that the primary task of an infant is to grow. She must focus on giving as much personal attention as possible in the form of handling, cuddling, holding and loving. This kind of care will prevent deprivation and promote healthy physical and emotional development.
- Accurate observation of the infant is extremely important as the infant cannot communicate its needs through speech. Cry is the infant's main method of communication. Restless movements of body parts are another way in which the infant communicates its needs.
- The nurse should know that the infant may cry when it is hungry, in pain, diaper is wet or feels uncomfortable for any other reason.
- The nurse should very closely observe infant's growth and development for any abnormalities.
- The nurse should also be aware of normal individual differences in an infant's development.
- It is important for the nurse to accept the infant as a unique individual.
- Parents should be encouraged to involve themselves in providing care and comfort to the infant.
- Sensory soothing measures such as stroking the skin, talking softly, giving pacifier, cuddling and hugging the child should be used to provide love, affection and care.
- The surroundings of the child should be pleasant and cheerful.
- Child should be given suitable toys for play.
- Use of force and violence should be avoided while dealing with the child.

2. Psychological Needs during Childhood

It includes love, recognition, security, acceptance, encouragement, protection, discipline, nutrition, etc.

Older children once they have recovered from an acute phase of illness enjoy the companionship of others in the ward. During illness a certain amount of regression may occur. For example, the child behaves in a manner more appropriate to a younger age. The nurse needs to recognize and help the child to return to a more mature behavior. The child should not be penalized or insulted for wetting the bed or resorting to baby talk.

Role of a Nurse

- Tender loving care and physical security continue to be important to the child during these years.
- It is important that the child's routine in hospital resembles normal life as far as possible. The child's day should be a well-established routine which includes a right time for play, stories, bath and rest.
- Accurate observation is important to identify physical or emotional problems.
- A cordial relationship should be established with the young patient by going down to his

level such as asking him—his nick name, likes and dislikes.

- Love and affection must be shown so as to make the children emotionally happier and less anxious.
- The nurse should be patient in dealing with children.
- The child should be encouraged to develop a spirit of independence.
- The child should be allowed to participate in care and help wherever possible (for example, taking medicine from a cup, holding a dressing).
- Medical procedures should be explained in simple terms and in relation to how it benefits the child.
- Choices should be provided wherever possible without causing excessive delays.
- The child must be praised for helping and attempting to co-operate and never shamed for lack of co-operation.
- Privacy must be provided from peers during procedures to maintain self-esteem.
- It is desirable that the child acts independently and does not remain in a dependent state for too long. He must be encouraged to do things for himself.
- It must be ensured that the child does not remain tense, moody, worried or sad on account of being subjected to new, sudden and harsh changes such as unexpected separation from parents or pre-operation fears.
- Opportunities for play should be provided. The child must be allowed to choose its own play if possible. Picture books and puzzles are favored when the child is old enough. Play will also allow the child to express its feelings of frustration by projecting them on its toys. Drawing or scribbling is excellent for the child to express emotions.
- Games and toys should be made available in the pediatric unit. If not, reading a story book or educational material to the child is a pleasant and useful amusement.
- Nurses can learn to use play therapeutically.

Handling Parent's Anxiety

Parents of sick children need to be helped too because of the acute anxiety they are going through. Some parents may become overcritical and resort to fault finding while exhibiting irrational behavior. They become annoyed and resentful when the nurse does not answer all their questions to satisfaction. A nurse should be sympathetic, tolerant and tactful when dealing with their questions and anxiety and not get upset or lose temper. There is a need to reassure parents and make them feel comfortable and cheerful.

Small children do not understand the meaning of sickness very clearly. They cannot understand cause and effect, symptoms and treatment. They may blame the nurse or doctor for their pain. It may be necessary to separate the functions of the nurse so that the nurse who gives the child its daily care is never associated with causing pain. Some children appear to associate nurse's uniform with the unpleasant experience of sickness and pain. The child's early experiences with sickness, pain, hospitalization, separation from its mother and being cared by nurses may influence attitude to sickness later in life.

3. Psychological Needs during Late Childhood

It includes love, affection, security, belonging needs, understanding, attention and physical care. The child needs opportunities to exercise its muscles and refine motor co-ordination. The child also requires protective environment, encouragement, discipline, provision for self-expression, guidance and direction to understand what behavior is expected.

Role of a Nurse

- Tender loving care and emotional support is important if the child is experiencing loneliness, pain or discomfort for any reason.
- The child needs guidance and direction to understand the expected behavior during hospitalization.
- The older child should be provided with explanation for procedures in simple terms

and in relation to how it benefits the child. Many questions may be asked which the nurse must clarify.

- Justification for hospital rules and regulations may be provided where necessary.
- Health teaching should be directly related to an illness or its prevention and in general encourage habits of personal hygiene too. Use of visual aids should be preferred for teaching. It is important to praise the child when successful in learning.
- Observation of the child's physical condition and behavior is important. Problems in emotional health may be reflected by signs of depression or sadness, withdrawal from others or lack of self-control.
- Intellectual development of the child can be evaluated by observing its ability to converse and reason, read, write or solve arithmetic problems.
- The child should be allowed to participate in care and help whenever possible.
- The child must be allowed to play. Word puzzles, jigsaw puzzles and quite games can be pleasant and amusing. The ambulatory child requires more physical exercise and should be encouraged to walk.
- The child might expect the nurse to share her time and attention with him. It may often be a challenge for the nurse to be fair and consistent as she relates with each one.

4. Psychological Needs of an Adolescent

These include need for status, independence, satisfying philosophy of life, a proper orientation to the opposite sex and guidance in selecting a vocation.

Role of a Nurse

- Relevant rules and regulations may be detailed.
- As the adolescent has a rapidly changing body and is extremely self-conscious about it, as much privacy as possible may be ensured while care is being provided.
- Encourage questions regarding fears, options and alternatives.
- Discuss how nursing procedure may affect appearance and what can be done to minimize it.
- Involve the adolescent in decision making and planning (for example, choice of time, place, individuals present during the procedure, etc.).
- Accept regression to more childish methods of coping. Adolescent may weep or become emotionally upset when facing an injection or unpleasant treatment. They should be given extra emotional support and loving care when this happens.
- Allow adolescents to talk with their peers who have undergone the same procedure.
- Adolescents will most likely be able to make decisions about caring for self and planning their health care for the future. In most cases, they will need their parents to accord permission for decisions which involve admission or discharge, surgery or other major hospital procedures.

5. Psychological Needs of Early Adulthood

It includes a balance of intimacy, commitment, freedom and independence. The adult too like the child and adolescent needs security, self-realization and recognition. Other needs are development of intimate relationships, marriage and status in the society.

Role of a Nurse

- Young adults are rarely hospitalized. When they are, it is usually for childbirth, injuries from accidents or problems of the digestive or genitourinary system. Emotional support and understanding will be of help for all parents when childbirth occurs.
- Young adults need teaching and assistance in handling the baby. The teaching should also include the importance of good nutrition, adequate sleep, proper exercise and prevention of venereal diseases.
- Personality characteristics of the patient should be recognized and respected. Major task of the nurse is to respond to the various needs of the different personalities.

- Explaining procedures and what is expected of the patient relieve anxiety. Answering questions about the diagnosis, treatment and care also relieve anxiety.
- Assist the patient in solving problems that are worrisome.
- Ultimate goal of the nurse patient relationship throughout adulthood is helping the patient to achieve independence. Independence should be encouraged by the nurse as soon as the patient is ready.

6. Psychological Needs of Middle Adulthood

It includes need for status in the society, launching children into their own lives, coping with changes due to sex hormones and need for accomplishment of family responsibilities.

Role of a Nurse

- The middle-aged adult is most likely to be hospitalized for cardiovascular problems or cancer. Higher blood pressure as well as high cholesterol level may be evident. Other common health problems at this age are diabetes, peptic ulcer and communicable diseases.
- When a middle adult is admitted to the hospital, he needs to feel welcome and secure. Hospital policies and procedures are to be explained clearly.
- Anxieties apart from illness are experienced on account of various responsibilities shouldered by the person. These include personal anxieties about other family members, responsibilities at home, possible loss of a job, etc. The nurse needs to guide the family members in helping the patient in each of these areas.
- Observation of emotional and physical health is necessary to recognize signs of physical decline.
- Persons of this age require better lighting to see well, repeated verbal directions so as to understand what is being said and remember what is being asked. Written instructions should be provided when needed.
- The nurse should recognize signs of her inability to deal with stress at both work and home. These signs include agitated body language, increased levels of vital signs, insomnia, irritability or depression.
- Health teaching should include the prevention and early diagnosis of most common diseases.
- The nurse should help patients take care of themselves. All healthcare members should encourage independence as soon as the patient is ready for it.

7. Psychological Needs of Late Adulthood

It includes need for improvement of self-image, need for normal roles and relationships, need for love and relatedness, need to improve sense of hopefulness and need for accomplishment of tasks.

Role of a Nurse

- Older adults may be hospitalized more often than any other age group. Nursing care of the elderly is called geriatric nursing.
- A special effort should be made to make the elderly person feel respected and valued as an individual. Insecurities and apprehensions should be relieved as much as possible by giving careful explanations to the patient and the family members.
- Terminal illness is often a part of care for the older adult. The nurses should be prepared to give care and support as the patient prepares to die. The patient must be allowed to express his emotions.
- The nurse should observe the patient's ability to hear, see and walk, and check the vital signs regularly.
- The elderly may not feel pain as readily as younger people and bedsores can quickly develop even with regular nursing care. If a patient cannot move easily without help, various parts of his body should be exercised regularly with assistance.
- The older adult also needs close observation on behaviors such as depression, lack of interest in others or environment, withdrawing from others, sleeping poorly,

expressing despair or sadness. All these reflect the inability to cope with changing life situations.
- Elderly people often express a longing for the warmth and personal touch of another person. Emotional help and support from others are much necessary in order for them to find the strength and inner resources to adapt to their changing lives and lifestyles. Personal relationships with others should be encouraged. Appropriate activities such as playing games or listening to music, entertainment, creative hand work may also be encouraged.
- The elderly person often need help to see well. Some methods help the older adults to see well such as reducing glare for reading, providing extra lighting where necessary, keeping things near the visual field and using large prints or magnifiers.
- Physical protection from harm and injury should be provided to the older person. This may include assistance in walking or moving, bedside rails especially at night and protection from tissue injury when compressors or other skin applications are used. The elderly person is easily disoriented in a new environment and if ambulatory should be protected from becoming lost.
- Health teaching should include personal hygiene, importance of exercise, good nutrition, etc. Teaching will be effective if pictures, diagrams and posters with large prints can be used.
- The most effective way of teaching for this group is to teach one thing at a time. The older adults can learn new things if presented in the right way and related to what is already familiar.
- Anything completely new and different may have to be repeated at regular intervals so as to help the person remember them. It can be very helpful to relate new concepts or ideas to previous experiences wherever possible.

INTRODUCTION TO CHILD PSYCHOLOGY AND ROLE OF A NURSE IN MEETING THE PSYCHOLOGICAL NEEDS OF CHILDREN

Child psychology deals with the study of psychological development in children. It encompasses the various stages of psychological development from birth till adolescence and how it differs from that of adults.

Child psychology focuses on understanding the normal stages of psychological growth in children and distinguishes them from abnormal signs. Child psychologists help parents understand how best to communicate and connect with their children, teach coping mechanisms to handle emotions, thrive and progress through each developmental stage.

Child psychologists not only identify abnormal behaviors early but also help to detect the root cause of common behavioral issues such as learning problems, hyperactivity, anxiety, etc. They also help children work through early childhood trauma, prevent, evaluate and diagnose developmental delays or abnormalities such as autism.

Role of a Nurse

Children have unique psychological needs that affect their physical, psychological, cognitive and social development. Early identification and support for psychological needs are important to improve health and wellbeing of children. A child's psychological needs include security, love, affection, warmth, comfort, acceptance, nourishment, discipline, providing opportunities to exercise his skills and physical contact.

Nurses are in a unique position to support and promote the wellbeing of children as they are involved in preventive, promotive, curative and rehabilitative care services. They act as a primary care provider, health educator, counselor, child care advocate, co-ordinator collaborator **(Figure 4.1)**. The main roles

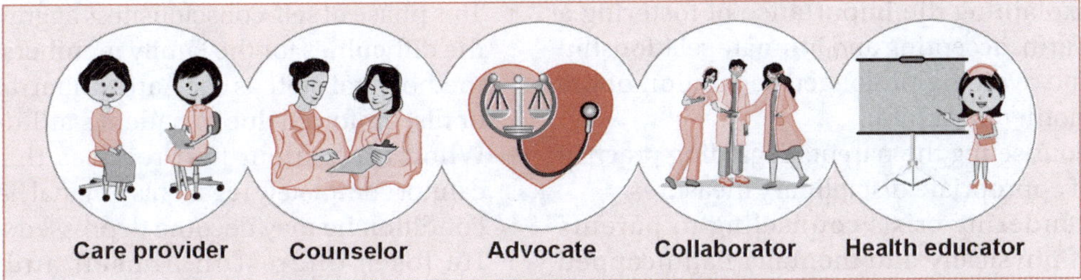

Figure 4.1: Role of a nurse to meet psychological needs of children

performed by nurses to meet psychological needs are as follows:

Primary care provider: As a primary care provider the nurse provides care for emotionally sick children in acute, rehabilitative care centers and community. The main responsibilities include:

- Providing a safe and comfortable environment.
- Meeting the physical and emotional needs of the children such as feeding, bathing, dressing and socialization.
- Assessing growth and development for any abnormalities.
- Assessing and monitoring psychological needs of children during their developmental period.
- Encouraging the parents to comfort the infant and provide sensory soothing measures.
- Identifying scholastic performance and emotional disturbances among school children and providing timely interventions.
- Providing preventive and screening services such as health education, assisting with decision making on health and immunization issues.
- Providing interventions for emotional problems, substance abuse and other mental health problems.
- Ensuring harmonious relationship among members of the family and teaching healthy adaptive techniques to counter stress.
- Providing crisis intervention services at mental hygiene clinics, psychiatric first-aid centers and walk-in-clinics for children passing through adolescence period.

Health educator: As a health educator her primary role is to provide information to parents, children and other significant members about prevention of illness and promotion of mental health. The main responsibilities include:

- Educating parents on safety and security needs of the child.
- Sensitizing parents and teachers on the various aspects of growth and development.
- Training the school teachers to recognize health related problems at an early stage and refer them to the appropriate agency.
- Teaching effective parenting practices and providing positive parenting tips such as responding to children in a predictable way. These may include:
  - Showing warmth and sensitivity
  - Having routines and household rules
  - Supporting health and safety
  - Using appropriate disciplinary measures without harshness
- Conducting mass health education programs through film shows, flash cards and appropriate audio-visual aids to sensitize on prevention of mental illnesses and promotion of mental health in the community.

Counselor: As a counselor the nurse is required to carry out many types of counseling interventions. The main responsibilities include:

- Counseling the parents of physically and mentally handicapped children with particular reference to the nature of defects. The parents need to accept and emotionally support the child and be satisfied with achieving limited goals.

- Explaining the importance of fostering a warm, accepting and intimate relationship and avoiding prolonged separation of the mother and child.
- Counseling the parents regarding practice of appropriate disciplinary measures.
- Rendering crisis counseling to parents of physically and mentally handicapped children.
- Promoting open healthy communication in families.

Care advocate: The nurse acts as an advocate to safeguard the child's rights and ensures best care from the healthcare team. The nurse acts as a representative for the child, family and the healthcare providers.

Co-ordinator and collaborator: The nurse co-ordinates nursing care services with the healthcare team which comprises of a psychiatrist, clinical psychologist, social worker, physiotherapist and a dietician.

PSYCHOLOGY OF VULNERABLE INDIVIDUALS—ROLE OF A NURSE

A vulnerable person belongs to a group within a society that is either oppressed or more susceptible to harm. Understanding the needs of vulnerable groups is very important as their needs are different from others. They require special care, support or protection due to their age, disability, risk of abuse or neglect. The knowledge of psychology of these people will help the nurses to deal with them in an effective way by providing appropriate nursing care.

Psychology of Challenged Individuals

- Chronic illness and prolonged disablement necessitate reconstruction of patient's idea of himself and a complete reorganization of relationships.
- A patient who realizes that he is permanently disabled becomes angry with himself and with others.
- He may express anger towards the family members and the hospital staff.
- He may refuse to meet people or go out.
- This phase of self-consciousness aggravates the difficulties for the family members and the hospital staff as they are embarrassed or discomforted due to patient's attitude.
- When the patient first realizes that he cannot completely regain his original health condition he may become depressed.
- He loses interest in himself and the surrounding and finds life not worth living.
- He refuses to take sufficient nourishment, treatment, neglects personal hygiene and loses interest in all activities.
- The will to live is essential to recover and the nurses must help the patient to see that in spite of his handicap he is needed by those who love him and that he can be useful to the community.
- Some health conditions are progressive causing dependence, disablement and suffering. The patient may feel obligated to pretend that he feels optimistic in order not to cause pain to his relatives.
- Some people who grow up with a disability (handicap) devote most of their time and energy in overcoming it and excelling in developing skills which are difficult to acquire. A few others cope with their disability by ignoring it and concentrating on achieving excellence in other areas.
- The greatest isolation occurs in those who lose sight, speech or hearing. Sometimes this isolation may lead to confusion, disorientation and a terrifying feeling of being lost leading to aggressive behavior. Blind people need constant interpretation of their environment while they are learning to use their other senses. It is important for the nurse to learn communication skills with the deaf such as gestures, mime, writing and demonstration.

The nursing care and rehabilitation of the disabled must aim at helping the patient to acknowledge his disability so that he can create a new idea of himself which includes his handicap.

Psychological Needs of Women

Just as physical disorders affect women differently than men, women's psychological needs are also different. In addition there are certain issues that are specific only to women due to the following reasons:

- Many women have been raised to be passive and place the needs of others before themselves. For example, a woman who is a wife and a mother may define her role as the giver and nurturer and disregard her own emotional needs. She may reach a point where she begins to experience anxiety and depression as she has lost her own identity.
- Women are twice as likely as men to experience depression.
- When an unwanted pregnancy occurs in woman's life, it can significantly alter her emotional development.
- Although infertility affects both men and women, women often feel the loss of not becoming pregnant and a psychological loss of not being a 'real woman'.
- More than 50% of women experience some form of violence from their spouses.
- Women who have been the victim of rape by a stranger, date rape or family member often experience a psychological effect known as rape trauma syndrome. Women experience low self-esteem or low level of confidence. There is lot of self-blame and self-attack. Other common feelings are depression and anger.

A nurse can help the woman uncover her strengths, needs and goals. The nurse will help her to understand the various options available and become more assertive when addressing difficult interpersonal situations.

Psychological Needs of Sick Person

The main aim of nursing care is to assist the patient in attaining the highest possible level of independence. Sickness interferes with self-care, interpersonal relationships, control over others, responsibilities and obligations particularly if admission to hospital is necessary. Inevitably illness results in disturbance of family and other social relationships. Illness also affects the emotional component in the individual.

- Short-term, non-life-threatening illness evokes a few emotional changes.
- Severe illness, particularly one that is life-threatening can lead to more extensive emotional reactions such as anxiety, shock, fear, anger, denial and depression.
- There may be anger about excess workload, occupational hazards or a dangerous lifestyle either of which may be held responsible for the illness.
- Communication problems among the patient and the family members may arise as they are not well-informed about the health issue. It is compounded when the doctors and nurses are not forthcoming due to seriousness of the aliment or poor communication skills. Such issues demand considerable amount of time, repeated contact, privacy and intimacy.
- Patients need to be stimulated by involving them in updates of current events and of people in the outside world. Visitors should be encouraged to share news rather than ask for it.
- The need to maintain family relationships and friendships during illness is important when small children are involved.
- Separation of children from their parents can cause a lot of anxiety. If the child is admitted, presence of the mother or the primary caregiver holds a lot of significance. When one of the parents is admitted in the hospital it is important that children should be allowed to visit them.
- During illness when patients remain at home they retain greater independence. Under such circumstances the nurse's job becomes all that more challenging as the patient may more readily exercise his right to deny care and forgo advice.
- Prolonged illness at home often results in isolation of the family due to the additional burden in providing health care to the patient.

Psychology of Caregivers during Illness

Illness in an individual also leads to considerable emotional disturbance among relatives who may feel guilty about not observing symptoms earlier or not taking complaints seriously.

If the illness is serious and the prognosis poor, relatives fear for patient's life which is accompanied by an anxiety about impending bereavement and a doubt about their own ability to cope.

The emotional and financial strain of chronic illness often results in a secret wish for early death. Such a wish is then followed by immediate regret and attempts to compensate for the guilt feeling. Relatives need someone who can help them to see that such thoughts are normal and understandable. When relatives can talk about their feelings they can often continue to shoulder the burden of care. When they cannot talk about their feelings they may detach themselves prematurely.

For many the pain of witnessing deterioration in their loved one may be too much to bear. They mourn the loss of the perfect image of the person they loved. By the time the patient dies their grief may already have been spent.

Loss and Grief

Patients who are terminally ill are often aware of the approach of death before anyone has discussed the subject with them. Glaser and Strauss (1965) have described three states of awareness that may surround the dying person and his family. These are closed awareness, mutual pretense and open awareness.

In closed awareness the patient and his family may be unaware of the impending death and may even lack a full appreciation of the illness. It may be that the relatives know but have decided that the patient should not be told. Conversely, the patient may know the truth but does not know if his closest relatives do. This creates problems for both the patient and his family and a dilemma for the nursing staff who may feel that the patient's trust in them may be threatened by less than honest communications.

In mutual pretense the patient, his family and the caregivers know that the prognosis is mortal but choose not to discuss the subject. Such mutual pretense is often motivated by a concern to protect against distress. But in reality it may lead to a sense of discomfort and burden created by the absence of anyone in whom to confide.

In open awareness all concerned know the truth and feel able to acknowledge and discuss the impending death. By doing so, the patient in particular is able to express his needs and desires and experiences a continuing sense of belonging and participating. It must be said however that open awareness is not an easy option and many still avoid it; some may feel able to discuss practical arrangements but need support and understanding to come to terms with their emotional responses.

Kübler-Ross (1969) having done extensive research with terminally ill patients identified five stages of feelings and behavior that individuals experience in response to a real, perceived or anticipated loss **(Figure 4.2)**:

- **Stage 1: Denial**—It is a stage of shock and disbelief. The response may be one of 'No, it can't be true!' Denial and shock is a protective mechanism that helps the individual survive the loss and cope within an immediate time frame while organizing more effective defense strategies. At this point, feelings that were once suppressed begin to resurface.
- **Stage 2: Anger**—It is a stage of frustration and irritation. 'Why me?' and 'It is not fair!' are comments often expressed during the anger stage. It is a natural response and perhaps a necessary one which may be directed at self or displaced on loved ones, caregivers and even God. It might be incomprehensible as to how something like this could happen. It is often due to a preoccupation with an idealized image of the lost entity. It is important to truly feel the anger as the more quickly it will dissipate, the more quickly the healing will happen.
- **Stage 3: Bargaining**—It is a stage of struggling to find meaning and telling one's story. 'I am ready to do anything to turn back time', 'If God will help me through this, I promise I will go to church every sunday

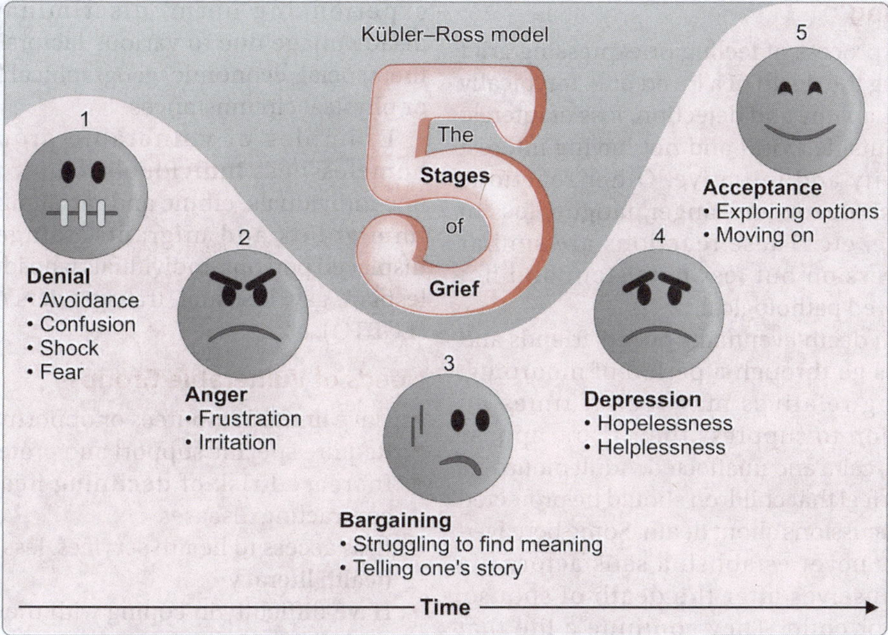

Figure 4.2: Stages of grief

and volunteer my time to help others' are the generally heard comments. During this stage, which is generally not visible or evident to others, a bargain is made with God in an attempt to reverse or postpone the loss. It is a stage of false hope where the individual falsely believes that he can avoid grief through a type of negotiation. 'If you change this, I'll change that'. There is a willingness to make a major life change in an attempt towards normality.

- **Stage 4: Depression**—It is a stage of helplessness. There is a feeling of hopelessness and thinking. 'What's the point in going on?', 'I am so sad' are the generally heard comments. Depression is a commonly accepted form of grief as it is a 'present' emotion. It is representative of the emptiness one experiences when there is a realization that the person or the situation is gone forever. During this stage the full impact of the loss is experienced. It is a time of quiet desperation and disengagement from all associations with the lost entity.
- **Stage 5: Acceptance**—It is a stage of exploring options and putting new plans in place. This final stage brings a feeling of peace with the grief event. 'It's going to be ok', I can take control of my future', are the generally heard comments. There is a perfect understanding that the loved one cannot be replaced and that one has to move on. Focus is on the reality of loss and its meaning for the individual affected by it. It is a time of adjustment and readjustment. Emotions begin to stabilize and the individual re-enters reality by coming to terms with the 'new' reality. There is renewed engagement with friends and formation of new relationships with passage of time.

All individuals do not experience each of these stages in response to a loss nor do they necessarily experience them in the same order. In some individuals grieving behavior may fluctuate and even overlap between stages. However, it is desirable to help the patient reach a state of acceptance rather than die in despair. It may be essential to help the patient through the earlier stages and encourage him to talk about his feelings. The nurse has to cope with the emotions of dying patients and their relatives and accept the feelings they express.

Mourning

It is the process of feeling or expressing grief following the death of a loved one. It typically involves apathy and dejection, loss of interest in the outside world and not having interest in activity and initiative. Other reactions may include anxiety, anger, fatigue, loss of appetite, etc. These reactions are similar to depression but less persistent and not considered pathological.

When death eventually occurs friends and relatives go through a period of mourning. Grieving relatives may feel at times an obligation to suppress their fears, appear tolerant, calm and unaffected. Adult mourners at times feel that children should be protected from discussions about death. Some bereaved persons never establish a satisfactory life for themselves after the death of spouse, parent or child. They continue a life that becomes progressively more isolated and depressed. Some may develop extreme hostility and resentment towards those with whom they were formerly associated through the deceased person. Especially in elderly, the death of the remaining spouse may occur soon after bereavement.

Worden (1983) described four tasks of bereaved. These are accepting the reality, accepting the pain that grief causes, adjusting to life without the loved one and being able to reinvest emotions in other relationships.

Nurses should be available to support the bereaved. The nurse should know the duration of grieving process. If prolonged or unresolved it may result in physical and psychological problems.

ROLE OF NURSE WITH VULNERABLE GROUPS

Vulnerable groups are subgroups of general population who are more susceptible to experiencing harm, discrimination or disadvantage due to various factors such as their social, economic, geographical location or physical circumstances.

Examples of vulnerable groups are homelessness individuals, below poverty line individuals, ethnic and racial minorities, immigrants and migrants, refugees and displaced persons, individuals who identify as lesbian, gay, bisexual, transgenders or queer (LGBTQ), etc.

Needs of Vulnerable Groups

- Have limited resources or opportunities
- Require specific support and protection
- Increased risk of declining health and contracting diseases
- Less access to health services, less optimal health literacy
- Have difficulty in coping with their health problems

Nurses' Role

- Nurses are in a unique position to help vulnerable groups by identifying the type of vulnerable groups a nurse may encounter at work or in the community.
- Promote healthcare awareness in society.
- Communicate with vulnerable groups and discuss their needs.
- Create a bond between all people while educating them on humanity and needs of vulnerable populations.
- Serve as an advocate to address the needs of vulnerable groups in schools, healthcare institutions and communities.
- Volunteer services in community clinics.
- Protect human rights and reduce health disparities.
- Provide quality care and advocacy to vulnerable individuals so as to improve equality in health and minimize health hazards.

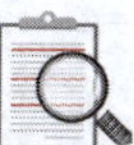

SYNOPSIS

- Development is the process of physiological maturation of the individual.
- Developmental psychology describes the process and factors that influence the growth and development of an individual in relation to his behavior from birth to old age.
- Physical development is continuous process from neonatal to adulthood.
- Psychosocial development refers to how individual's needs interact with demands of the society.
- Cognitive development refers to how individuals organize their ideas and make sense of the world they live in.
- Nurses play an important role in identifying individual, family and group needs across the lifespan.
- On admission to hospital, children experience many distressing events.
- The nurse should very closely observe infant's growth and development for any abnormality.
- Nurses can learn to use play therapeutically.
- Parents of sick children need to be helped to handle their emotions.
- Child psychology deals with the study of psychological development in children.
- Children have unique psychological needs that affect their physical, psychological, cognitive and social development.
- Nurses are in a unique position to support and promote the wellbeing of children.
- Chronic illness and prolonged disability necessitate a reconstruction of patient's idea of himself and a complete reorganization of relationship.
- Women psychological needs are different from men.
- Common psychological needs of women are body image, assertiveness, depression, teen pregnancy, infertility, domestic violence and rape.
- Sickness interferes with self-care, interpersonal relationships, control over others and responsibilities.
- Illness in an individual leads to disturbance among caregivers.
- According to Kubler-Ross there are 5 stages of grief: denial, grief, bargaining, depression, acceptance.

Review Questions

Long Essays

1. Describe psychological needs at different age levels—role of a nurse.
2. Describe psychological needs of patients—role of a nurse.
3. What is the meaning of physical development? Describe physical development across the lifespan.
4. What is the meaning of psychosocial development? Describe psychosocial development across the lifespan.
5. What is the meaning of cognitive development? Describe cognitive development across the lifespan.

Short Essays

1. Vulnerable individuals.
2. Psychological development during adolescence.
3. Developmental stages of an individual.
4. Explain stages of development.
5. Describe the role of a nurse in supporting normal growth and development across the lifespan.

Short Answers

1. Meaning of growth
2. Meaning of development

Short Notes

1. Geriatric problems
2. Psychological needs of infants
3. Grief
4. Mourning and loss
5. Psychological reactions of terminal illness

Multiple Choice Questions

1. Growth implies:
   a. Physical changes in the individual
   b. Quantitative changes in the individual
   c. Changes in structure
   d. All of the above

2. Development refers to:
   a. Qualitative change
   b. Quantitative change
   c. Both a and b
   d. Changes in height and weight

3. Puberty:
   a. Typically begins earlier in boys than in girls
   b. Typically begins later in girls living in affluent homes
   c. Is the period at which maturation of the sexual organs occurs
   d. Is a consequence of heredity and not affected by culture or class

4. Which of the following is continuous?
   a. Growth
   b. Development
   c. Both growth and development
   d. None of the above

5. Which of the following factor/factors influence growth and development?
   a. Heredity
   b. Cultural factors
   c. Environmental factors
   d. All of the above

6. Which of the biological factors influences physical growth?
   a. Family economic status
   b. Intelligence
   c. Endocrine glands
   d. Both b and c

7. Growth and development in any one dimension affects the growth and development in other dimensions too. This principle is known as:
   a. Principle of integration
   b. Principle of uniformity
   c. Principle of interaction
   d. Principle of interrelation

8. Which stage of the life is characterized by rapid growth and development?
   a. Infancy b. Toddler
   c. Preschooler d. Adolescent

9. Which of the following is a psychological need for the infant?
   a. Love
   b. Education
   c. Encouragement
   d. Provision for self-expression

10. Neonatal period refers to:
   a. First 4 weeks after birth
   b. First 12 months after birth
   c. First 1 week after birth
   d. First 2 weeks after birth

11. Which of the following is the infant's main method of communication?
   a. Body movement
   b. Crying
   c. Smiling
   d. Restless movements

12. Which of the following nursing interventions is more appropriate for an infant?
   a. Personal attention such as handling, cuddling, holding
   b. Providing physical security
   c. Praising the child for his co-operation
   d. Providing privacy

13. Which of the following nursing intervention is more appropriate for an adolescent?
   a. Personal attention such as handling, cuddling, holding
   b. Providing physical security
   c. Explaining each procedure with scientific rationale
   d. Using sensory soothing measures

14. Elisabeth Kübler–Ross observed that people facing death move through five stages in the following order:
   a. Denial, anger, bargaining, depression, acceptance
   b. Denial, depression, anger, bargaining, acceptance
   c. Anger, bargaining, denial, depression, acceptance
   d. Bargaining, anger, denial, acceptance, depression

15. Adolescent period starts from onset of puberty and ends with attainment of maturity. True/False

16. Development of habits, attitudes, manners are called moral development. True/False

17. Developmental psychologists are interested in the effects of both ________ and ________ on development.

18. Growth is the process of physical maturation. True/False

19. Which of the following concept best suits cognitive development?
   a. How individuals meet challenges and opportunities in each developmental stage?
   b. How individuals need to interact with needs or demands of the society?
   c. How individuals organize their ideas and make sense of the world they live in?
   d. How individuals change their behavior based on society demands?

20. Which of the following is termed as prenatal period?
   a. Starts at conception and ends at birth
   b. Starts at birth and continues up to two years of age
   c. Starts at two years of age and continues until six years of age
   d. Starts at six years of age and continues until the onset of puberty

ANSWER KEY

1. d	2. a	3. c	4. b	5. d	6. c
7. d	8. a	9. a	10. a	11. b	12. a
13. c	14. a	15. True	16. True	17. Heredity, environment	18. True
19. c	20. a				

CHAPTER

5 Personality

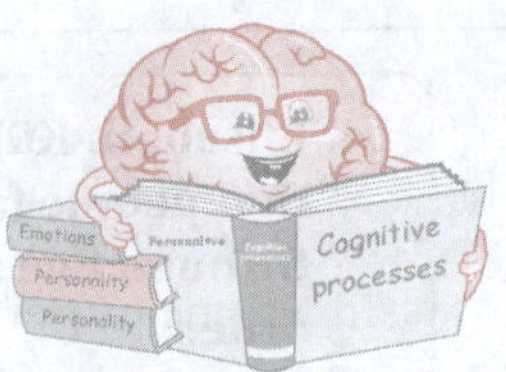

CHAPTER OUTLINE

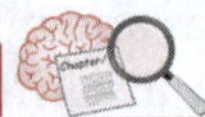

- Characteristics and classification of personalities
- Theories of personality development—psychoanalytic theory, theory of psychosocial development, humanistic approach theory, trait and type theories of personality, learning theories of personality
- Measurement and evaluation of personality—interview method, observation method, personality inventories, projective techniques
- Alterations in personality due to illness
- Role of nurse in identification of individual personality and improvement in altered personality

Etymologically, the word personality has been derived from the Latin word 'persona' meaning a theatrical mask usually worn by performers or actors. While a mask is generally worn to conceal one's identity, the theatrical mask worn by Roman and Greek actors was used to represent or project a specific personality trait of a character to the audience. The mask thus gave the actor his characteristic features.

Meaning and Definitions

Personality is the total quality of an individual behavior as it is shown in the habits, thinking, attitudes, interests, the manner of acting and the personal philosophy of life. It is the totality of one's being. It includes physical, mental, emotional and temperamental makeup and how it shows itself in behavior.

- 'Personality consists of the distinctive patterns of behavior including thoughts and emotions that characterize each individual's adaptation to the situations of his or her life.'

  —Walter Mischel (1976)
- 'Personality is the sum of activities that can be discovered by actual observations over a long enough period of time to give reliable information.' **—Watson**
- Personality refers to deeply ingrained patterns of behavior which include the way one relates to, perceives and thinks about the environment and oneself.

  —American Psychiatric Association (1987)

CHARACTERISTICS OF PERSONALITY

- One of the most important characteristics of personality is that it is a product of heredity and environment. A child though not born with a personality develops the same in course of continuous interaction with his environment. The social and cultural factors as well as the various experiences influence the development of personality.
- Personality includes the cognitive, affective and psychomotor behaviors and covers all the conscious, subconscious and unconscious also.
- It is specific and unique for each and every individual.
- It is not static, but dynamic in nature. Personality of an individual keeps adjusting itself to the environment on a continuous basis.

CLASSIFICATIONS OF PERSONALITIES

Personalities are classified based on individuals who share a common collection of traits. Classifications of personalities are depicted in **Figure 5.1**.

1. Hippocrates Classification

Hippocrates tried to classify all human beings into four characteristic groups according to their temperament. These are: sanguine, phlegmatic, melancholic, and choleric.

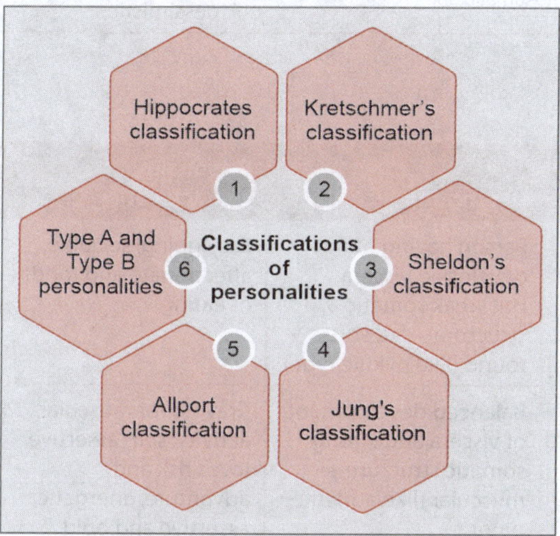

Figure 5.1: Classifications of personalities

Their personality characteristics are listed in **Table 5.1**.

2. Kretschmer's Classification

Kretschmer classified all human beings into certain biological types according to their physical structure. These are: pyknic, athletic, and leptosomatic. Their personality characteristics are listed in **Table 5.2.**

3. Sheldon's Classification

Sheldon classified human beings into certain types according to their physical structure and attached certain temperamental characteristics to them. These are—endomorphic mesomorphic, and ectomorphic. Their personality characteristics are listed in **Table 5.3.**

4. Jung's Classification

Dr Karl G Jung proposed to classify all individuals into two main groups. These are: extrovert and introvert. Their personality characteristics are listed in **Table 5.4**.

There are very few people who are purely extroverted or introverted. Most of us have a balance of extrovert and introvert features in our personality and can flip into either depending on the mood, context and goals. In other words we are ambiverts.

Table 5.1: Hippocrates classification of personality

Personality type		Fluids in the body	Personality characteristics
Sanguine	Sanguine	Blood	Optimistic, happy, hopeful, accommodating and light-hearted
Phlegmatic	Phlegmatic	Phlegm	Cold, calm, slow and indifferent
Melancholic	Melancholic	Black bile	Sad, depressed, pessimistic, dejected, deplorable and self- involved
Choleric	Choleric	Yellow bile	Irritable, passionate, strong, active, imaginative

Table 5.2: Kretschmer's classification of personality

Personality type		Description	Personality characteristics
Pyknic	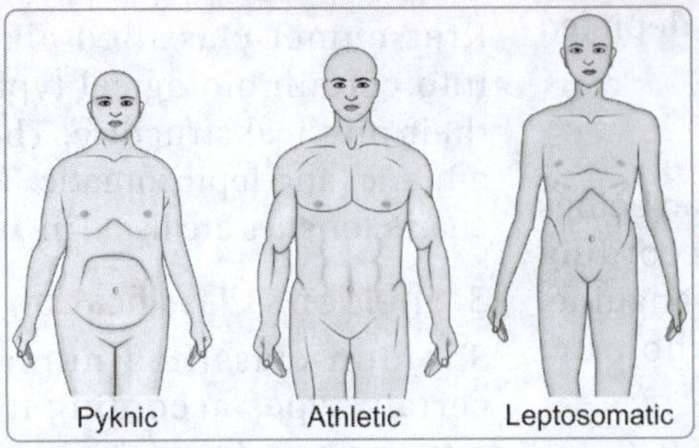 Pyknic Athletic Leptosomatic	Having fat body	Sociable, jolly, easy going and good natured
Athletic		Having balanced body	Energetic, optimistic and adjustable
Leptosomatic		Having lean and thin body	Unsociable, reserved, shy, sensitive and pessimistic

Table 5.3: Sheldon's classification of personality

Personality type		Description	Personality characteristics
Endomorphic	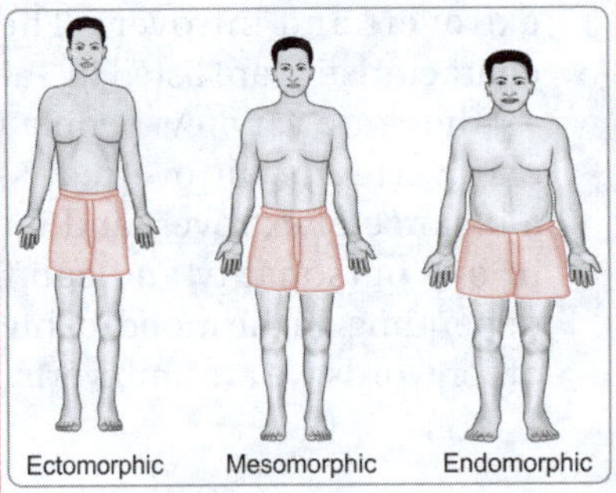 Ectomorphic Mesomorphic Endomorphic	Person having highly developed viscera, but weak somatic structure—fat, soft, round (like pyknic type)	Easy going, sociable, affectionate and fond of eating
Mesomorphic		Balanced development of viscera and strong somatic structure—muscular (like athletic type)	Craving for muscular activity, self- assertive, loves risk and adventure, energetic, assertive and bold tempered
Ectomorphic		Weak somatic structure as well as undeveloped viscera—thin, long, fragile (like leptosomatic type)	Pessimistic, unsociable, reserved, brainy, artistic and introvert

Table 5.4: Jung's classification of personality

Personality type		Personality characteristics
Extrovert	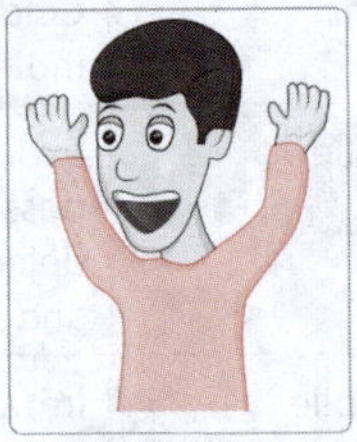	◆ Extroverts are interested in the world around them ◆ They are sociable, friendly, not easily upset by difficulties ◆ They are men of action rather than reflection ◆ They are successful in adjusting to the realities of their environment, are socially active and more interested in leaving a good impression on others ◆ Their behavior is influenced more by physical stimulation than by their inner thoughts and ideas ◆ Politicians, social workers, lawyers, insurance agents, salesmen, etc., fall in this category

Contd...

Contd...

Personality type	Personality characteristics
Introvert	• Introverts are interested in themselves, their own feelings and emotions, and are unable to adjust easily to social situations • Socially they are aloof, withdrawn, shy and reserved • They prefer to work alone and avoid social contacts. They are inclined to worry and get easily embarrassed • They seek manifestation of their life through inner activities by going inward or dragging up things from within themselves • Philosophers, scientists, writers, etc., fall in this category. There are very few people who are purely extroverted or introverted.

5. Allport Classification

Allport classifies all individuals into two types viz. ascendants and descendants **(Table 5.5)**.

'Type psychologists' assume that human personalities can be classified into a few clearly defined types. Our observation, careful and detailed measurements of personality traits show that this assumption is wrong. We cannot classify people only as tall or short, thin or fat, intelligent or stupid, sociable or unsociable. Most of us possess qualities or traits which are somewhere between these two extremes.

6. Type A and Type B Personality

Two specific behavior pattern types are known to be associated with increased or decreased likelihood of coronary artery disease. These are: Type A and Type B personalities. Their personality characteristics are listed in **Table 5.6**.

Table 5.5: Allport's classification of personality

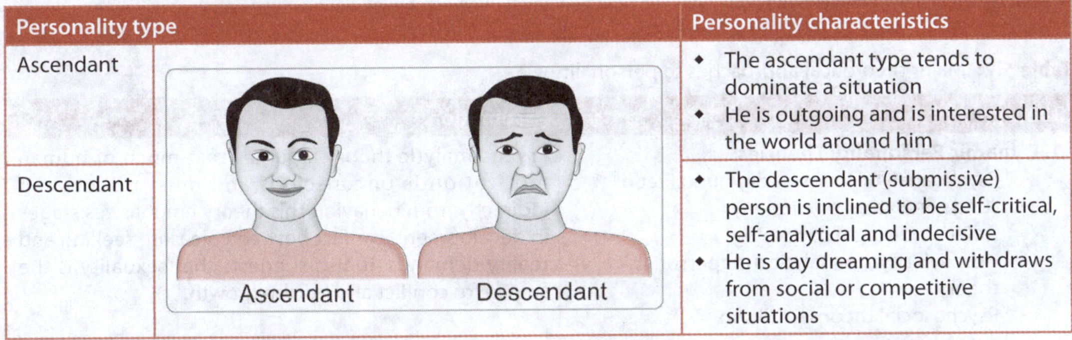

Personality type	Personality characteristics
Ascendant	• The ascendant type tends to dominate a situation • He is outgoing and is interested in the world around him
Descendant	• The descendant (submissive) person is inclined to be self-critical, self-analytical and indecisive • He is day dreaming and withdraws from social or competitive situations

Table 5.6: Characteristics of type A and type B personality

Personality type	Personality characteristics
Type A personality	• Type A persons are hard-driving and competitive, seek recognition and advancement and take on multiple activities with deadlines to meet • They live under constant pressure largely of their own making. Under stressful conditions they find it difficult to control themselves and are likely to become hostile, impatient, anxious and disorganized • Given a task to do, Type As' tend to perform any task near their maximum capacity no matter what the situation calls for

Contd...

Contd...

Personality type	Personality characteristics
Type B personality	• Type B persons are quite the opposite. They are easy going, non-competitive, placid and unflappable • They bear stress easily. They are likely to live longer than type A persons • Type Bs' work harder when given a deadline

THEORIES OF PERSONALITY DEVELOPMENT

Developmental theories identify behaviors associated with various stages through which individuals pass thereby specifying what is appropriate or inappropriate at each developmental level.

The major theoretical approaches to understand personality include psychoanalytic theory, humanistic theories, trait theory and learning theory **(Table 5.7).**

Despite the shortcomings of each of the major perspectives on personality theory each point of view has enlarged our understanding of human behavior. Psychoanalysis broadened our awareness of the continuity between infant and the adolescent. Learning theory provided insight into how behavior is acquired, maintained and extinguished. Humanistic theory enlarged our horizons by emphasizing human strivings towards self-fulfillment and growth.

Table 5.7: Major theoretical approaches to personality

Theory	Assumption
1. Dynamic Personality Theories – Psychoanalytic theory—Sigmund Freud – Jung's analytical psychology – Adler's individual psychology – Horney's psychoanalytic interpersonal theory – Psychosocial theory—Erikson	Psychoanalytic theory assumes that much of human motivation is unconscious and must be inferred indirectly from behavior. This theory emphasizes stages in development, conflict between pleasure seeking and reality demands. It also suggests that sexuality is the source for conflict and human growth.
2. Humanistic Theories—Personality as the Self – Roger's self-theory – Maslow's self-actualization theory	Humanistic theories of personality are concerned with the individual's personal view of the world, self-concept, and push towards growth or self-actualization.
3. Type and Trait Theories of Personality – Type theories—Eysenck's hierarchical theory – Trait theories – Allport's theory	The basic assumption of the trait theories is that individual personalities can be described in terms of a limited number of dimensions.
4. Learning and Behavioral Theories of Personality – Dollard and Millers early social learning theory – Skinner's radical behaviorism – Bandura and Watsons—later social learning theory	Social learning theory assumes that personality differences result from variations in learning experiences. Responses may be learned through observation without reinforcement. However, reinforcement is important in determining whether the learned responses will be performed. Emphasis is on situation—specific behavior rather than on broad characterizations of personality across diverse situations.

I. Psychoanalytic Theory

Sigmund Freud (1856–1939), an Austrian neurologist is considered as the father of psychoanalytic theory **(Figure 5.2)**. He emphasized the unconscious processes or psychodynamic factors as the basis for motivation and behavior. Freud categorized his personality theory according to structure, dynamics and development. Freud organized the structure of personality into three major components: id, ego and superego **(Figure 5.3)**.

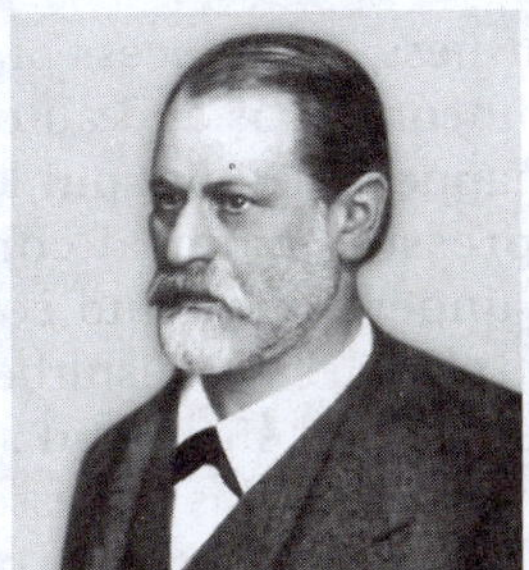

Figure 5.2: Sigmund Freud—founder of psychoanalytic theory

The id contains all our biologically based drives and operates according to the 'pleasure principle'. Id driven behaviors are impulsive and may be irrational. The ego functions on the basis of 'reality principle'. It maintains harmony between the external world, the id and the superego. The superego is referred to as the 'perfection principle'. The superego is important in the socialization of the individual as it assists the ego in the control of id impulses **(Figure 5.3)**.

A person who is well-adjusted or mentally healthy has all the three components of personality. Freud would expect anyone in whom many of the components are absent or out of balance to display maladaptive behaviors. Defense mechanisms have been associated strongly with Freud's theories.

One of the Freud's main beliefs is that abnormal behaviors result from ineffective personality development and unconscious processes. He believed that ineffective personality development was in some way related to the relationship of the child with the

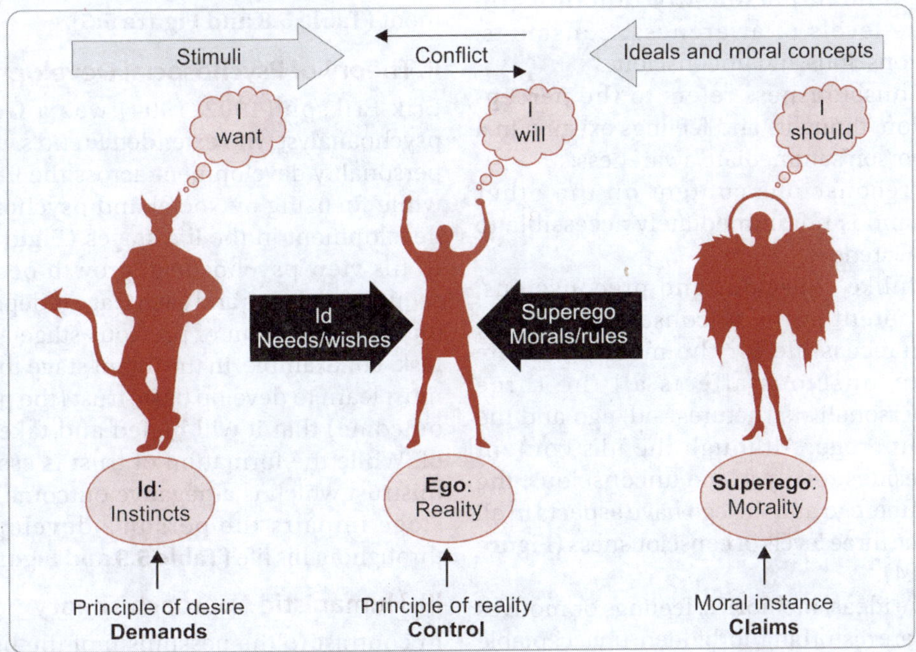

Figure 5.3: Freud's components of personality: Id, ego and superego

parent and that it was related to what he called psychosexual development.

Dynamics of Personality

- Freud believed that 'psychic energy' is the force or impetus required for mental functioning. Originating in the id, it instinctually fulfills basic physiological needs. As the child matures, psychic energy is diverted from the id to form the ego and then from the ego to form the superego.
- Psychic energy is distributed within these three personality components with the largest share required to maintain a balance between the id (impulsive behavior) and the superego (idealistic behavior). If an excessive amount of psychic energy is stored in one of these personality components, behavior will reflect that part of the personality. For instance, an impulsive behavior will prevail when excessive psychic energy is stored in the id.
- Over investment in the ego will reflect self-absorbed or narcissistic behaviors and an excess within the superego will result in rigid, self-deprecating behaviors.
- The human personality functions on three levels of awareness: conscious, preconscious and unconscious.
    1. Consciousness refers to the perception, thoughts and feelings existing in a person's immediate awareness.
    2. Preconscious content on the other hand is not immediately accessible to awareness.
    3. Unlike conscious and preconscious, content in the unconscious remains inaccessible for the most part. The unconscious affects all the three personality structures—id, ego and the superego. Although the id's content resides totally in the unconscious, the superego and the ego have aspects in all the three levels of consciousness **(Figure 5.4)**.
- Some ideas, memories, feelings or motives that are disturbing, forbidden, unacceptable and anxiety producing are repressed from consciousness. The process of repression itself is unconscious and automatic and simply happens without our knowledge. This repressed material continues to operate underground and converts the repressed conflicts into disturbed behavior and unexplained signs and symptoms. According to Freud this repressed material is also responsible for some of our dreams, accidental slips of tongue, etc.

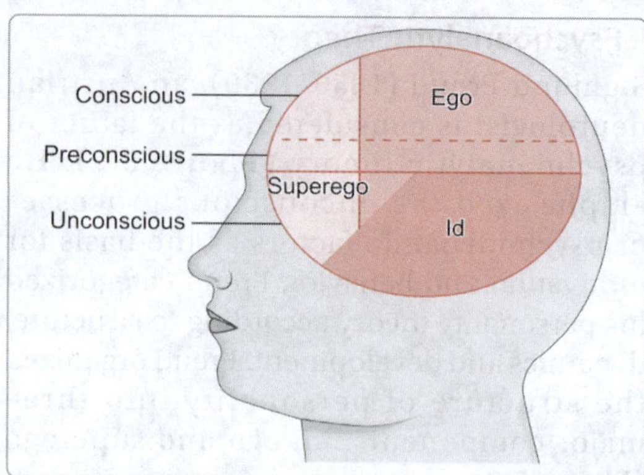

Figure 5.4: Freud's structure of personality

Freud's Stages of Personality Development

Freud described formation of personality through five stages of psychosexual development **(Table 5.8 and Figure 5.5)**.

II. Theory of Psychosocial Development

Erik Erikson (1902–1994) was a German psychoanalyst who extended Freud's work on personality development across the life span while focusing on social and psychological development in the life stages **(Figure 5.6)**. In his view psychosocial growth occurs in sequential phases and each stage is dependent on the completion of previous stage and life task. For example, in the infant stage the baby must learn to develop basic trust (the positive outcome) that it will be fed and taken care of. While the formation of trust is essential, mistrust which is a negative outcome of this stage impairs the person's development throughout his life **(Table 5.9 and Figure 5.7)**.

III. Humanistic Approach Theory

In contrast to the pessimism of the psychodynamic perspective, the humanistic

Table 5.8: Freud's stages of personality development

Stage of development	Focus of libido	Main characteristics	Successful task completion	Examples of unsuccessful task completion
Oral				
Birth–2 years	Mouth	Primary focus is on oral stimulation, use mouth and tongue to deal with anxiety (e.g., sucking, feeding)	Oral gratification	Smoking, alcoholism, obesity, nail biting, drug addiction, difficulty in trusting others
Anal				
2–3 years	Anus	Primary focus is on controlling bladder and bowels—eliminating/retaining feces, anus provides sensual pleasure, toilet training can be a crisis	Bowel and bladder control	Constipation, perfectionism, obsessive compulsive disorder
Phallic				
3–7 years	Genitalia	◆ Primary focus is on differences between male and female genitals ◆ Child becomes aware of anatomical sex differences giving rise to conflict between erotic attraction, resentment, rivalry and jealousy—Oedipus complex (in boys) and Electra complex (in girls) ◆ It is resolved through the process of identification—child represses the urge and adopts the characteristics of the same sex parent	Becomes aware of sexuality	Homosexuality, transsexuality, sexual identity problems in general, difficulty in accepting authority
Latency				
7–11 years	None	A quite stage in sexual development with greater focus on intellectual and social pursuits	Learns to socialize	Inability to conceptualize, lack of motivation in school or job
Genital				
11 years–adulthood	Genitals (for reproduction)	Sexual maturity and satisfactory relationships with the opposite sex	Sexual maturity	Frigidity, impotence, premature ejaculation, unsatisfactory relationships

approach optimistically argues that people have enormous potential for personal growth. When personality development focuses upon the development of self, it is called humanism. Humanists like Carl Rogers and Abraham Maslow reject the internal conflicts of Freud's view and the mechanistic nature of behaviorism. They believe that each person is creative and responsible, free to choose and strives for fulfilment or self-actualization.

Humanistic theories emphasize the importance of people's subjective attitudes, feelings and beliefs especially with regard to the self. Carl Rogers's theory focuses on the impact of

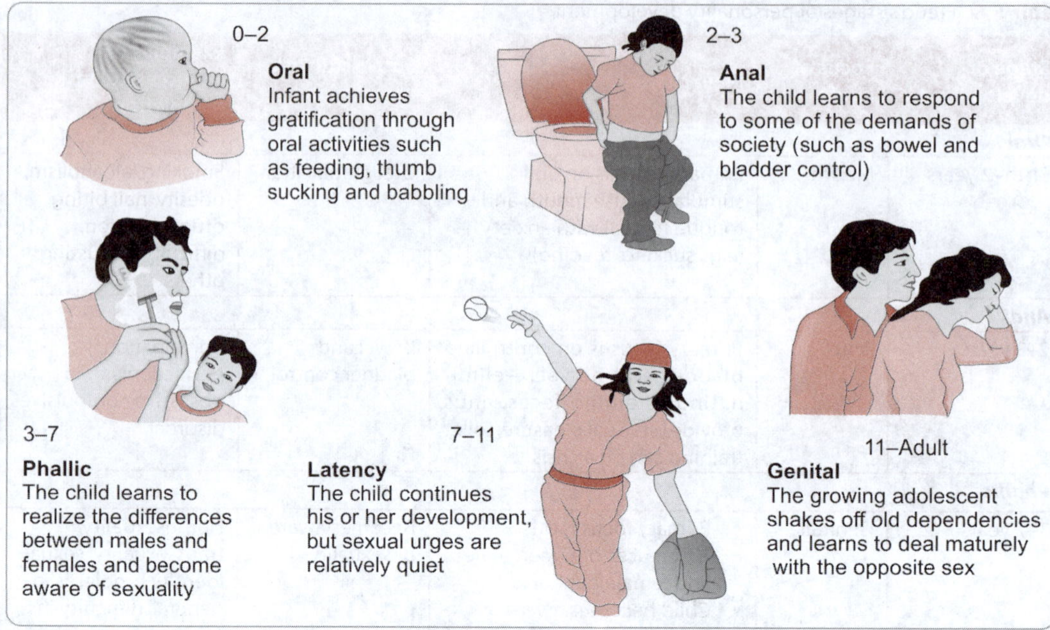

Figure 5.5: Freud's stages of personality development

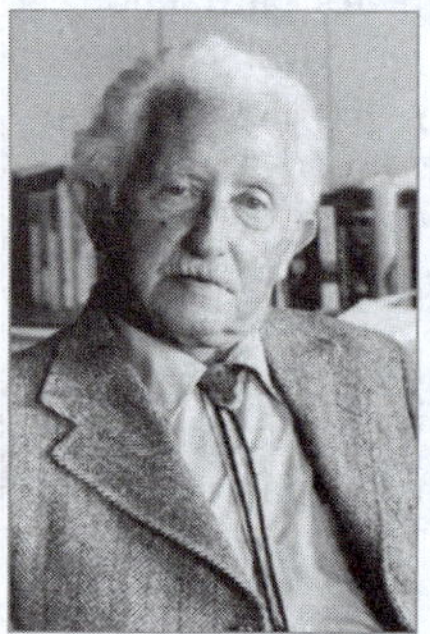

Figure 5.6: Erik Erikson—founder of psychosocial theory

Table 5.9: Erikson's eight stages of psychosocial development

Stage and approximate ages	Virtue	Task	Positive resolution	Consequences of unsuccessful task completion
Infant Trust vs. Mistrust (Birth–18 months)	Hope	Viewing the world as safe and reliable, relationships as nurturing, stable and dependable	Sense of security	Suspiciousness, trouble with personal relationships
Toddler Autonomy vs. Shame and doubt (1–3 years)	Will	Achieving a sense of control and free will	Sense of independence	Low self-esteem, dependency (on substances or people)

Contd...

Contd...

Stage and approximate ages	Virtue	Task	Positive resolution	Consequences of unsuccessful task completion
Preschool Initiative vs. Guilt (3–6 years)	Purpose	Beginning development of a conscience, learning to manage conflict and anxiety	Balance between spontaneity and restraint	Passive personality, strong feelings of guilt
School age Industry vs. Inferiority (6–12 years)	Competence	Emerging confidence in own ability, taking pleasure in accomplishments	Sense of self-confidence	Unmotivated, unreliable
Adolescence Identity vs. Role confusion (12–18 years)	Fidelity	Formulating a sense of self and belonging	Unified sense of self	Rebellion, substance abuse, difficulty in keeping personal relationships. May regress to child play behaviors
Young adult Intimacy vs. Isolation (18–25 years)	Love	Formulating adult, loving relationships and meaningful attachments to others	Form close personal relationships	Emotional immaturity may deny need for personal relationships
Middle adult Generativity vs. Stagnation (25–45 years)	Care	Being creative and productive, focus is on establishing family and guiding the next generation	Promote well-being of others	Inability to show concern for anyone but self
Maturity Ego integrity vs. Despair (45 years to death)	Wisdom	Accepting responsibility for one's self and life	Sense of satisfaction with life, well lived	Has difficulty in dealing with issues of ageing and death, may have feelings of hopelessness

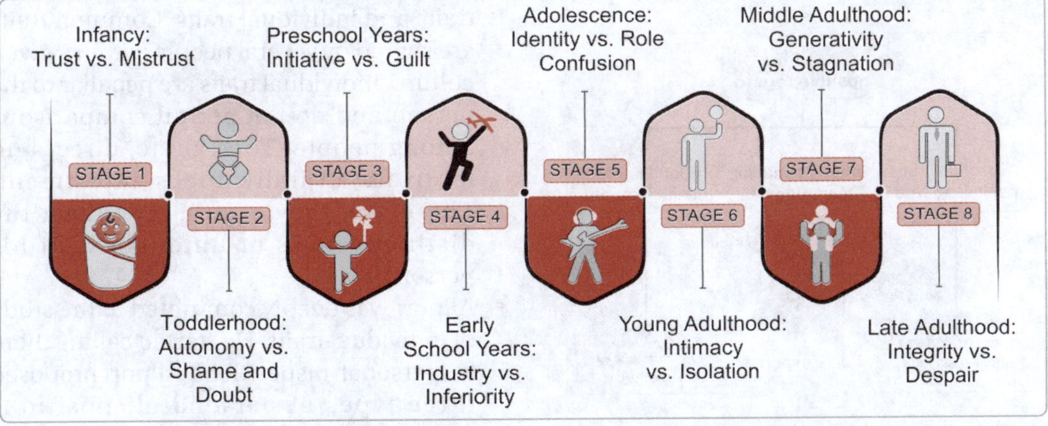

Figure 5.7: Erikson's eight stages of psychosocial development

disparity between a person's ideals, self and perceived real self. Maslow focuses on the significance of self-actualization.

1. Rogers Person-centered Approach (1980)

Carl Rogers (1902–1987) emphasized that each of us interprets the same set of stimuli differently. Hence there are many different 'real worlds' as there are people on this planet

Self-actualization

Carl Rogers used the term self-actualization to capture the nature underlying the tendency of humans to move forward and fulfill their true potential. He argued that people strive towards growth even in less favorable surroundings. According to the humanistic view of Carl Rogers, people have a basic need to be loved and respected. An unconditional positive regard from others will help to develop more realistic self-concepts. However, if the response is conditional it may lead to anxiety and frustration.

Personality development

Carl Rogers proposed that even young children need to be highly regarded by other people. Children also need positive self-regard to be esteemed by self as well as others. Rogers believed that everyone should be given unconditional positive regard. It should be non-judgmental and genuine love without any strings attached **(Figure 5.8)**.

2. Maslow's Hierarchy of Needs

- One of the basic themes underlying Maslow's theory is that motivation affects the person as a whole rather than just in part. Maslow believed that people are motivated to seek personal goals which make their lives rewarding and meaningful.
- Abraham Maslow suggested that five basic classes of needs or motives influence human behavior. According to Maslow, needs at the lowest level of the hierarchy must be satisfied before people can be motivated by higher-level goals *(Refer Chapter 7 - Page No. 192 for further details)*.

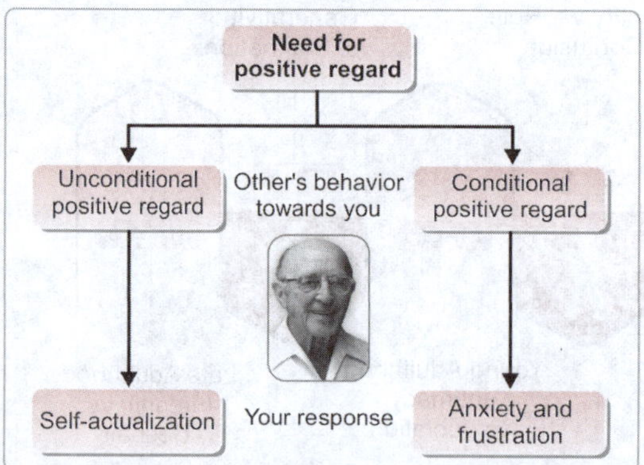

Figure 5.8: Humanistic view of Carl Rogers

IV. Trait and Type Theories of Personality

'Personality is the dynamic organization within the individual of those psychophysical systems that determine his unique adjustments to his environment.' **—Gordon Allport (1937)**

Two major themes that underlie trait and type theories of personality are:

1. No two individuals are alike.
2. People possess broad predispositions or traits to respond in certain ways in diverse situations. This suggests that people display consistency in their actions, thoughts and emotions across time, events and experiences.

1. Gordon Allport's Theory (1937)

- Gordon Allport's (1897–1967) an exponent of trait and type theories of personality asserts that no two individuals are alike. Allport regarded 'traits' as being responsible for these individual differences. According to Allport, trait is a predisposition to act in the same way in a wide range of situations.
- Allport distinguished between common traits and individual traits. Common traits are shared by several people within a given culture. Individual traits are peculiar to the person and do not permit comparisons among people. They guide, direct and motivate an individual's adjustment. Therefore, they accurately reflect the distinctiveness or uniqueness of his personality.
- Allport was deeply committed to the study of individual traits. He started calling them as 'personal' dispositions. Allport proposed three types of personal dispositions **(Figure 5.9)**.

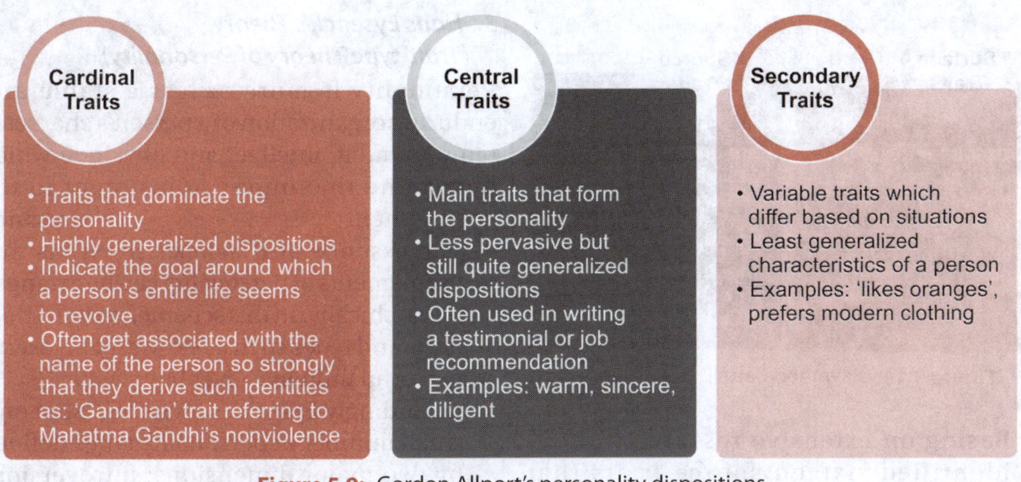

Figure 5.9: Gordon Allport's personality dispositions

1. ***Cardinal disposition:*** A cardinal disposition is so dominant that all actions of the person are guided by it to the point that the person becomes known specifically for these traits. Very few people possess cardinal dispositions. For example, Ms Nightingale whose actions were driven by compassion for people.
2. ***Central disposition:*** These are not as dominant as cardinal dispositions. However, as they influence a person's behavior in a very prominent way they are called the building blocks of personality. For example, a person may have such central dispositions as punctuality, responsibility, attentiveness, honesty, loyalty, etc.
3. ***Secondary disposition:*** These are not very consistent and are thus less relevant in reflecting the personality of the individual. These are sometimes related to attitudes or preferences and often appear only in certain situations or under specific circumstances. For example, food and clothing preferences, specific attitudes, etc., may be considered as secondary dispositions.

2. Raymond Cattell's Theory (1965)

- Raymond Cattell (1905-1998) spoke of the multiple traits that comprise the personality, the extent to which these traits are genetically and environmentally determined and the ways in which genetic and environmental factors interact to influence behavior.
- According to Cattell, personality is that which permits us to predict what a person will do in a given situation. In line with his mathematical analysis of personality, prediction of behavior can be made by means of a specification equation:

$$R = f(S, P)$$

- According to this formula, response (R) of a person is a function (f) of stimulus (S) at a given point of time and of the existing personality structure (P). This equation conveys Cattell's strong belief that human behavior is determined and can be predicted.
- Traits are a major part of Cattell's theory which he defined as the individual's stable and predictable characteristics.
- Cattell divided traits into surface traits and source traits. Surface traits are not consistent over time and do not have much value in accounting for the individual's personality. Source traits are the basic building blocks of personality which determine the consistencies of each person's behavior over an extended period of time **(Figure 5.10)**.

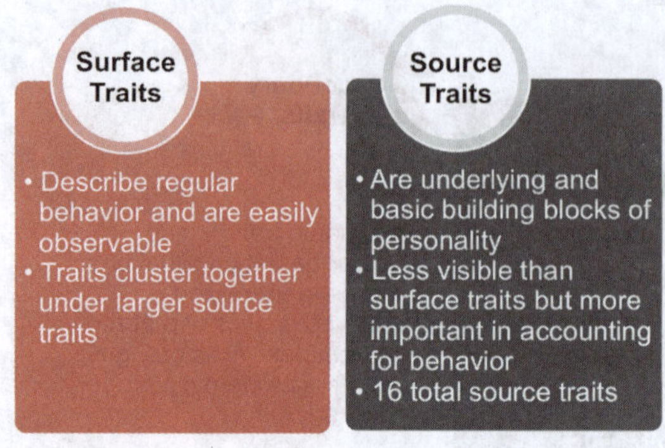

Figure 5.10: Raymond Cattell's trait theory

- Basing on extensive research, Cattell identified sixteen source traits that constitute the underlying structure of personality (such as outgoing-reserved, stable-emotional, self-sufficient-group dependent, etc.) He constructed a scale to measure these source traits which came to be known as 'Sixteen Personality Factor Questionnaire' (16 PF Questionnaire).

3. *Hans Eysenck's Theory (Trait-type Theory of Personality)*

Personality is more or less a stable and enduring organization of a person's character, temperament, intellect and physique which determine the unique adjustment to the environment. —**Eysenck**

- The essence of Eysenck's theory is that the elements of personality can be arranged hierarchically. In this scheme, certain super traits and types such as extroversion exert a powerful influence over behavior.
- Accordingly Eysenck's focus has been on a small number of personality types defined by two major dimensions: introversion-extroversion, stability-instability (neuroticism).
- Based on these personality types, Eysenck proposed four separate categories of people (**Figure 5.11**).
- Later, he added a third type of dimension to personality called the psychoticism-

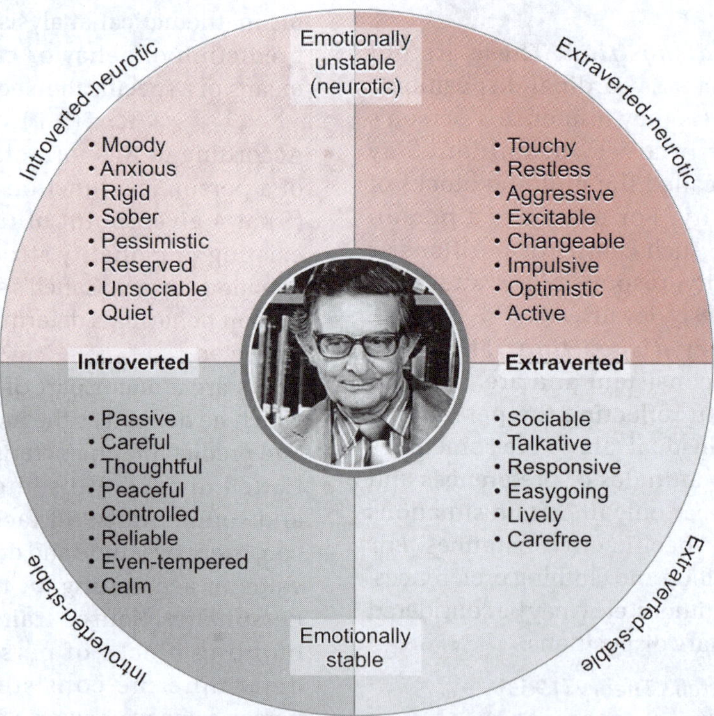

Figure 5.11: Eysenck's trait-type theory of personality

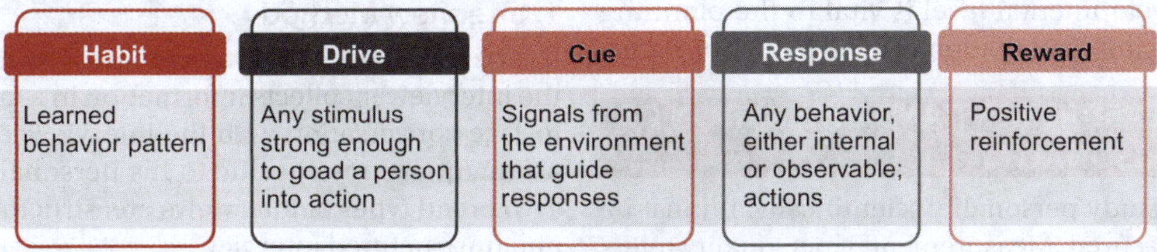

Figure 5.12: Concepts of Dollard and Miller's learning theory of personality

superego strength. People belonging to this category are selfish, impulsive and opposed to social customs.

- Basing on his categorization of personality types, Eysenck constructed an inventory called Eysenck Personality Questionnaire (EPQ). It covers items from each of the personality types identified by him.
- Throughout his writings Eysenck consistently emphasized the role of genetic factors and neurophysiological factors, role of the cerebral cortex, autonomous nervous system, limbic system, reticular activating system (RAS) in explaining individual differences in behavior.
- Cattell and Eysenck have been called as factor analytic trait theorists.

V. Learning Theories of Personality

These theories emphasize the importance of learning and objectivity to understand personality.

1. Dollard and Miller's Learning Theory of Personality

This theory emphasizes the development of personality on the basis of responses and behavior learnt through the process of motivation and reward. It stresses on habit formation through learning as a key factor in the development of personality. Habits are formed by stimulus response connections through learning. As one's fondness for learning grows on the basis of experiences and interaction with one's environment, habits are reorganized, new habits are learned and consequently the personality is modified and developed in terms of learning new behavior and picking up new threads or styles of life. Concepts of Dollard and Miller's learning theory of personality are described in **Figure 5.12**.

2. Bandura and Walter's Social Learning Theory

Albert Bandura and Richard Walter (1963) came out with an innovative approach to personality in the form of their social learning theory. They advanced the view that what an individual presents to the world at large as his personality is acquired through a continuous process of structuring and restructuring of experiences gathered by means of social learning and later imitated in corresponding situations **(Figure 5.13)** *(Refer Chapter 6 - Page No. 140 for details)*.

Implications to Nursing

Nurses must have a basic knowledge of human personality development to understand maladaptive behavioral responses commonly seen in the mentally ill. Knowledge of the appropriateness of behavior at each

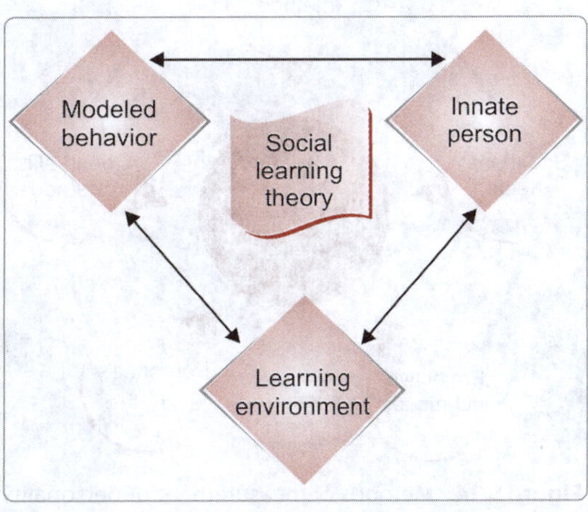

Figure 5.13: Social learning theory

developmental level is vital to the planning and implementation of quality nursing care.

MEASUREMENT AND EVALUATION OF PERSONALITY

To study personality scientifically, it must be measured. Measurement of personality refers to the assessment of personal characteristics of an individual using various psychological tests.

Importance of Personality Assessment

- Provides a means for studying personality.
- Helpful in assessment of personality for the purpose of employment or selection for education.
- Helpful for an individual to assess his own personality so that he can better understand himself and others, choose a career wisely and therefore find greater happiness in life.
- To refine clinical diagnosis and psychological interventions.

Methods of Measuring Personality

As personality is complex and varies from person to person, it is very difficult to form a correct idea of one's personality by a single method or technique. There are number of procedures and techniques that are being used for proper evaluation. Commonly used methods of measurement or evaluation of personality traits are presented in **Figure 5.14.**

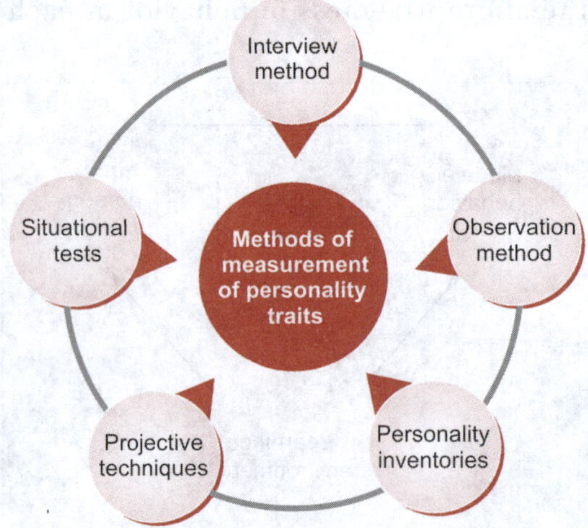

Figure 5.14: Methods of measurement of personality traits

1. Interview Method

Interview can be defined as a process in which the interviewer collects information in a face-to-face conversation with the interviewee by asking questions specific to his personality. Two broad types of interviews are: structured and unstructured interview.

i. In 'structured interview' predetermined questions are asked for which answers are highly specific. This type of interview is used where exact quantification is required. For example, industrial psychologists use structured interviews to select employees for a job.

ii. 'Unstructured interview' is an open interrogation where the interviewer questions or lets the individual speak freely so as to get a clear picture of the individual. From what he says, the interviewer knows about his interests, problems, strengths and limitations. Interviewee gives detailed answers and scoring is often subjective. For example, clinical psychologists, counsellors use unstructured interviews to assess personality traits.

Merits

- Highly flexible tool which can be used with a wide variety of population.
- The person can be observed for body language in addition to what is said.

Demerits

- Highly subjective
- Results can get influenced by the personal qualities of the interviewer
- Time consuming and at times costly too
- Requires a well-trained and competent person to conduct the interview
- Interview must be long and comprehensive to give a true picture of the individual's personality.

Example

The seven-point plan (Rodger, 1974) is a structured interview schedule for job interviewing. It includes physical characteristics, attainments, overall ability, special aptitudes, interests, personality attributes and circumstances. It provides a framework within which interviewers can work and explore in the context of matching the candidate with the job.

2. Self-report Techniques/Personality Inventories

A personality inventory is a printed form containing statements, questions or adjectives which apply to human behavior. The individual provides information about his/her personality by responding to statements/questions on the inventory. Responses are scored in quantitative terms and interpreted on the basis of norms that are developed for the test.

Merits

- Inventories are less time consuming and easy to administer when compared to other assessment procedures.
- Good validity opinions are sought directly
- Can be easily replicated—reliable.
- Closed questions are quantifiable as they can be summarized into tables and graphs and compared.
- Used for counseling, research purpose and in employment selection and promotion process.

Demerits

- There is a prospect of the subject creating false impression about himself or hiding his weaknesses if he wishes to do so
- Low response rate
- Misunderstanding of questions can lower reliability
- Lower validity as fixed choice of questions lack flexibility thereby forcing people to answer
- Subject may be ignorant of his own traits

Example

'Minnesota Multiphasic Personality Inventory' (MMPI) developed by Starke R Hathaway and J Charnley McKinley is the most commonly used clinical testing instrument to help diagnose mental health disorders. It is a self-report inventory with 567 true-false questions about oneself dealing with various personality traits such as attitudes, emotional reactions, physical and psychological symptoms. In this form of inventory answers are measured quantitatively and personality assessment done based on the scores. The test takes 60-90 minutes to complete.

Some examples of questions used in personality inventories or questionnaires are given in **Table 5.10.**

Other personality inventory measurements are Eysenck Personality inventory, Cattell's Sixteen personality factor Inventory (16 PF), California Personality Inventory, Bell Adjustment Inventory etc.

3. Observation Method

It involves the observation and recording of activities of a person by the observer in a controlled or natural situation. Based on the recordings inferences about the personality are drawn.

In this method the individual is observed in various situations (such as observing a person at work or play) for several days before coming to certain conclusions. Direct observation is most accurate if the observers are well trained in this activity. Observer may use several devices such as tape recorder, camera, telescope, etc. Observation is recorded by means of a rating scale which is used to rate the various personality traits, emotions, interests, attitudes, etc. The categories may be numerical or graphic.

Merits

- Most common and simplest method of data collection as it does not require technical knowledge.

Table 5.10: Personality questionnaire

Questions	Answers	
Do you adapt yourself easily to new conditions?	Yes	No
Do you have frequent ups and downs in mood?	Yes	No
Do you usually take the initiative in making new friends?	Yes	No
Do you prefer to work alone rather than with people?	Yes	No

- Data collected is more reliable than those collected through interview or questionnaire.
- It is the only appropriate tool to understand behavior in infants, deaf and dumb persons, cases of serious abnormality, non co-operative individuals and those who do not understand the language of researcher.

Demerits

- Some occurrences may not be open to observation
- Lack of reliability
- Faulty perception
- Personal bias of the observer
- Time consuming and expensive

Evaluation by observing can be made more accurate and objective if the observer uses a list of behavioral traits as a guide and rates the person on a scale. Having more than one observer helps to improve accuracy and prevent bias in making assessments.

4. Projective Techniques

Projective techniques are based on the principle that responses to unstructured stimuli reveal a subject's underlying motives, attitudes, fears and aspirations. In projective tests an individual is presented with a relatively unstructured or ambiguous task like a picture, inkblot or incomplete sentence which permits a wide variety of interpretations by the subject. The basis of assumption underlying projective tests is that individual's interpretation of the task will project the characteristic mode of responses, personal motives, emotions and desires and thus enable the examiner to understand more subtle aspects of the personality. The most commonly used projective techniques are listed in **Figure 5.15**.

A. Rorschach Inkblot Test

It was developed by Swiss psychiatrist, Herman Rorschach in 1921. This test consists of ten abstract inkblots (5 black and white, 2 black and red and white, 3 multicolored) that are shown to the subject one at a time in a prescribed order, who reports what is seen or whatever they bring to his mind. The subject's statements yield a great deal of information about his personality style, structure, quality of thinking and affect, diagnostic issues and also facilitate treatment, planning and evaluation. **(Figure 5.16)**.

B. Thematic Apperception Test

Thematic apperception test (TAT) was developed by CD Morgan and Henry A Murray in 1935. Assumption underlying the TAT is that the meaning which we see in a picture reveals something of our past experience, feelings, attitudes and motives.

In this test, subject is shown ambiguous pictures and asked to make up a story for each one. The themes in these stories are likely to involve conflict, affection, fear, contentment or achievement assumed to be determined partly by the subject's underlying concerns **(Figure 5.17)**.

C. Word Association Test

In this test the examiner utters a series of words, one word at a time and the subject immediately utters the first word that comes to his mind. There are no right or wrong answers. The examiner then records the reply to each word spoken by him, the reaction time and any unusual speech or behavior manifestations which might accompany a given response. Based on subject response the examiner evaluates the individual's personality. In this

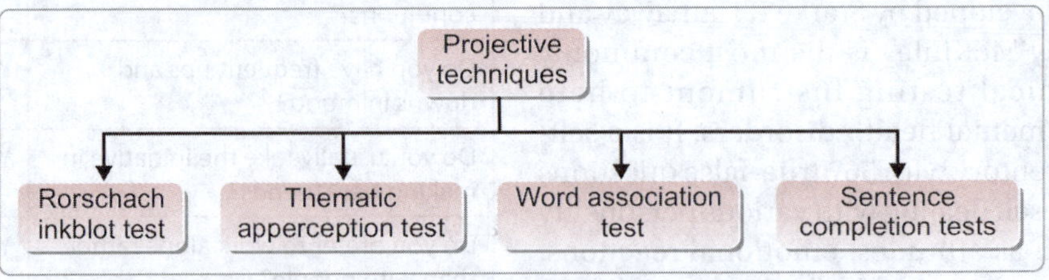

Figure 5.15: Commonly used projective techniques

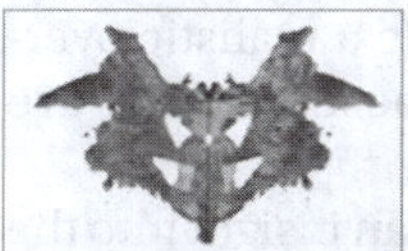

Card 1

Popular responses
bat, butterfly, moth

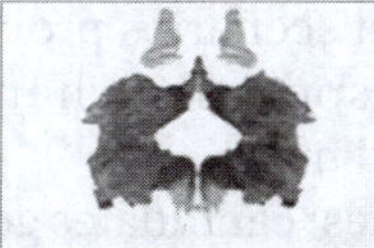

Card 2

Popular responses
two humans, four-legged animal, dog, elephant, bear

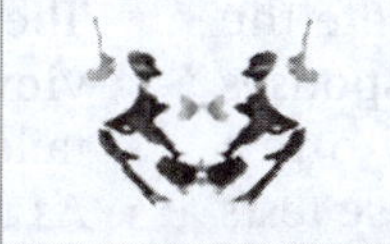

Card 3

Popular responses
two humans, human figures

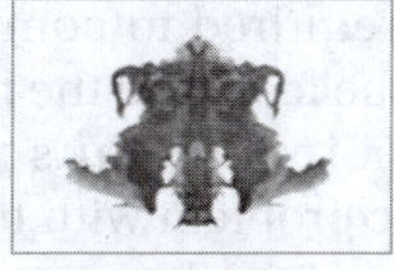

Card 4

Popular responses
animal hide, skin, rug

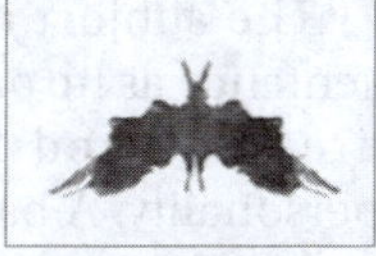

Card 5

Popular responses
bat, butterfly, moth

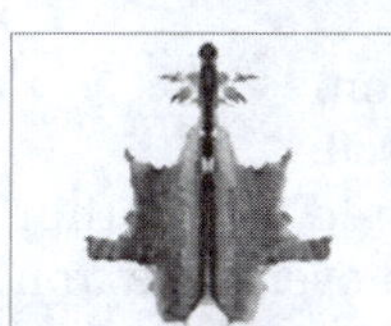

Card 6

Popular responses
animal hide, skin, rug

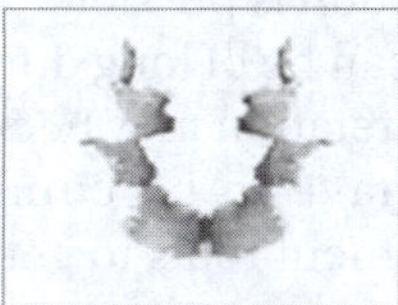

Card 7

Popular responses
human heads or faces

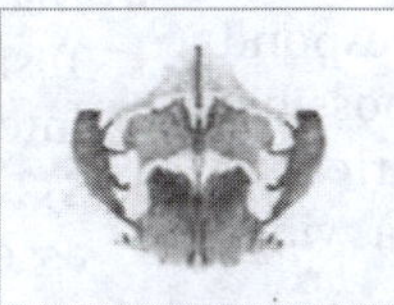

Card 8

Popular responses
animal: not cat or dog four-legged animal

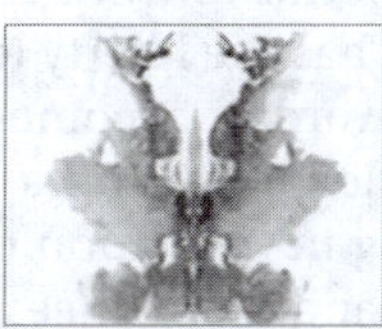

Card 9

Popular responses
human

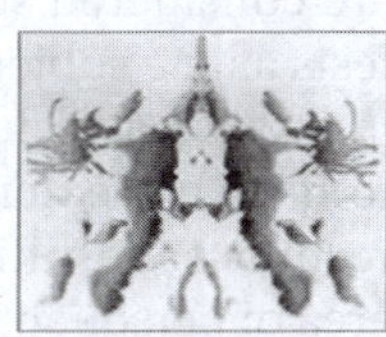

Card 10

Popular responses
crab, lobster, spider rabbit head, caterpillars, worms, snakes

Figure 5.16: Inkblots used in Rorschach test

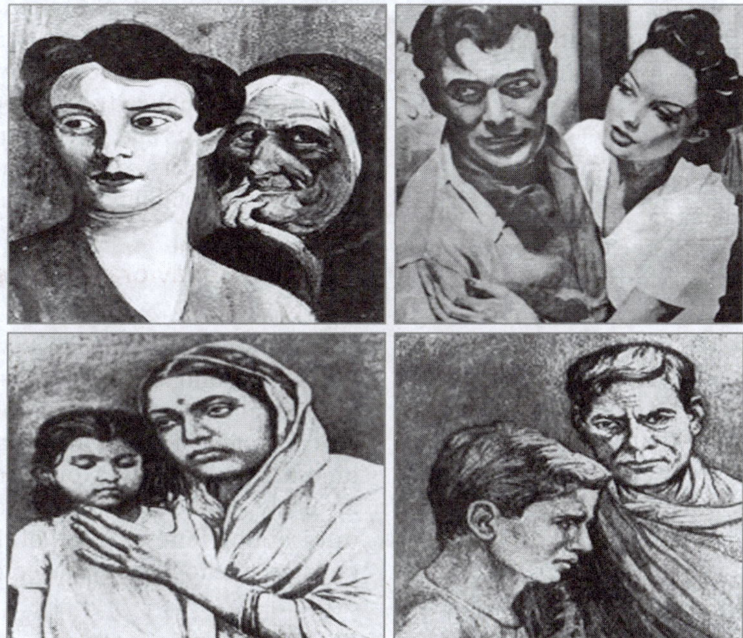

Figure 5.17: Sample pictures from thematic apperception test (TAT)

test people are read a standard array of 100 terms, e.g., 'head,' 'to sin,' 'to pray,' 'bride,' 'to abuse' with an instruction to respond to each term as quickly as possible with the first word that occurs to the subject's mind.

D. Sentence Completion Test

In this test a number of incomplete sentences are given and the subject is required to complete them. For example, I often feel I am............

The subject is required to complete the sentence as he or she feels and the responses are analyzed for indications of one's personality. A basic problem with these tests is that the interpretation of response is very subjective and based on the experience of the examiner.

The sentence completion tests however are considered superior to word association tests as the subject has the liberty to respond in more than one word. It becomes possible to have a greater flexibility and a variety of responses resulting in revelation of a wider area of personality and experiences.

Merits

- Powerful tool for understanding the unconscious processes in human mind
- Used to test unconscious thoughts and feelings about an object or event
- Often used in psychotherapy

Demerits

- Needs highly qualified and experienced professionals to implement and interpret the results
- Time consuming

E. Situational Judgement Tests (SJTs)

These tests involve real life situations where the subjects have to perform certain given activities. Subject's performance and behavior with respect to such situations helps in understanding his personality. In this test, subject's behavior is evaluated by trained judges. For example, a child's aggressiveness can be measured by letting it play with dolls and observing the number of times he is aggressive or does something destructive with them.

Merits

- Used to assess communication skills, interpersonal skills, team work and other abilities.
- Help in selection and recruitment by saving time and resources.
- Predictive validity is higher than in personality tests.
- Less expensive and a cost-effective tool for screening processes.
- The test scenarios provide a realistic overview especially when assessments are tailored made.
- As the test candidates get an insight into the profession's requirements, difficulties and intricacies beforehand, the staff turnover is significantly low.

Demerits

- Deception is possible.
- Tests can be of long duration.
- Interpretation may be biased.
- SJTs have to be combined with other assessment tools to get an overall view on applicants.

ALTERATIONS IN PERSONALITY DUE TO ILLNESS

Illness is a highly personal state in which the person's physical, emotional, intellectual, social, developmental or spiritual functioning is thought to be diminished or impaired compared to the previous experience.

How people behave when they are ill is highly individualized and affected by many variables such as age, sex, occupation, socio-economic status, religion, ethnic origin, psychological stability, personality and mode of coping.

Common Behavioral Changes due to Illness

Behavioral changes associated with short-term illness are generally mild and short lived. An individual may become irritable resulting in lack of energy or desire to interact with family members or friends. More acute responses are likely with severe life-threatening, chronic or disabling illness. Some of the behavioral changes due to illness are depicted in **Figure 5.18.**

Withdrawn Behavior

Illness particularly long-term or severe may cause patients to withdraw. Regardless of whether patients are in a hospital or at home they may avoid interaction, remain in their rooms or resort to solitary activities. They may become apathetic and depressed and try to close themselves off from their surroundings.

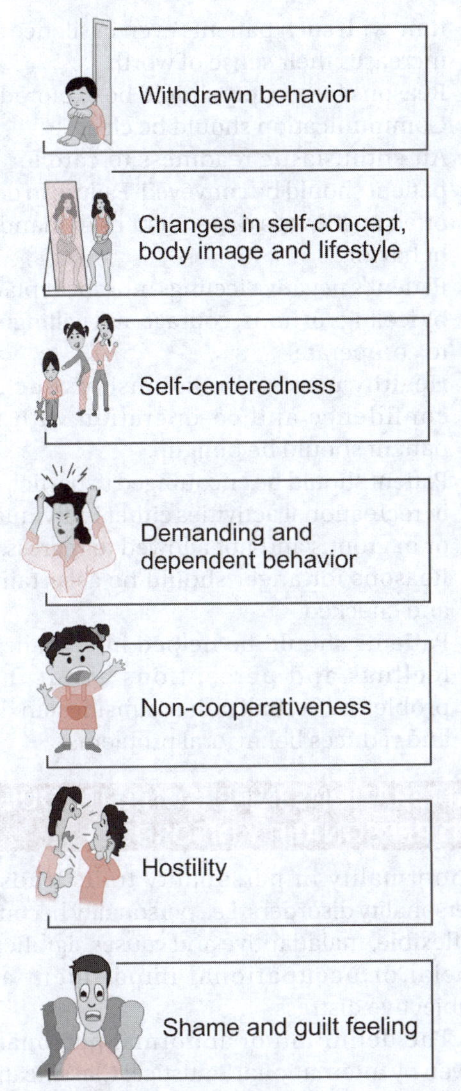

Figure 5.18: Behavioral changes due to illness

All these increase their loneliness and feelings of rejection.

Illness may weaken a patient's feeling of security. The factors which cause insecurity are delayed diagnosis and uncertainty of recovery, strangeness of place and people surrounding him, change of daily routine.

Changes in Self-concept, Body image and Lifestyle

Certain illnesses can change the patient's body image or physical appearance especially severe scarring or loss of a limb or a special sense organ. These patient's self-esteem and self-concept may also be affected.

Self-concept is important in relationship with other family members. A patient whose self-concept changes because of illness may no longer meet family expectations leading to tension or conflict. As a result the family members may change their level of interaction with the patient.

Illness imposes a certain amount of restriction on the patient regardless of his age, socioeconomic status or profession. Normal activities have to cease for some time, normal interests and responsibilities have to be given up.

Self-centeredness

An individual experiencing illness gets too personal. The threat posed by illness typically causes the patient to become preoccupied with himself and his health. The individual notes the changes in himself and shows much concern about his illness. As the seriousness of an illness increases even less attention is paid to the outside world or the concerns of others. He finds himself to be important and tries to be more careful about his health every time. Self-centeredness interferes with quick recovery.

Demanding and Dependent Behavior

Many patients tend to regress to a more childish level of behavior as a reaction to illness. This is reflected in the behavior of adult patients who are highly demanding or anxious or excessively dependent on others. Adult patients who seem to be afraid of taking the treatment and react timidly are also regressed.

Non-cooperativeness

Individuals react to illness in many different ways. Some patients are non-cooperative and show reluctance towards healthcare. Patients who do not follow advice of their caregivers are often labeled as resistive or non-compliant or non-cooperative. Sometimes such patients fail to enter a treatment program or dropout early. They often fail to keep follow up or referral appointments. Non-cooperative patients do not take prescribed medications regularly and fail to alter their lifestyle or activities. The mutual effort towards recovery becomes a tug of war between the nurse and the patient.

Hostility

Hostility is a type of aggression oriented to cause purposeful harm because of anger or provocation. Patient may be angry about the helplessness of the situation, unfair fate, etc. Hostility may in many circumstances be inwardly directed by persons having feeling of worthlessness and manifest itself in self-deprecating and self-punishing behavior.

Shame and Guilt Feelings

When a patient believes his illness is a punishment for sin or wrong doing (either imagined or real), he may react with feelings of shame and guilt. Certain diseases may make an individual feel disgraced or ashamed depending upon his family and cultural background. Some people feel that they shamed their family by having certain unacceptable conditions, e.g., mental disorders, venereal diseases, epilepsy, etc. They may feel unrealistically responsible for having brought on the condition. Such feelings of shame and guilt related to illness are damaging to the self-concept. Illnesses that are socially unacceptable, e.g., communicable diseases, AIDS, etc., cause the patient to be rejected.

ROLE OF NURSE IN IDENTIFICATION OF INDIVIDUAL PERSONALITY AND IMPROVEMENT IN ALTERED PERSONALITY

- Nurses need to help patients express their thoughts and feelings and provide care that helps the patient effectively cope with change.
- Feelings of insecurity should be lessened by straight forward explanations of hospital conditions and procedures including details of routine by being warm and reassuring in her manner and through sincerity of personal interest in the patient.
- Withdrawn patients should be given gentle encouragement to talk, express feelings and relate to the nurse. The nurse should spend time with such patients even in silence as it increases their sense of worth.
- Reasons for anxiety should be explored.
- Communication should be clear.
- An enthusiastic readiness to care for the patient should be conveyed. Failure to do so often aggravates dependent or demanding behavior.
- Patient's negative feelings must be replaced by feelings of hope, courage and willingness to co-operate.
- Healthy personal relationships such as confidence and co-operation with the patient should be built up.
- Patient should be encouraged to participate in recreational activities either individually or in groups and not allowed to regress.
- Reasons for anger should be ascertained and checked.
- Patients should be helped in verbalizing feelings and perceptions about their problems. Verbalization subsides anxiety and reduces behavioral problems.

ALTERATIONS IN PERSONALITY DUE TO PERSONALITY DISORDERS

Abnormality in personality traits leads to personality disorders, i.e., personality becomes inflexible, maladaptive and causes significant social or occupational impairment and subjective distress.

The definition of abnormal personality given by International Statistical Classification of Diseases and Related Health Problems— 9th revision (ICD9) is as follows:

'An abnormal personality is one in which there are deeply ingrained maladaptive patterns of behavior recognizable by the time of adolescence or earlier and continuing through most of the adult life. It results in patient suffering and also that of significant others with an adverse effect on the individual or the society'.

Classification of Personality Disorders

- Paranoid personality disorder
- Schizoid personality disorder
- Dissocial (antisocial) personality disorder

- Histrionic personality disorder
- Narcissistic personality disorder
- Borderline personality disorder
- Anxious personality disorder
- Dependent personality disorder
- Obsessive compulsive (anankastic) personality disorder

The exact cause of personality disorders is unknown as they most likely represent a combination of genetic, biological, social, psychological, developmental and environmental factors.

Clinical Features of Abnormal Personalities

Individuals with 'paranoid personality disorders' are marked by a distrust of other people and a constant unwarranted suspicion that others have sinister motives. Persons with paranoid personality disorder search for hidden meanings and hostile intentions in everything others say and do.

'Schizoid personality disorder' is characterized by detachment and social withdrawal. People with this disorder are commonly described as loners with solitary interests and occupations and no close friends. Typically they maintain a social distance even from family members and seem unconcerned about praise or criticism.

'Antisocial personality disorder' is characterized by chronic antisocial behavior that violates others rights or social norms which predisposes the affected person to criminal behavior. The person is unable to maintain consistent, responsible functioning at work, school or home.

Individuals with 'histrionic personality disorder' characteristically have a pervasive pattern of excessive emotionality and attention seeking behavior and are drawn to momentary excitements and fleeting adventures.

Individuals with 'narcissistic personality disorder' are self-centered, self-absorbed and lacking in empathy for others. They typically take advantage of people and use them without regard to their feelings to achieve their own ends.

'Borderline personality disorder' is marked by a pattern of instability in interpersonal relationships, mood, behavior and self-image.

'Anxious personality disorder' is marked by feelings of inadequacy, extreme social anxiety, social withdrawal and hypersensitivity to others opinions. People with this disorder have low self-esteem and poor self-confidence. They dwell on the negative and have difficulty viewing situations and interactions objectively.

'Dependent personality disorder' is characterized by an extreme need to be taken care of which leads to submissive, clinging behavior and fear of separation or rejection. People with this disorder let others make important decisions for them and have a strong need for constant reassurance and support.

'Obsessive compulsive (anankastic)' personality disorder is marked by a pervasive desire for perfection and order at the expense of openness, flexibility and efficiency. The individual places a great deal of pressure on himself and others not to make mistakes. He may have a constant sense of righteous indignation and feelings of anger and contempt for anyone who disagrees with him. He believes his way of doing something is the only right thereby forcing himself and others to follow right moral principles and conform to extremely high standards of performance while insisting on literal compliance with authority and rules.

Personality disorder is often difficult to treat. Drug treatment has a very limited role and may be used if associated with mental illness like depression or psychosis. Individual and group psychotherapy, therapeutic community and behavioral therapy may be beneficial. Manipulation of the social environment can be tried.

IMPLICATIONS TO NURSING

An understanding of personality will help the nurse to predict her behavior as well as the behavior of others. Major decisions in life depend upon this knowledge. For example, selection of a career or spouse, relationship with friends and relatives depends upon her expectations of their behavior by understanding their personalities.

A nurse should not only acquire skills and knowledge but also develop a strong and pleasing personality if she should be successful. Patients, doctors, co-workers and other important members of the society expect certain qualities and behavioral patterns from them. Patients appreciate a nurse who with her skills brings physical comfort, is prepared to understand their emotional reactions and difficulties caused by illness.

Besides possessing such professional qualities as integrity, dignity, mental alertness, self-confidence, caring attitude, empathy, approachability, respect for the patient, ability to build trust and accepting the patient as he is, she ought to have such personal qualities as sympathetic understanding, friendliness of spirit, gracious manner, kindliness, adaptability, genuineness, optimism, sincerity and self-awareness. Also, good health, fresh and neat appearance, a strong purpose and will power, a high standard of values, healthy work habits, sense of humor, teaching as well as managerial abilities and the ability to control one's emotions and a healthy and friendly interpersonal relationship are important traits that the professional nurse should cultivate.

As a nurse deals with patients from different age groups she should be aware of their personalities. A sick person is very emotional, sensitive, dependent and demanding. A warm, sincere outlook can help them.

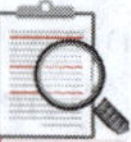

SYNOPSIS

- Personality includes cognitive, affective and psychomotor behavior and covers all the conscious, subconscious and unconscious activities.
- Personalities are classified based on individuals who share a common collection of traits.
- Psychoanalytic theory assumes that much of human motivation is unconscious and must be inferred indirectly from behavior.
- Humanistic theories of personality are concerned with the individual's personal view of the world and self-concept.
- Trait theories assume that individual personalities can be described in terms of a limited number of dimensions.
- Social learning theory assumes that personality differences result from variations in learning experiences.
- There are a number of procedures and techniques being used for personality evaluation.
- In interview method face-to-face conversation is carried out with some basic goals.
- In observation method, the individual is observed in various situations for several days before coming to conclusion.
- Personality inventory contains statements or questions. The individual indicates his reaction to the various items and then the test is evaluated.
- In projective technique the individual is exposed to unstructured stimuli to reveal underlying motives, attitudes, fears and aspirations.
- Behavioral changes associated with short-term illness are generally mild and short-lived.
- Behavioral changes due to illness are withdrawn behavior, self-centeredness, demanding and depending behavior, non-cooperativeness, hostility, shame and guilt feeling.
- An understanding of personality will help the nurse to predict her behavior as well as the behavior of others.

Review Questions

Long Essays

1. Define personality and theories of personality.
2. Define personality. List out types of personality. Explain Freud's psycho-analytic theory.
3. Write an essay on different types of personality.
4. Elucidate factors influencing the development of personality and its characteristics.
5. Define personality. Discuss the determinants of personality.
6. What is personality? Explain any three theories of personality with its evaluation.
7. What are the different types of personality? How is personality assessed?
8. Explain the trait theory of personality. Discuss the various trait compositions necessary to have effective nurse-patient relationship.
9. What are the personality changes due to illness?
9. Discuss the personality traits of an effective teacher.
10. Explain the importance of personality in nursing.
11. What is nature of personality? What factors contribute to development of personality?
12. What are projective tests? Explain their role in personality assessment.

Short Essays

1. Types of personality tests.
2. Assessment of personality.
3. Discuss Freud's theory of psychosexual development.
4. What effect does acute illness have on personality?
5. Role of questionnaire in personality assessment.
6. Discuss various trait compositions necessary to have effective nurse-patient relationship.
7. Briefly describe organization of personality.
8. Personality traits and an ideal nurse.

Short Notes

1. Id
2. Ego
3. Trait
4. Projection
5. Introverts
6. Development of personality
7. Physical traits
8. Social traits
9. What are 'traits' and 'types'?
10. Give two examples for projective tests of personality.
11. Superego

Multiple Choice Questions

1. Personality is unique for every individual because it is the result of the person's:
   a. Intellectual capacity, race and socioeconomic status
   b. Genetic background, placement in family and autoimmunity
   c. Biological constitution, psychological development and cultural setting
   d. Childhood experiences, intellectual capacity and socio-economic status

2. A relationship that is of extreme importance in the development of personality is that of the:
   a. Peer
   b. Sibling

c. Parent—child
d. Heterosexual

3. For an emotional balance the individual always needs:
a. Family, work and play
b. Financial security and social recognition
c. Biological satisfaction and social acceptance
d. Individual recognition and group acceptance

4. Family is most important in the emotional development of an individual because it:
a. Provides support for the young
b. Gives rewards and punishment
c. Helps one to learn identity and roles
d. Gives good educational background

5. Groups are important in the emotional development of the individual because peer group:
a. Always protects its members
b. Are easily identified by their members
c. Go through the same developmental phases
d. Identify acceptable behavior for their members

6. Problems with dependence versus independence develop during the stage of growth and development known as:
a. Infancy b. Toddler
c. Preschool d. School age

7. The basic emotional task for the toddler is:
a. Trust b. Industry
c. Identification d. Independence

8. ______ originated psychoanalytic theory in the early 1900s.
a. Erik Erikson
b. Alfred Adler
c. Sigmund Freud
d. Carl Jung

9. According to Freud, which component of personality operates according to the reality principle?
a. Id b. Ego
c. Superego d. Libido

10. Freud argued that exhibiting unusual rigidity or extreme disorderliness may be a sign of fixation at the ______ stage of personality.
a. Oral
b. Anal
c. Phallic
d. Latency

11. The ______ pushes the person towards greater virtue while the ______ pushes the person towards thoughtless pleasure-seeking.
a. Superego, id
b. Id, ego
c. Superego, ego
d. Ego, id

12. During the oedipal stage of growth and development the child:
a. Loves and hates both parents (ambivalence)
b. Loves parent of same sex and hates parent of opposite sex
c. Loves parent of opposite sex and hates parent of same sex
d. Loves both parents

13. Resolution of the oedipal complex takes place when the child:
a. Rejects parent of same sex
b. Introjects behaviors of both parents
c. Identifies with parent of the same sex
d. Identifies with parent of the opposite sex

14. An elderly client tells the nurse 'I am useless to everyone, even myself'. The nurse recognizes that the client has probably failed to accomplish Erikson's developmental task of:
a. Identity vs. role confusion

b. Generativity vs stagnation
c. Ego integrity vs despair
d. Autonomy vs shame and doubt

15. The ability to tolerate frustration is an example of one of the functions of the:

a. Id
b. Ego
c. Superego
d. Unconscious

16. Superego is that part of the psyche which:

a. Contains the instinctual drives
b. Is the source of creative energy
c. Operates on the pleasure principle and demands immediate gratification
d. Develops from internalizing the concepts of parents and significant others

17. Another term for superego is:

a. Self
b. Ideal self
c. Narcissism
d. Conscience

18. A person has a mature personality if the:

a. Ego responds to the demands of the superego
b. Society sets demands to which the ego responds
c. Superego controls the ego
d. Ego acts as a balance between the pressures of the id and superego

19. Which of the following represents the proper order of personality development according to Freud?

a. Oral, phallic, latency, anal, genital
b. Anal, oral, phallic, latency, genital
c. Oral, anal, phallic, latency, genital
d. Anal, oral, phallic, genital, latency

20. Psychosocial theory of personality was proposed by:

a. BF Skinner
b. Abraham Maslow
c. Erik Erikson
d. Sigmund Freud

21. Which approach to personality emphasizes the innate goodness of people and their desire to grow?

a. Humanistic
b. Psychoanalytic
c. Learning
d. Biological

22. Personality has been described in terms of traits by:

a. Cattell
b. GW Allport
c. Maslow
d. Karn Horney

23. Which stage of Erikson's psychosocial development theory deals with adolescence?

a. Ego integrity vs. Despair
b. Generativity vs. Stagnation
c. Intimacy vs. Isolation
d. Identity vs. Role confusion

24. The later childhood stage of Erikson's psychosocial development theory is:

a. Autonomy vs. Shame and doubt
b. Industry vs. Inferiority
c. Initiative vs. Guilt
d. Trust vs Mistrust

25. ______ are enduring dimensions of personality characteristics along which people differ.

a. Traits
b. Quirks
c. Factors
d. Profiles

26. According to ______ approach the ultimate goal of personality growth is self-actualization.

a. Neo-Freudian
b. Psychoanalytic
c. Psychosocial
d. Humanistic

27. The tests of personality that best reflect the unconscious are:

a. Self-administered questionnaires
b. Rating scales and checklists
c. Projective techniques
d. Observation for prolonged periods

28. Classification into endomorphic, mesomorphic and ectomorphic was proposed by:
a. Hippocrates b. Ernst Kretschmer
c. Sheldon d. Jung

29. Classification into introvert and extrovert types was proposed by:
a. Hippocrates
b. Ernst Kretschmer
c. Sheldon
d. Jung

30. What is an ambiguous stimuli in a Rorschach test?
a. Visual illusions
b. Stories without endings
c. Inkblots
d. Slightly blurred pictures

31. Which of the following is a similarity between the Rorschach test and the thematic apperception test (TAT)?
a. Both tests are examples of projective personality tests
b. Both tests are examples of the learning approach to studying personality
c. Both tests have evolved from and are similar to the MMPI
d. Both tests are biological in nature

32. Being impatient, irritable, always in a hurry and working under deadlines are traits associated with:
a. Oral stage fixation
b. Latency stage fixation
c. Type A personality
d. Type B personality

33. Sixteen personality factor questionnaire was developed by ________.

34. Expand TAT.

35. Which type of personality people are more prone to coronary artery disease?

36. Expand MMPI.

37. Erikson's theory of ________ development involves a series of eight stages each of which must be resolved in order for a person to develop optimally.

38. A person shown a picture and asked to make up a story about it would be taking a ________ personality test.

39. ________ therapies assume people should take responsibility for their lives and the decisions they make.

40. Which of the following is a function of personality which deals with determination and augmented effort in overcoming obstacles and difficulties?
a. Attitude b. Attribution
c. Will d. Character

41. Which of the following refers to judgment of an individual based upon certain qualities?
a. Attitude b. Attribution
c. Will d. Character

ANSWER KEY

1. c	2. c	3. d	4. c	5. d	6. b
7. d	8. c	9. b	10. b	11. d	12. c
13. c	14. c	15. b	16. d	17. d	18. d
19. c	20. c	21. a	22. b	23. d	24. b
25. a	26. d	27. c	28. b	29. d	30. c
31. a	32. c	33. Raymond Cattell	34. Thematic Apperception Test	35. Type A	36. Minnesota Multiphasic Personality Inventory
37. Psychosocial	38. Projective	39. Humanistic	40. c	41. d	

CHAPTER

6 Cognitive Process

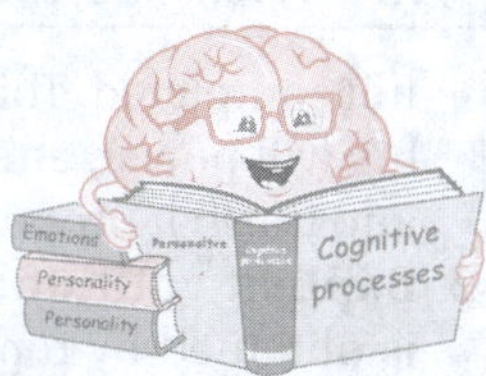

CHAPTER OUTLINE

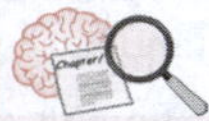

- Types and determinants of attention
- Duration and degree of attention
- Alterations in attention
- Principles of perception
- Factors affecting perception
- Effects of heredity and environment on intelligence
- Intelligence—uses, theories
- Learning—nature, types, factors influencing laws, theories
- Learner and learning
- Learning process
- Habits—characteristics, formation, breaking of habits
- Role of habits in health and illness
- Memory—types, influencing factors, theories, methods
- Forgetting—types, causes, theories
- Thinking—types, levels, elements, errors, stages
- Thinking in relation to language and communication
- Aptitude—concepts, types, individual differences
- Psychometric assessment of cognitive process
- Application in nursing profession

ATTENTION

Attention is the focus of consciousness on a particular object or idea at a particular time, to the exclusion of other objects or ideas.

Definitions

- Attention is defined as a process which compels the individual to select some particular stimulus according to his interest and attitude out of the multiplicity of stimuli present in the environment.
  —**Sharma RN (1967)**
- Attention is the concentration of consciousness upon one object rather than upon another. —**Dumville (1938)**

TYPES OF ATTENTION

There are two main types of attention: Voluntary (volitional) and involuntary (nonvolitional) (**Flowchart 6.1**).

Flowchart 6.1: Types of attention

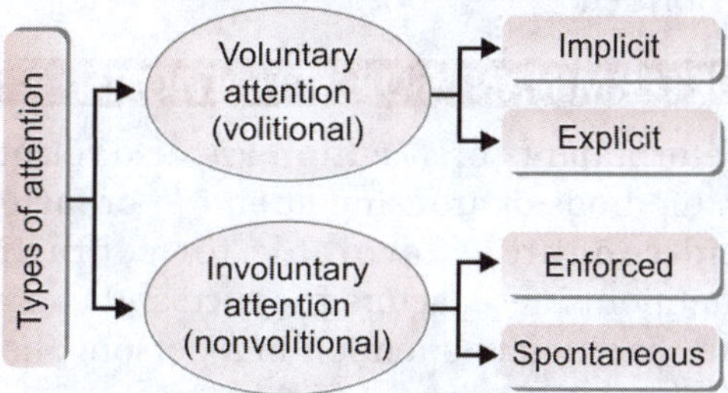

Voluntary Attention

Voluntary attention demands a conscious effort on our part. For example, solving an assigned problem in mathematics or answering a question in an examination needs voluntary attention. It is further subdivided into two categories:

1. **Implicit volitional attention:** A single act of will is responsible for arousing attention. For example, a teacher assigns practice work to a child and warns of punishment, if

not completed. This can make him exercise his will power, attend to the assigned task and finish it properly.

2. **Explicit volitional attention:** Attention is obtained by repeated acts of will. Hard struggle is essential to keep oneself attentive. It requires strong motives, willpower and keen attention for accomplishment of the task. For example, the attention paid during examination days for securing good grades.

Involuntary Attention

This type of attention is aroused without the play of will or without making a conscious effort on our part. For example, we give involuntary attention to loud sounds, bright lights and strong odors, etc. It is further divided into two categories:

1. **Enforced non-volitional attention:** It is aroused by the instincts is called enforced non-volitional attention. For example, giving attention out of curiosity.
2. **Spontaneous non-volitional attention:** It is aroused by sentiments is called spontaneous non-volitional attention. For example, we give an automatic or spontaneous attention to an object, idea or a person around which our sentiments are formed.

DETERMINANTS OF ATTENTION

Determinants of attention are also termed as methods of arousing attention or factors and conditions favorable for capturing attention. These factors produce and control the condition of attention in a person. These can be classified as:

- External (objective)—those found in one's environment and
- Internal (subjective)—those within the person himself

Methods of securing attention are based upon these external and internal factors of attention **(Table 6.1)**.

Table 6.1: Determinants of attention

External factors	Internal factors
Nature of stimulus	Interest and attention
Intensity of stimulus	Motives
Size of stimulus	Mental set-up
Contrast, change and novelty	Past experience
Location of stimulus	Emotion
Repetition of stimulus	Habit
Movement of stimulus	Aim
Definite form of the object	Meaning
Isolation of stimulus	Disposition and temperament

External Factors or Conditions

1. **Nature of stimulus:** All types of stimuli do not evoke the same degree of attention. An attractive stimulus should always be chosen for capturing maximum attention. A picture attracts attention more readily than words. Among pictures, that of human beings (especially beautiful women or handsome men) capture more attention than those of animals or objects. It has been found that in comparison to other sensations, color and sound attract more attention.
2. **Intensity of stimulus:** In comparison to a weak stimulus, an intense stimulus attracts more attention of an individual. Our attention becomes easily directed to a loud sound, a bright light or a strong smell.
3. **Size of stimulus:** As a general rule larger objects in the environment are more likely to catch our attention than smaller objects. A small object or a picture on a large background also attracts attention.
4. **Contrast, change and novelty:** Change and variety strike attention more easily than routine. The use of maps and charts attracts student's attention instantly when compared to the routine verbal talk. Though we do not notice the ticking of a clock in the regular course, no sooner it stops than it catches our attention. Any change in the stimulation to which we have become adapted captures our attention immediately. Novelty means something new or different. It attracts attention very easily and is closely related to change. A new building, a new teacher

are all examples of common novelty. It is thus always better to introduce a change or novelty for breaking monotony and securing attention.

5. **Location of stimulus:** The location of stimulus also affects attention. In the case of visual stimuli, the most effective location is to be right in front of the eyes. For example, advertisements given on the front page or on the upper half of any page attract more attention.
6. **Repetition of stimulus:** A repeated stimulus attracts our attention. Though we may ignore a stimulus at the first instance, when repeated several times it captures our attention. A misspelt word is more likely to be noticed if it occurs twice in the same paragraph than if it occurs only once. But this practice of repetition should be carefully used. Too much repetition of a stimulus may bring diminishing returns.
7. **Movement of stimulus:** A moving stimulus catches our attention more quickly than a stimulus that does not move. This is why the pictures on a television screen or those in a cinema hold our attention for hours at time.
8. **Definite form of the object:** A sharply defined object attracts our attention more than a broad indefinite object. Also a figure attracts more attention than the background.
9. **Isolation of stimulus:** Isolation is an important external determinant of attention. A student sitting alone in the corner of the class is seen first (attracts more attention than others).

Internal Factors or Conditions

A person's attention to a stimulus depends not only upon the characteristics of the stimulus or the favorable environmental conditions but also upon his interest, motives, basic needs and urges, etc.

1. **Interest and attention:** Interest is a very helpful factor in securing attention. We attend to objects in which we are interested than those in which we are not interested.
2. **Motives**: The basic drives and urges of the individual are very important in securing attention. Thirst, hunger, sex, curiosity, fear are some of the important motives that exercise definite influence upon attention. When hungry we savor even distasteful food but when the belly is full we may not attend to even the tastiest one.
3. **Mental set-up:** A person always attends to those objects towards which his mind has a leaning. For example, on the day of examination the slightest thing concerning the examination easily attracts the attention of the students.
4. **Past experience:** Learning and previous experiences facilitate attention. If we know by our past experience that a particular person is sincere to us, we pay attention to whatever he advices.
5. **Emotion:** The emotional state of a person determines the level of attention. For example, a person attends only to bad qualities of his enemy.
6. **Habit:** It is also an important determinant of attention. A man develops the habit of attending to necessary and desirable things and on the other hand also develops a habit of not attending to unnecessary and undesirable things.
7. **Aim:** Every man has some immediate and ultimate aims. Thus a student whose aim is to pass the examination will attend to textbooks and notes regularly.
8. **Meaning:** In comparison to meaningless stimuli, meaningful stimuli attract more attention.
9. **Disposition (natural tendency) and temperament:** Both are important internal factors which attract attention. For example, a man with religious disposition and spiritual temperament will attend to religious matters sincerely.

Besides the conditions described above many other factors influence attention such as heredity, education, family, school, society, training, etc., which have a wide influence on attention.

DURATION AND DEGREE OF ATTENTION

There are five major conditions of attention that are referred to as duration and degree of attention (**Figure 6.1**):

Span of Attention

Maximum amount of material that can be attended to in one period of attention is called span of attention. This can either be visual or auditory attention.

- **Span of visual attention:** Experiments have been carried out to measure the span of visual attention by making brief exposures to a number of objects. The time of exposure is very short, ranging from 1/100 to 1/5 of a second. Objects exposed to the eye are simple like dots, lines, letters or complex words or triangles, etc. The mind can attend to a maximum four or five separate units if the items are not grouped into familiar units. But if the items are combined into meaningful wholes, for example, letters are arranged into words, a larger number of items can be perceived in a single instance.
- **Span of auditory attention:** The number of auditory impressions perceived at a single instance is called span of auditory attention. An adult can perceive eight sounds made in rapid succession, but when sounds are made in a rhythm, a much larger number of sounds can be perceived.

Duration of Attention

It refers to how long one can attend to an object without a break. If we attend to a single, simple object such as a dot, it will remain in the focus of our consciousness for utmost a second, then something in the margin will crowd it out or memory of a past event will intrude.

The duration of attention depends upon the nature of the material, the interest of the observer and other conditions.

Sustained Attention (Act of Fixation of Mind)

To sustain attention is to concentrate one's activity continuously upon some object or a happening or a problem. The individual attention always remains on track and the activity proceeds systematically without any serious distraction. All internal as well as external factors of getting attention can be helpful in this track.

Shifting Attention

While paying attention towards an object or an event, it is not possible to hold attention continuously with the same intensity for a longer duration. It is constantly shifting from one object to another, from one aspect of the situation to another. We can perform only one voluntary act at a time and not two or more acts at a time. However, we can quickly shift attention from one voluntary act to another.

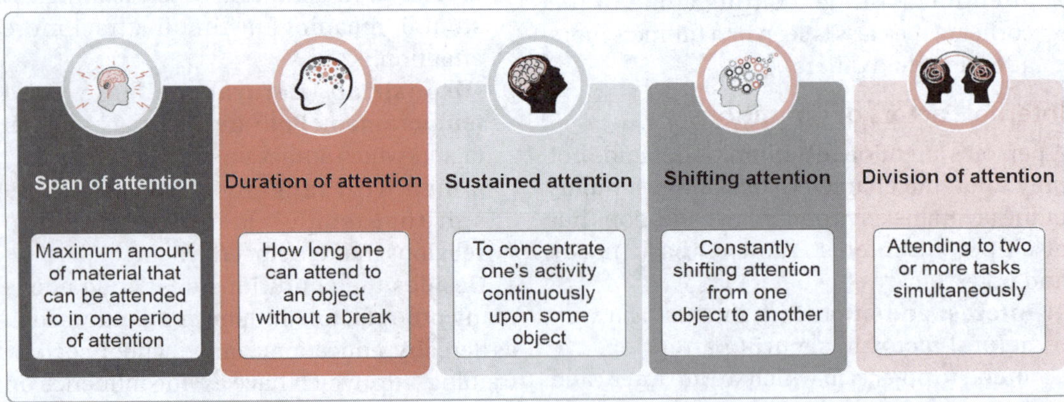

Figure 6.1: Major conditions of attention

Division of Attention

Division of attention means to attend to two or more tasks simultaneously. Psychologists opine that one cannot attend to two things at a given time and that there is no possibility of division of attention.

The reason for being able to pay attention to more than one task at a given time may be due to one of the following reasons:

- In performing two tasks simultaneously one of the two activities requires no attention at all.
- Attention rapidly shifts from one task to the other.

ALTERATIONS IN ATTENTION (DISTRACTION)

Distraction means any stimulus whose presence interferes with the process of attention or draws away attention from the object which we wish to attend.

—HR Bhatia (1968)

These alterations in attention reduce the efficiency of work.

Sources of Distraction

The sources of distraction vary very much. They affect the individual according to his own mental set-up and personality characteristics. The sources of distraction can be classified into:

- **External factors:** Noise, music, improper lighting, uncomfortable seats, unfavorable temperature, inadequate ventilation, defective methods of teaching, defective voice of the teacher, etc.
- **Internal factors:** Emotional disturbances, ill health, boredom, lack of motivation, fatigue, etc.

The nurse should take great care to get away all possible causes of distractions in working area so as to sustain attention.

Types of Distraction

- **Continuous distraction**: The distraction is continuous in nature. For example, the sound of radio played continuously, the noise at the market place, etc. Experiments have shown that adjustment to continuous distraction takes place quickly.
- **Discontinuous distraction:** The distract is irregular in nature. For example, the hearing of somebody's voice every now and then. It interferes with work because of the impossibility of adjustment.

Some major means of removing distractions are:

- Being active in work
- Disregard for distraction
- Making the distraction a part of the work

PERCEPTION

Sensation is the initial response of an individual to a stimulus and precedes perception. Perception is the interpretation of sensory stimuli reaching the sense organs and the brain. When our sense organs come in contact with the world, are stimulated by external stimuli and receive sensations it results in perception. Interpretation gives meaning to sensation thereby making us aware of objects.

Definitions

- Perception is the experience of objects, events or relationships obtained by extracting information from and interpreting sensations.

  —JH Jackson, O Desiderato and DB Howieson (1976)

- Perception is an individual's awareness aspect of behavior, for it is the way each person processes the raw data he receives from the environment into meaningful patterns.

  —RE Silverman (1976)

PRINCIPLES OF PERCEPTION (PERCEPTUAL ORGANIZATION)

When we perceive the world there are many different stimuli coming in at the same time. Individuals tend to organize these stimuli into a meaningful pattern or whole according to certain principles. These principles try to explain when and how our minds perceive different visual components as being part

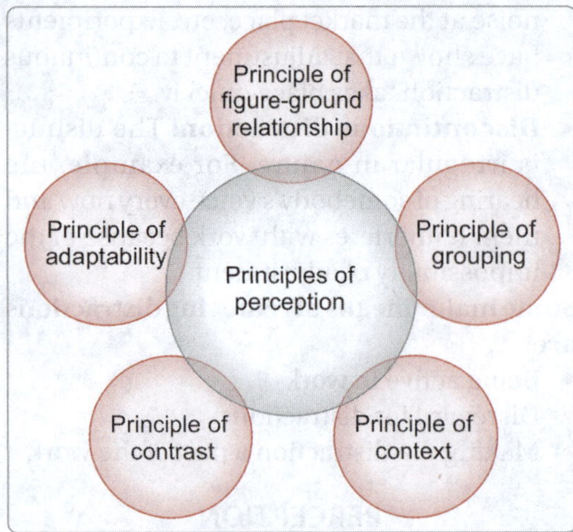

Figure 6.2: Principles of perception

of the same group. The principles explained below are a combination of those proposed originally by Max Wertheimer (1923), Stephen Palmer (1999, 2002), and other contemporary Gestalt theorists **(Figure 6.2)**.

1. Principle of Figure-ground Relationship

According to principle of figure-ground relationship, a figure is perceived in relationship to its background. The perception of the object or figure in terms of color, size, shape and intensity, etc. depends upon the figure ground relationship. We perceive a figure against a background or background against a figure depending upon the characteristics of the perceiver as well as the relative strength of the figure or ground. A proper figure-ground relationship is quite important from the angle of perception of the figure or the ground. In case where such relationship does not exist we may witness ambiguity in terms of clear perception.

Sensory experiences other than visual experiences may also be perceived as figure and ground. Sometimes, when equally balanced qualities are present in various parts within the general field of awareness, there could be a conflict resulting in formation of two or more figures. In such a case there will be a shifting of the ground and the figure. One part may be the ground at one moment and at the next moment the ground may become the figure. In this picture either the colored faces or the white vase may become the figure. Moreover it is impossible to perceive both figure and background at the same time **(Figure 6.3)**.

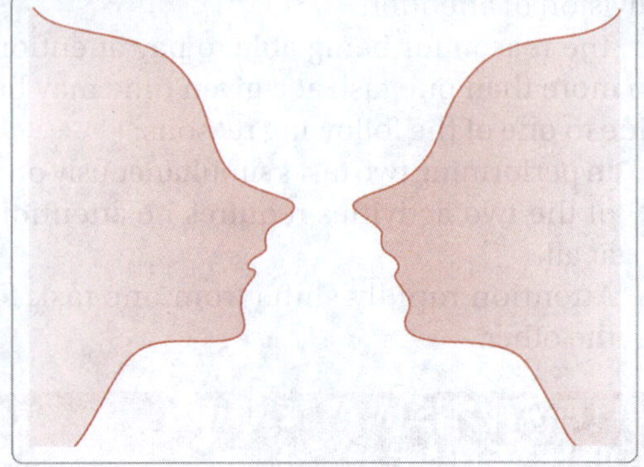

Figure 6.3: Figure-ground relationship

2. Principle of Grouping

The main founder of Gestalt psychology is Max Wertheimer. According to Gestalt principle, objects can be perceived meaningfully when they are grouped together. This school of thought looks at the human mind and behavior as a whole. (Gestalt is a German word which means 'shape, figure or form.' It is also interpreted as 'pattern' or 'configuration'). The following principles make our perception more meaningful:

- **Principle of proximity:** Proximity means nearness. The objects which are nearer to each other can be perceived meaningfully by grouping them. In **Figure 6.4A** we see three sets of two lines each and not six separate lines.
- **Principle of similarity:** There is a tendency to perceive objects of a similar size and shape or color as a unit or figure. In **Figure 6.4B**, we see vertical columns of circles and squares.
- **Principle of continuity:** Any stimulus which extends in the same direction or shape is perceived as a whole. Our attention is held more by continuous patterns rather than discontinuous ones. In **Figure 6.4C,** we see a curved line and a straight line. We do not see a straight line with small semi-circles above and below.

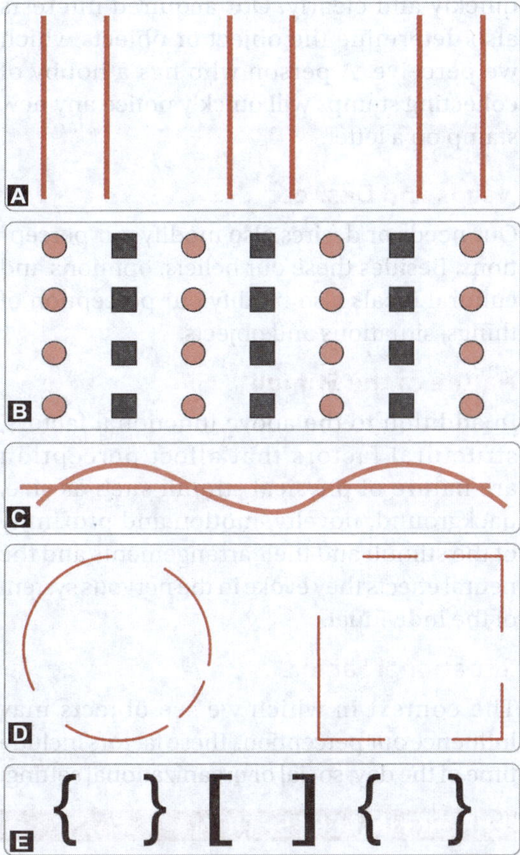

Figures 6.4A to E: (A) Principle of proximity; (B) Principle of similarity; (C) Principle of continuity; (D) Principle of closure; (E) Principle of symmetry

- **Principle of closure:** While confronting an incomplete pattern one tends to complete or close the pattern or fill in sensory gaps and perceive it as a meaningful whole. This type of organization is extremely helpful in making valuable interpretation of various incomplete objects, patterns or stimuli present in our environment. The lines in **Figure 6.4D** may well be perceived as a circle and a square.
- **Principle of symmetry:** Objects having symmetrical shape are perceived as groups. For example, brackets of different shapes shown in **Figure 6.4E** are perceived meaningfully because the symmetrical ones are grouped together.

3. Principle of Context

Perceptual organization is also governed by the principle of context, i.e., an examiner may award higher marks to the same answer book in a pleasant context than in an unpleasant one.

4. Principle of Contrast

Perceptual organization is much affected through contrast effects as the stimuli that are in sharp contrast to nearby stimuli may draw our maximum attention and carry different perceptual affects. For example, in **Figure 6.5A and B** the surrounding circles in **Figure 6.5A** make the central circle seem larger than the central circle in **Figure 6.5B** even though the two are of the same size.

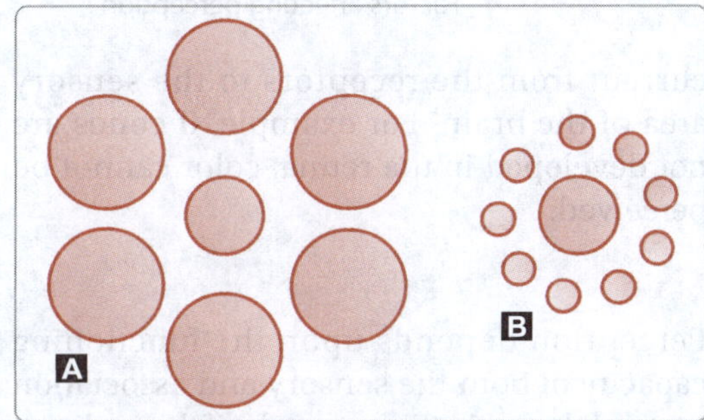

Figures 6.5A and B: Principle of contrast

5. Principle of Adaptability

Perceptual organization for some stimuli depends upon the adaptability of the perceiver to perceive similar stimuli. An individual who adapts himself to work before an intense bright light will perceive normal sunlight as quite dim.

FACTORS AFFECTING PERCEPTION

There are individual differences in perceptual abilities. Two people may perceive the same stimulus differently. Factors affecting perception are presented in **Figure 6.6**.

Sense Organs

Perception depends upon the sense organs or receptors on which the stimuli act and the sensory neurons that transmit the nerve

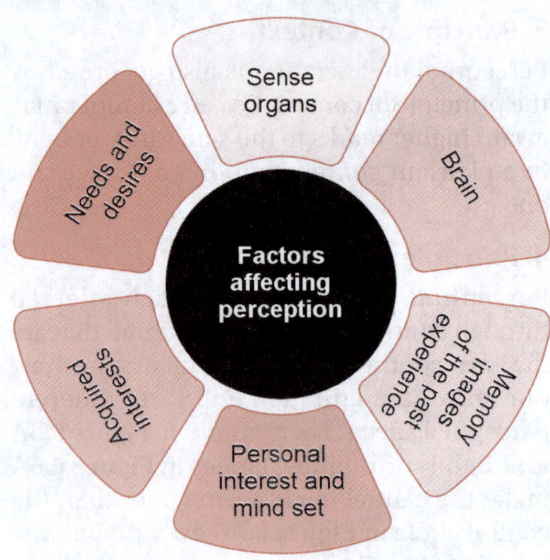

Figure 6.6: Factors affecting perception

current from the receptors to the sensory area of the brain. For example, if cones are not developed in the retina, color cannot be perceived.

Brain

Perception depends upon the functioning capacity of both the sensory and association areas of the brain. For example, if the auditory area is destroyed we cannot have auditory perception.

Memory Images of the Past Experience

Memory images help us in the comprehension of the object or stimulus before us. Generally, perception involves the integration of sensory experience in the light of past experience and present psychological conditions. Experiments have shown that whenever we come in contact with new stimuli we are inclined to interpret them in terms of our experiences with similar stimuli in the past. For example, a child has come in contact with a horse for the first time. He has already seen a cow. When he is asked what it (horse) is, he may say it is a cow or like a cow.

Personal Interests and Mind Set

We perceive those concerning our interests, attitudes, motives, expectations and mindset quickly and clearly. Our acquired interests also determine the object or objects which we perceive. A person who has a hobby of collecting stamps will quickly notice any new stamp on a letter.

Needs and Desires

Our needs or desires also modify our perceptions. Besides these our beliefs, opinions and cultural ideals also modify our perception of things, situations and objects.

Nature of the Stimuli

In addition to the above functional factors, structural factors that affect perception are nature of physical stimuli such as size, background, novelty, motion and proximity of the stimuli and their arrangements and the neural effects they evoke in the nervous system of the individual.

Situational Factors

The context in which we see objects may influence our perception. These factors include time of the day, social or organizational setting.

ERRORS IN PERCEPTION

Perceptual processes enable an individual to perceive things accurately and facilitate smooth functioning. However, some errors creep into this process under certain circumstances leading to impaired perceptions. These are—illusions and hallucinations.

- **Illusion:** It is a misinterpretation of actual perception. When the interpretation of a particular stimulus goes wrong, it gives rise to a wrong perception or illusion. For example, a rope in the dark is perceived as a snake or vice-versa. The voice of an unknown person is mistaken as a friend's voice. An unknown person standing at a distance may be perceived as a known person.
  Illusions are caused by inadequacies of our sense organs, distance of the object from the sense organ which perceives it, misleading stimuli in the environment, our perceived notions and expectancy.

- **Hallucination:** Hallucination is identified as one of the major errors of perception. It is a sensory perception that occurs in the absence of any corresponding external sensory stimuli. Hallucinations are imaginary perceptions in which one sees or hears something that is not seen or heard by others around him. An alcoholic may see 'pink elephants,' a paranoid schizophrenic may hear voices, experience foul odors in the absence of any sensory stimulation. Hallucinations are more common in mentally ill people.

Depending upon the sensory modality involved people experience different types of hallucinations. For example, visual, auditory, kinesthetic, olfactory and gustatory.

Accurate perception is absolutely necessary in order to record an accurate observation. It is possible to make errors in perception due to a number of reasons.

Causes for Inaccurate Perception

Reality is determined through perception. It affects how one processes, interprets, remembers, synthesizes and decides about reality. Various causes for inaccurate perception are presented in **Figure 6.7.**

1. **Defective functioning of sense organs**: Sensory defects like myopia, deafness and anesthesia can cause inaccurate perception.
2. **Inadequate stimulus**: Our receptors may not be stimulated adequately if the stimuli are vague, indefinite or not strong enough. A very weak light or soft sound will make it difficult to perceive correctly.
3. **Too many stimuli at one time**: When too many stimuli are present at one given time, perceiving each stimulus separately is difficult. For example, in the presence of loud noises it may be difficult to perceive the call of a patient.
4. **Poor health**: Sense organs cannot function correctly and adequately as a result of illness. For this reason perceptions of patients may be inaccurate.
5. **Limited attention**: If we try to apprehend more things than we can at a time, we are liable to have an inaccurate perception.
6. **Figure merges in the ground**: Sometimes objects are perceived with difficulty because they resemble their surroundings. For example, a white patch is difficult to detect on a white wall. The nurse learns to perceive signs of illness or wellness in patients only when she learns what these signs are.

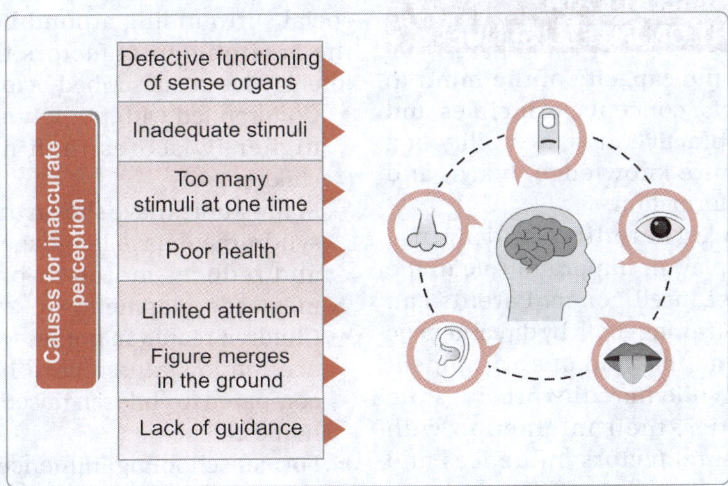

Figure 6.7: Causes for inaccurate perception

7. **Guidance**: Perception is inaccurate when we do not know what to perceive.

INTELLIGENCE

Intelligence is the general capacity for comprehension and reasoning that manifests itself in various ways. It consists of an individual's mental or cognitive ability which helps the person in solving his actual life problems and leading a happy and well-contended life.

DEFINITIONS

- Intelligence is the aggregate or global capacity of an individual to think rationally, act purposefully and deal effectively with the environment. **—Wechsler (1944)**
- Intelligence is the ability to master the information and skills needed to succeed within a particular culture. **—Lolurto (1991)**
- Intelligence can be defined as a sort of mental energy in the form of mental or cognitive abilities available with an individual which enables him to handle his environment in terms of adaptation to face novel situations as effectively as possible. **—Mangal (1993)**

EFFECTS OF HEREDITY AND ENVIRONMENT ON INTELLIGENCE

Intelligence is the capacity of the mind to understand facts, concepts, principles and apply them in practice. It is the ability of a person to acquire knowledge, learn, and comprehend information.

Both nurture (heredity) and nature (environment) play an important role in the development of intelligence. Parents can influence their offsprings both by direct genetic transmission and the kind of environment they provide. While heredity provides the inherent abilities, their interaction with the environmental factors influences and further shapes those abilities. Differences and similarities in intelligence among individuals are explained by the level at which heredity and environmental factors have influenced the development of intelligence.

Intelligence abilities run along with families. Genes concerned with intelligence are passed from parents to their children. Children born of parents with high IQ are likely to have a high IQ. Some of the cognitive domains such as processing information, speed of receiving information, verbal comprehension, working memory and perceptual organization of information are determined by genetic factors.

Twins and adoption studies explain the role of heredity and environmental factors in development of intelligence. Some of the facts revealed by research studies are:

- Identical twin studies showed similar IQ for the twins even when they were reared up in different environments. This implies that genetic factors act as the primary factor for development of intelligence.
- Adoption studies showed that adopted children exhibited intelligence similar to their biological parents.

Intelligence is not entirely influenced by genetic factors. Environment in which a child is raised, prenatal infections, care and affection also have a profound effect on the level of intelligence. These may also include schooling and play, nutrition, socio-economic status of the family, physical and social surrounding around home. Some of the environmental factors that influence intelligence are described below:

- Children fed with proper nutrition exhibit higher IQ scores than malnourished children.
- Many studies have shown that fetal alcohol syndrome delays language development and reduces motor co-ordination and mental development.
- Children reared in homes with high socio-economic status record high IQ scores compared to children raised in low income homes.
- Formal schooling influences intelligence. Many studies have reported that attending regular school promotes intellectual growth through acquisition of cognitive process.

- Studies have also shown that IQ of school dropouts declines year after year with every missed academic year.

Both heredity and environment play an important role in determining intelligence. These can be compared to land and seeds used to grow a crop. While the seed represents heredity, land represents the environment. If the land is not fertile even a good seed cannot help harvest a good crop. Similarly with fertile land and poor quality seeds one cannot achieve good results. As both fertile land and good quality seeds are required for a good crop both heredity and stimulating environment are required for achieving higher intelligence.

CLASSIFICATION OF INTELLIGENCE

Intelligence can be classified into three types **(Figure 6.8)**:

1. **Concrete intelligence:** This is related to concrete materials. This type of intelligence is applicable when an individual is handling concrete objects or machines. It is best put to use by engineers and mechanics operating tools and instruments.
2. **Social intelligence:** It is the ability of an individual to react to social situations in daily life. It includes the ability to understand people and act wisely in human relationships. Individuals having this type of intelligence know the art of winning friends and influencing them. Leaders, ministers, salesmen, diplomats are endowed with this type of intelligence.
3. **Abstract or general intelligence:** It is the ability to respond to words, numbers, letters, etc. This type of intelligence is acquired by study of books and related literature. Mostly good teachers, lawyers, doctors, philosophers exhibit this type of intelligence.

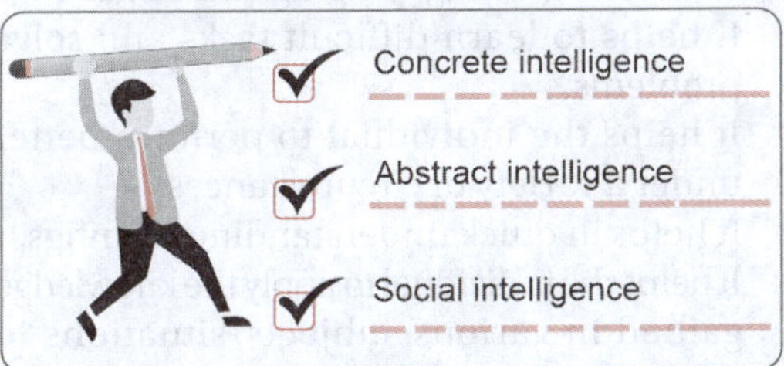

Figure 6.8: Classification of intelligence

Gardner's Multiple Intelligence

According to Howard Gardner there are eight major kinds of intelligence **(Figure 6.9 and Table 6.2)**.

Intelligence Quotient

The idea of intelligence quotient was utilized for the first time in 1916 for formulation of Stanford-Binet tests. Intelligence quotient is the ratio between mental age (MA) and chronological age (CA). While chronological age is determined from date of birth, mental age is determined by intelligence tests.

$$IQ = \frac{MA}{CA} \times 100$$

Imagine a 10-year-old boy scores a mental age of 12. His IQ will be:

$$IQ = \frac{MA}{CA} \times 100 = \frac{12}{10} \times 100 = 120$$

Classification of Individuals According to IQ

There exists a wide difference among individuals with regard to intelligence. No two individuals, even the identical twins nurtured almost in similar environment have same level of intelligence. This is an important fact that every nurse must understand. It is due to

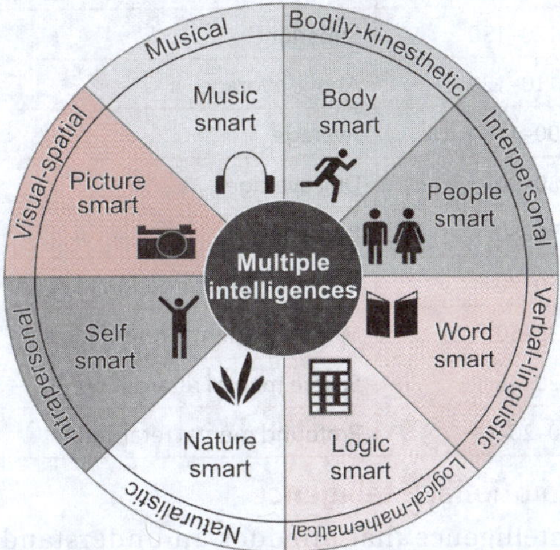

Figure 6.9: Gardner's eight major kinds of intelligences

Table 6.2: Gardner's eight major kinds of intelligence

Type of intelligence	Description
1. Musical intelligence	Skill in tasks involving music. *Example*: Musicians
2. Bodily-kinesthetic intelligence	Skill in using the whole body or its parts to resolve problems or construction of products. *Example*: Dancers, athletes, actors, surgeons, etc.
3. Logical-mathematical intelligence	Skills in problem solving and scientific thinking. *Example*: Scientists
4. Linguistic intelligence	Skills involved in the production and use of language. *Example*: Literati
5. Spatial intelligence	Skills involving spatial configurations such as those used by artists and architects
6. Interpersonal intelligence	Skills in interacting with others such as sensitivity to the moods, temperaments, motivations and intentions of others
7. Intrapersonal intelligence	Knowledge of the internal aspects of oneself; access to one's own feelings and emotions
8. Naturalist intelligence	Ability to identify and classify patterns in nature

(*Source:* Adapted from Gardner, 2000).

these individual differences that some patients understand the instructions of the nurse without much difficulty while others cannot in spite of their best efforts. Individuals can be classified between genius to mentally retarded based on their IQ **(Table 6.3)**.

Table 6.3: Classification of individuals according to IQ

IQ range	IQ classification
140 and above	Genius
130–140	Very superior
120–130	Superior
110–120	Above average
90–110	Average
80–90	Dull average
70–80	Borderline
50–70	Mild mental retardation
35–50	Moderate mental retardation
20–35	Severe mental retardation
0–20	Profound mental retardation

Emotional Intelligence

Intelligence that provides an understanding of what other people are feeling and experiencing, and allowing us to respond appropriately to their needs is called emotional intelligence. It is the basis of empathy for others, self-awareness and social skills. High emotional intelligence might enable an individual to tune into other's feelings thus permitting a high degree of responsiveness to others.

Abilities in emotional intelligence might help to explain why people with even moderate intelligence quotient (IQ) scores can be quite successful despite their lack of traditional intelligence.

USES OF INTELLIGENCE

- Intelligence helps the individual to adjust to changing situations quickly and correctly.
- It helps to carry on higher mental processes such as reasoning, judging and criticizing.
- It helps to learn difficult tasks and solve problems.
- It helps the individual to perform better under a variety of circumstances.
- It helps in quick understanding of things.
- It helps the individual to apply the knowledge gained in various subjects/situations in dealing with the present situation.

MEASUREMENT OF INTELLIGENCE

Intelligence can be assessed through a series of tasks designed to measure the capacity to learn, construct thoughts and deal with novel situations. Alfred Binet (1875–1911) was the first psychologist to device an intelligence test. Intelligence tests can be classified into two broad categories: Individual and group intelligence tests **(Flowchart 6.2)**.

Individual Intelligence Tests

Individual intelligence tests are administered individually in a closed setting with no other individuals present. The Wechsler Intelligence Scale for Children (WISC) and the Stanford Binet-Intelligence scale are examples of individualized intelligence tests. Individual intelligence tests can further be classified into verbal and non verbal tests:

- **Individual verbal intelligence tests**: These tests make use of language and test one individual at a time. *Example*: Stanford-Binet scale.
- **Individual non-verbal intelligence tests**: These tests involve the manipulation of objects (e.g., picture arrangement, picture completion, block design, etc.) with minimum use of paper and pencil. Instructions are generally given by demonstrations and gestures. These tests are used in infants, mentally retarded, foreigners and those who do not understand language in which the tests are conducted. Example: Bhatia's Battery of Performance Test.

Group Intelligence Tests

Group intelligence tests are administered in groups to measure how a child's intellectual performance compares with that of other children in the same age group. Otis-Lennon School Ability Test (OLSAT) is an example of group intelligence test. These can further be classified into verbal and non-verbal tests:

- **Group verbal intelligence tests**: These tests use language and are applied to a group of individuals at a time. *Examples*: Army Alpha Test, Army General Classification Test.
- **Group non-verbal intelligence tests**: These tests are applied to a group of individuals at a time and do not necessitate the use of language. They employ pictures, diagrams and geometrical figures printed in a booklet and do not contain words or numerical figures. The subject is required to perform such activities as to fill in some empty spaces, draw some simple figures, point out similarities and dissimilarities, etc. *Examples*: Army Beta Test, Raven's Progressive Matrices Test.

Comparison between individual and group tests is given in **Table 6.4**.

Flowchart 6.2: Classification of intelligence tests

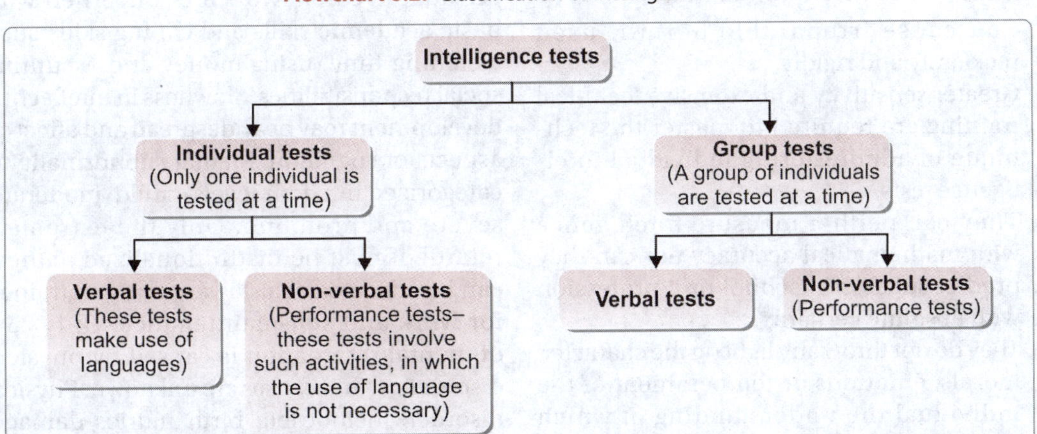

Table 6.4: Comparison between individual and group tests

Individual tests	Group tests
They test one individual at a time; mainly done to observe characteristic of an individual	A group of children are tested at the same time; mainly done to meet the practical needs
These tests involve one to one consultation with the individual	These tests include multiple choice items
These are uneconomical in terms of time, labor and money	Comparatively more economical in terms of time, labor and money
These are applicable both for children and adults	These tests cannot be administered to children below the age of 10 years
These bring the tester and child closer and establish a better relationship between the two	Personal contact between the two is not possible

Uses of Intelligence Tests

- Intelligence testing is used to predict how well a person will learn in a program of study.
- They help teachers to classify each student based on his learning ability.
- They help to separate the slow learner from the gifted learner enabling the use of suitable methods to train these two different groups.
- They are used in selection for admission to different courses of study and for awarding scholarships and vocational guidance.
- They are used in selection of candidates for different jobs.
- Intelligence tests are also useful in child guidance as they help in identifying educational backwardness and other related difficulties.

Limitations of Intelligence Tests

- Can cause irreparable harm if used recklessly and rigidly.
- Greater sensitivity and extensive technical training are required to master the technique of administering individual intelligence tests.
- They can neither measure intelligence with mathematical accuracy nor can they predict success in school or a profession with absolute certainty.
- They do not throw any light on the character, morals, emotions or temperament of the individual the understanding of which is so essential in comprehending one's personality.

Mental Deficiency (Mental Subnormality)

It refers to subaverage intellectual functioning which originates in the developmental period and is associated with impairment in adaptive behavior. A person is regarded as mentally subnormal if:

- IQ attained is below 70 on standard psychological tests of intelligence.
- Their adaptive skills are inadequate to cope up with the daily routines.

Adaptive skills are those behaviors by which an individual makes adjustments and independent living in the society. In childhood these refer to self-help activities such as eating and dressing independently. Later on the adaptive behaviors are concerned with basic academic skills and coping skills such as telling time, using money and assuming social responsibilities. Slowness in intellectual development may be widespread and affect all aspects of cognition. Mental subnormality is categorized into four levels—mild, moderate, severe and profound. Only the extremely retarded must be institutionalized. Others can be educated at a slower pace and trained for work and self-maintenance. Only 25% of mental retardation is caused by physical disorders. Other causes are unknown. Physical disorders include fetal birth injuries, damage, genetic abnormalities and metabolic disorders. These are phenylketonuria, microcephaly, hydrocephaly, cretinism and Down syndrome.

Mentally Gifted Children

These are individuals with IQs of 140 or higher. In early childhood a gifted child is generally found to be a misfit in his class because the level of teaching in normal class room is for an average child whereas the gifted child is able to comprehend much faster. As a consequence they often indulge in behavioral irregularities. They have been found to be gross underachievers and extremely unhappy. One problem seems to be that such extremely bright children find themselves intellectually misfit with children of their own age and physically misfit with elders who are their intellectual equals. But things improve by adulthood and they appear to be happier and better adjusted than most others of their age. With the right type of training their superior potential is channelized in constructive task.

The most common mental disorders that affect cognitive functions mainly memory processing, perception and problem solving are amnesia, dementia and delirium. Others include anxiety disorders such as phobias, panic disorders, obsessive-compulsive disorder, generalized anxiety disorder and post-traumatic stress disorder. Mood disorders such as depression and bipolar disorder are also cognitive mental disorders. Psychotic disorders such as schizophrenia and delusional disorder are also classified as cognitive mental disorders.

Cognitive disorders affect thinking and perceptual processes and acquisition of knowledge and new information. Cognitive disorders have an enormous social impact because special educational resources are required and independent living often cannot be achieved. Learning problems may lead to behavioral disorders at home and community. Severe cognitive impairment is usually accompanied by physical abnormalities.

THEORIES OF INTELLIGENCE

Attempts from psychologists in analyzing components of intelligence have resulted in the development of various theories. Every approach to thinking comes up with its own different perspective and assumptions, often contradicting at least one earlier theory. Some of the common theories relating to intelligence are: factor theories of intelligence, process-oriented theories of intelligence and information-processing theory.

1. Factor Theories of Intelligence

Two-factor theory or general intelligence (G-factor) theory: It was advocated by Charles Spearman (1927), a British psychologist.

Spearman proposed the involvement of a broad general intelligence factor (G) in every intellectual activity an individual undertakes. Every individual possesses general intelligence factor (G) in varying amounts. This determines the individual's overall ability. 'G' is a universal inborn ability. Higher the 'G' in an individual greater is the success in life. In addition to the G-factor there are specific abilities which allow an individual to deal with specific kind of problems. Specific intelligence factor (S) is learned and acquired from the environment and varies from activity to activity even in the same individual. Examples of these specific abilities can be language ability, mathematical ability, musical or drawing skills and so on. These specific abilities may be represented as S1, S2, S3, etc.

Thus, an individual's total ability or intelligence (A) is the sum of the general factor and all his specific abilities. This can be expressed as:

$$A = G + S1 + S2 + S3 + \dots\dots\dots$$

Group factor or multifactor theory: This theory was expounded by LL Thurstone in 1938. Thurstone explained that certain mental operations have a common primary factor which gives them psychological and functional unity and also differentiates them from other mental operations. These mental operations constitute a group factor. There are many groups of mental abilities with each group having its own primary factor. Thurstone and his associates have identified seven such factors. They are:

1. **Verbal factor (V):** Comprehension of verbal ideas or words.
2. **Spatial factor (S):** Ability to imagine an object in space.
3. **Numerical factor (N):** Ability to perform mathematical calculations rapidly and accurately.
4. **Memory factor (M):** Ability to memorize quickly.
5. **Reasoning factor (R):** Ability to reason and think things out.
6. **Perceptual factor (P):** Ability to perceive objects accurately.
7. **Problem-solving factor (PS):** Ability to solve problems independently.

2. Process-oriented Theories of Intelligence

These theories have focused on intellectual processes—the pattern of thinking that people use when they reason and solve problems. These theorists prefer to use the term cognitive processes in place of intelligence. They are more often interested in how people solve problems and how many get the right solution. They have focused on the development of cognitive abilities. Piaget's work is a significant contribution in this area.

- **Piaget's theory (Jean Piaget, 1970):** According to Piaget, intelligence is an adaptive process involving interplay of biological maturation and interaction with the environment. He viewed intelligence as an evolution of cognitive processes such as understanding the laws of nature, principles of grammar and mathematical rules.
- **Bruner's theory (Jerome Bruner, 1973):** According to Bruner, intelligence is a growing dependence on internal representation of objects or situations. These growing abilities are influenced by the environment especially the rewards and punishments people receive for using particular intellectual skills in particular ways.
- **Information-processing theory (Robert Sternberg, 1984):** The most recent acceptable theory of intelligence has been put forward by the American psychologist Robert Sternberg by adopting an information processing approach to cognition or problem-solving. The information processing approach is the manner in which one proceeds to perform a mental task or solve a problem from the time one comes across it, gathers information and makes use of this information for completing the task or solving the problem in hand. The theory propagated by Sternberg identified the following steps in the way one processes information:
  - *Encoding*: Identifying the relevant available information in the mind
  - *Inferring*: Drawing necessary inference
  - *Mapping*: Establishing a relationship between the previous and present situations
  - *Application*: Applying the inferred relationship
  - *Justification*: Justifying the analyzed solution to the problems
  - *Responding*: Providing the best possible solution

LEARNING

One of the most important characteristics of human beings is their capacity to learn. An individual starts learning immediately after his birth or in a strict sense even earlier in the womb of the mother. Our personality which is a combination of habits, skills, knowledge, attitudes, interests and character is largely the result of learning. It is the key process in human behavior. All our adaptive as well as maladaptive, cognitive as well as affective behavior are formed by learning processes. These are of vital importance in helping the individual to adapt to his changing environment.

DEFINITIONS

- Learning is the acquisition of habits, knowledge and attitudes. It involves new ways of doing things and operates on individual's attempts to overcome obstacles or adjust to new situations. It represents progressive changes in behavior. It enables him to satisfy interests to attain a goal.

—Crow and Crow (1973)

- The term learning covers every modification in behavior to meet environmental requirements. **—Gardner Murphy (1968)**

NATURE OF LEARNING

- Learning is a process not a product.
- It involves all those experiences and trainings of an individual (right from his birth) which helped him produce a change in his behavior.
- Learning though brings changes in behavior it does not necessarily guarantee an improvement or development in the positive direction. One has equal chances to drift to the negative side of human personality.
- Learning prepares an individual for the necessary adjustment and adaptation.
- All learning is purposeful and goal oriented. Without purpose there would hardly be any learning.
- The scope of learning is too wide to explain in words. It is a very comprehensive process which covers nearly all the domains—conative, cognitive and affective of human behavior.
- Learning is universal and continuous. Every creature that lives learns. In human beings it is not limited to any age, sex, race or culture. It is a continuous never-ending process that goes from womb-to-tomb.
- Learning does not include the changes in behavior on account of maturation, fatigue, illness or drugs, etc.
- Learning is transferable from one situation to another.
- Learning helps in proper growth and development.
- Learning helps in balanced development of personality.

TYPES OF LEARNING

An individual is constantly interacting with and influenced by the environment. This experience induces a change or modifies his behavior so as to deal with it effectively. All learning involves activities which may either be physical or mental. What activities are learned by the individual is referred to as types of learning. These include:

1. Stimulus Response Learning

Conditioning learning involves the conditioning of respondent behavior through a process of stimulus association and substitution. In this type of learning establishment of connections between sensory systems and motor systems occurs.

- **Classical conditioning:** Association between two stimuli viz. unconditioned stimulus (US) and conditioned stimulus (CS). It involves pairing a previously neutral stimulus with an unconditioned stimulus.
- **Instrumental conditioning:** Association between a response and a stimulus. It allows an organism to adjust its behavior according to the consequences of that behavior. For example, reinforcement (positive, negative) and punishment.

2. Perceptual Learning

Sight, hearing, taste, smell and touch are considered as the five gateways of knowledge. The individual receives information from sense organs and interprets them in the light of previous experience. The attaching of meaning to sensation is called perception. It is the foundation for all higher forms of learning as it depends on sensation. Hence sensation is the first physiological factor which is involved in the learning process. Learning is dependent on the relative perception of the senses. This learning is confined to the presentation of a concrete object **(Figure 6.10)**.

3. Verbal Learning

All learning taking place in formal education is verbal learning. Learning of this type helps in the acquisition of verbal behavior. The

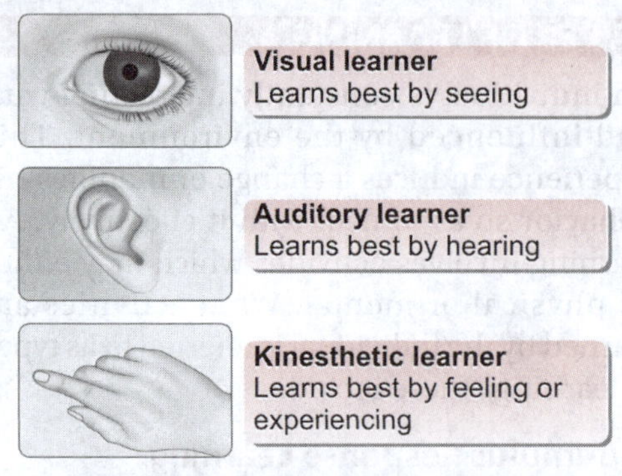

Figure 6.10: Types of perceptual learning

language we speak, communication devices we use are the result of such learning. Signs, pictures, symbols, words, figures, sounds and voices employed by individuals are essential instruments in the process of verbal learning.

4. Motor Learning

When learning involves primarily the use of muscles it is called motor learning. In this type the individual acquires new muscular co-ordinations as a mode of response to asimilar situation. Learning to walk, swim, play throw ball, piano are examples of motor learning.

5. Concept Learning

A concept is a form of a mental image that denotes a generalized idea about things, persons or events. In learning a concept, an individual tries to find out some common property among a group of objects. This learning implies that the individual starts thinking in abstract terms. He understands about the object without its concrete form. These abstract concepts gradually multiply and become a part of the mental makeup.

For example, our concept of a 'car' is a mental image that throws up similarities or common properties of all the different cars we know. We will call a thing 'car' when it has some specific characteristics, the image of which we have already acquired in our mind on account of our previous experience, perception or exercise of imagination. The formation of such concepts on account of previous experience or training is called concept learning. Concept learning proves very useful in recognizing, naming and identifying things. Once a concept is formed, the individual manipulates it in language and thinking.

6. Problem-solving Learning

It is a higher type of learning. This learning requires the use of cognitive abilities like thinking, reasoning, generalization, imagination, etc.

7. Attitude Learning

Much of our learning is based on attitudes. Because of formation of attitudes we show favorable or unfavorable responses to various objects, persons or situations. The individual learns a subject based on his attitude towards the subject.

8. Paired-associate Learning

In this type of learning the learning tasks are presented in such a way that they may be learned by reason of their associations. Krishna, a boy's name may be easy to remember in a paired association with Lord Krishna. Much of the verbal or motor learning may be acquired by means of the technique of paired or multiple association.

9. Other Types of Learning

Visual learning, auditory learning, kinesthetic and tactile learning **(Figure 6.11)**.

These types do not always occur independently. Two or more of the above types of learning are involved in many situations. For example, in typing both motor and verbal learning are involved. In playing chess problem solving, concept learning and verbal learning are involved.

FACTORS INFLUENCING LEARNING

Learning is a process of bringing relatively permanent change in behavior of the learner through experience or practice. The learning process is centered on three elements:

1. The learner whose behavior is to be changed or modified.
2. The type of experience or training required for modification in the learner's behavior.

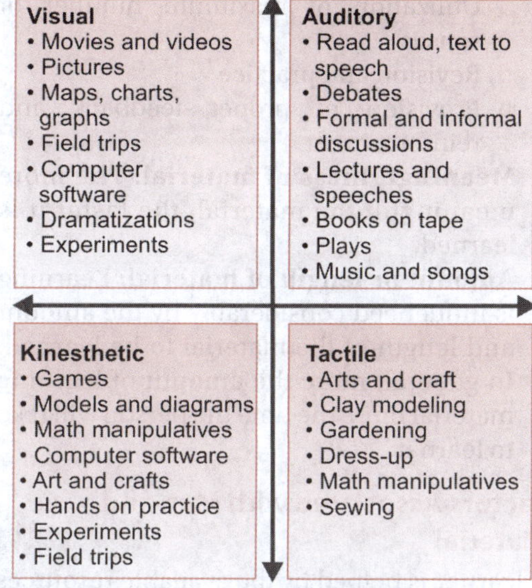

Figure 6.11: Types of learning

3. The men and material resources needed for providing desired experiences and training.

The success or failure in the task of learning depends upon the quality as well as control and management of the factors associated with the above elements **(Table 6.5)**.

Factors Associated with Learner

- **Learner's physical health:** Physical health of the learner is an important factor. Fever, sensory defects particularly of the eyes or the ears, malnutrition, loss of sleep and fatigue are some of the physical handicaps that hinder effective learning. The learner should have sound health for learning.
- **Learner's mental health:** Experiments have shown that worries, fears, persistent day dreams; feelings of loneliness and inferiority affect learning. If the learner has no self-confidence, self-reliance or self-respect due to the attitudes of teachers or others it is very difficult for him or her to learn well. Hence, the necessity of building up the learner's self-confidence, self-respect, self-reliance through praise and approval for the work well done or well attempted is essential.
- **Basic potential of the learner:** It includes
  - Learner's innate abilities and capacities for learning.
  - Learner's general intelligence, knowledge, understanding skills, etc.
  - Learner's basic interest, aptitudes and attitudes related to the learning of a particular thing or area.
- **The level of motivation:** The stronger and clearer the motive in learning anything, the greater is the effort and interest shown by the learner in learning it. The result is greater and more permanent learning.
- **Goals of life:** The philosophy of immediate as well as ultimate goals of one's life affects the process and product of learning.
- **Readiness and will power:** A learner's readiness and will power to learn are great deciding factors in his learning results. If the learner has a will to learn he will ultimately find a way for effective learning.
- **Maturation:** Maturation helps in the process of learning. We learn things when we are mature to learn them. Maturation

Table 6.5: Factors influencing learning

Factors associated with learner	Factors associated with type of learning experience	Factors associated with men and material
• Physical health • Mental health • Basic potentials • Motivation • Goals of life • Readiness and will power • Maturation • Age • Emotions • Sex	• Nature of learning experience • Methodology of learning • Meaningfulness of material • Amount or length of material	• Quality of teaching • Learning material • Textbooks • Teaching learning aids • Library and laboratory facilities • Conducive environment

and learning are closely related to each other. Learning can only take place if the stage for that type of learning has been achieved through a process of maturation. For example, the child has to be physically mature before he can learn to walk or run.

- **Age:** Age is also an important factor in learning. There are certain limitations that old people face in learning new things. They are physically weak and their ability to learn is slow. They have poor recent memory and low reasoning speed. Learning ability for verbal material increases till the age of twenty. Later there is a slow decline till the age of fifty followed by a sharp drop in the later years.
- **Emotions:** Tension or anxiety is a double edged emotion. It has a positive as well as a negative effect on learning. Some amount of stress or anxiety is essential for learning. It provides the drive to learn. Our learning improves with moderate amount of stress. But after a certain optimal level, learning efficiency declines with further increase in stress.
- **Sex:** Although no sex is superior to the other, certain differences in interests and aptitudes are found between the two sexes. Females like to learn things that involve people while men are more object-oriented.

Factors Associated with Type of Learning Experience

- **Nature of learning experience:** Learning is influenced by the nature of the subject matter and the learning experiences presented to a learner such as formal or informal, incidental or well-planned, direct or indirect.
- **Methodology of learning:** Learning depends upon the methods, techniques and approaches employed for the teaching and learning of the selected contents. Some of these techniques are:
  - Linking the recent learning with those of the past
  - Correlating learning in one area with that of another
  - Utilization of maximum number of senses
  - Revision and practice
  - Provision of proper feedback and reinforcement
- **Meaningfulness of material:** The more meaningful the material, the faster it is learned.
- **Amount or length of material:** Learning is influenced considerably by the amount and length of the material to be learned. In general, more the amount of learning material more the time the person will take to learn it.

Factors Associated with Men and Material

A learner is helped by the available resources for bringing desirable changes in his behavior. Certain factors which affect learning are:

- Quality of teaching.
- Availability of appropriate learning material and facilities like teaching-learning aids, textbooks, library and laboratory facilities, project works, etc.
- Availability of conducive environment like proper seating arrangement, calm and peaceful environment, absence of distractions, co-operative and competitive group situations, congenial learning environment at home, provision of opportunity for creativity and self-expression.

LEARNING PROCESS

Learning is a sequence of mental events leading to a change in the learner.

Steps in Learning Process

Learning process has continuity and is carried over through the following steps:

1. **Motive:** These are the dynamic forces that energize behavior and compel the individual to act. The direction of learning will depend upon the relative strength of motives. Unsatisfied motives or needs compel the individual to satisfy them which initiates a learner to learn something.

2. **Goal:** For satisfaction of needs the individual sets definite goals for achieve-ment. The setting of goal helps in making the learning purposeful and interesting. The goal attracts the individual to learn.
3. **Block to the attainment of the goal:** If the individual faces no difficulty in attaining the goal he will not change his present behavior meaning there is no necessity to learn. If a block or barrier obstructs the individual in reaching a goal the individual will then try to change or modify his behavior. This means he learns something to change his behavior or reach a goal.

Along with the above steps individual readiness is important for learning, i.e., physical and mental maturity. Some other aspects involved in learning are reinforcement, integration and learning situation.

Reinforcement: If the response is successful in action and satisfying the need, that response is reinforced and on subsequent occasions the individual will tend to repeat it.

Integration: In this process the individual integrates the successful responses with the individual's previous learning so that it becomes a part of a new functional whole.

Learning situation: It provides opportunity for learning. The quality, speed and effectiveness of learning depends much upon the kind of learning situation and environment available to the learner. Healthy and favorable learning environment brings satisfactory results in learning while the poor and unfavorable learning environment proves an obstacle in the path of learning.

The process of learning does not end only with the acquisition of certain knowledge, skill and changes in behavior in one particular situation. Learning is a never ending process and the change once acquired or the learning once accomplished gets its fixation in other likewise situations. It stands for its modification and thus seems always in a process of continuous change and development.

HABIT

A habit is the tendency of an individual to behave in the same way as he has behaved earlier. It is the repetition of a similar action in similar circumstances. Habits may either be good or bad.

Characteristics of Habits

- It is learned or acquired through repetition.
- A habitual action is automatic meaning it requires little effort or attention once it has been acquired.
- It is performed in a uniform way only under similar circumstances.

Formation of Habits

Steps in habit formation are as follows:

- **Enthusiastic or strong start:** A new habit forms quickly if strong motivation is present.
- **Voluntary repetition of new work/habit:** Voluntary repetition of a new habit helps to make it firm.
- **Absence of exception:** Another important principle in the formation of habit is the absence or avoidance of any exception in the process of formation.
- **Acquainting with situations that will help in habit development:** Relate with only such situations that will encourage habit formation and avoid all other alternate situations.
- **Practice the new habit:** Practice new habit until it becomes routine.

Breaking of Habits

- In order to remove a bad habit it must be replaced with a good habit.
- Start with a strong desire to change.
- Do not allow exceptions while practicing a good habit.
- Seek support from others for practicing the new good habit.
- Practice the new habit continuously.

Some other rules for breaking bad habits are:

- Breaking of habits by voluntary practice and conscious repetition tends to give us a control over habits thus facilitating their cessation at will.
- Formation of a contradictory habit to break it.
- Breaking of habit by doing it to excess.

Role of Habits in Health and Illness

- Some habits and practices involve risk factors for health. Habits can have positive or negative effects on health. Habits with potential negative effects such as sedentary lifestyle, overeating or poor nutrition, insufficient rest and sleep and poor personal hygiene are risk factors.
- Other habits that put a person at risk for illness include alcohol or drug abuse, unsafe sex, multiple sex partners, etc.
- Some habits are risk factors for specific diseases. For example, excessive sun bathing increases the risk of skin cancer, excessive eating of certain foods increases the risk of cardiovascular diseases.
- Good habits like regular exercises, balanced diet and good personal hygiene improve health.

It is important for the nurse to understand the impact of specific habits on health status. Nurses can educate patients and the public on developing good habits to improve health.

Study Habits

A student nurse must bear in mind the following points for her learning to be effective:

- **Being self-prepared:** Sound physical and mental healths are pre-requisites for good study. Besides this the student nurse should also have capacity for hard work.
- **Wholeness:** It is recommended to have a bird eye-view of the complete subject before going into details of the study. Dr Buchanan has suggested that the entire course outline be skimmed so as to identify the main idea underlying the whole course and locate the sections that deserve close study.
- **Planning and organization:** The student nurse should have a time-table for the whole day with a definite period for study. The time selected for study should be such that the chances for disturbance are minimum.
- **Clarity of purpose:** The student nurse should be clear about what she is learning and associate it with as many issues as possible. In particular she must know how the piece of learning will help her in the career.
- **Prompt start:** When one has to study he should get down to it without delay and avoid wasting time in trivia.
- **Search for essentials in an assignment:** The students must always look for the basic facts of the subject study and give due importance to the general principles as well as details.
- **Note-taking:** Students should cultivate the habit of taking notes while studying. Intelligent note-taking lends seriousness to the study and helps the student to think and reason. Notes should be brief and concentrate on the vital ideas.
- **Review and over learn**: The rate of forgetting is far in excess of what is retained. Therefore, constant review is required to retain the essentials of any subject. Besides one must learn more than what is necessary. It is advisable to read the same topic from many books and also recall what has been learned. If the recall is unsatisfactory the lesson should be revised. Over learning is helped by repetition and recitation.
- **Paying attention towards charts, tables and formulae**: During the course of study meaning of new words should be noted down as and when they appear and an effort made to use them effectively. The student nurse should also be able to study the charts and tables and remember the formulae when required.
- **Proper physical surroundings**: If the place of study is fixed and the hours of study regular, one can easily get into the mood for study. The surroundings should invariably be sober, clean and adequately illuminated. Poor light, bad ventilation, extreme heat and cold reduce efficiency while learning.
- **Interrelationship**: Interrelationship and correlation among various subjects such as anatomy, physiology, chemistry is conducive to effective learning. The student nurse should also know how it is useful in studying the patient. All old knowledge must be related with the new.

Studying for Examination

Points to be kept in mind while studying for examinations are:

- Attitude should be positive and thinking hopeful.
- All nervousness should be avoided and it is better not to study anything few hours before the examination.
- Keeping awake the previous night should be avoided as lack of sleep and nervous exhaustion distorts one's judgment.
- Cramming should be avoided as there is no intelligent learning or grasp. It is mechanical in nature. Useful study consists of constant review and should be reflective.

LAWS OF LEARNING

Psychologists have identified several principles of learning that are applicable to the learning process. Also referred to as laws of learning they have been discovered, tested, and used in practical situations. They provide additional insight into what makes people learn most effectively. The various laws of learning are as under **(Figure 6.12)**:

1. Law of Readiness

Learning takes place best when a person is ready to learn. For this to happen some sort of preparatory attitude or mindset is necessary. If the nervous pathway is ready for action response quickly follows. If it is exhausted and not quick for action, the response does not follow readily. Learner's reaction depends upon the readiness of the sensory and motor neurons.

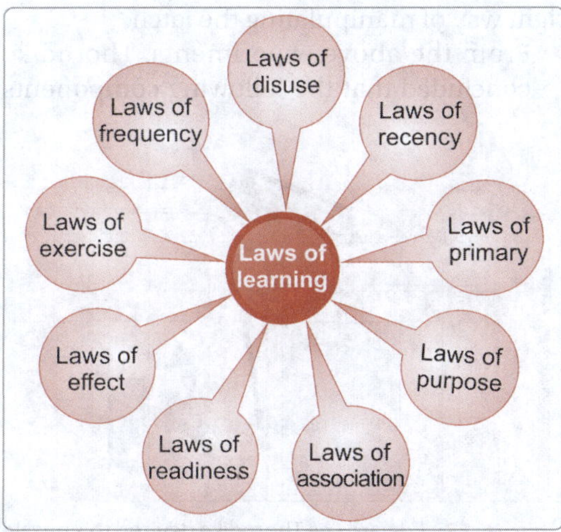

Figure 6.12: Laws of learning

2. Law of Effect

A successful reaction gives satisfaction to the individual and the same reaction tends to be repeated. An unsuccessful reaction annoys the individual and tends to inhibit. Thus, pleasure and pain have their effects on learning reactions.

3. Law of Exercise/Use

Native reactions are strengthened by practice. The use of a response strengthens it and makes it more prompt, easy and certain.

4. Law of Frequency

The law of frequency is correlated to law of use. If one response strengthens the situation-response connection, two responses will strengthen it further, three still further and so on. The more frequently a connection is exercised the stronger the connection becomes.

5. Law of Disuse

Any learning process which is not practiced for some time gradually decays. Use strengthens a situation-response connection. Disuse weakens the connection. Material without any meaning like irrelevant syllables is quickly forgotten. Material with meaning as in poetry is not so quickly forgotten.

6. Law of Recency

The law of recency is correlated to law of disuse. The more recent is the exercise, the stronger is the connection between the situation and the response. The connection between a situation and the response is weakened gradually through disuse.

7. Law of Primacy

The first experiences and acts are novel and apt to attract attention. They are readily impressed in the mind. The first day at school, the first act in learning to solve a puzzle are easily impressed.

8. Law of Purpose

With a clear or definite goal in mind the student works towards a definite purpose.

9. Law of Association

It is on the basis of association of ideas that we can explain how one idea gives way to the other and so on. When we recall a name we usually remember other objects associated with it. For example, when somebody refers to the Taj Mahal we recall it as being made of marble as these ideas are closely associated with one another. Laws which govern the association of ideas are:

- The law of similarity
- The law of contrast

THEORIES OF LEARNING

During the early part of the 20th century a number of psychologists became increasingly interested in turning psychology into a more scientific endeavor. To be more scientific they argued that psychology needed to study only those things that could be measured and quantified.

A number of different learning theories emerged to explain how and why people behave the way they do. The learning theories of development are centered on the influence of environment on the learning process. Such environmental influences include associations, reinforcements, punishments and observations. Some of the primary learning theories include, trial and error theory of learning, learning by conditioning, theory of operant conditioning, theory of insightful learning, observational learning.

1. Trial and Error Theory of Learning

This theory was propagated by Edward Lee Thorndike (1874–1949). According to Thorndike, learning consists of making bonds or connections between stimuli and responses. These bonds are made in the nervous system. According to Thorndike, learning is nothing but the stamping in of the correct responses and stamping out of the incorrect responses through trial and error. To support his point of view Thorndike conducted the following experiment.

A hungry cat was placed in a box. There was only one door for exit which could be opened by correctly manipulating a latch. A fish was placed outside the box which worked as a strong motive for the cat to come out of the box. Consequently the cat made a number of random movements such as biting, clawing and scrambling around as it struggled to come out the box. In one of the random movements the latch was manipulated and the door opened. The cat came out and got its reward.

The process was repeated in the subsequent trial. However, this time around the cat took much lesser time in coming out. In subsequent trials incorrect responses like biting and clawing gradually diminished until the cat reached a stage where it manipulated the latch as soon as it was put in the box and came out immediately to eat the fish. The cat by this technique gradually learned the art of opening the door. Thorndike named the learning of his experimental cat as 'trial and error learning' **(Figure 6.13)**. He maintained that learning is nothing but the stamping in of the correct responses and stamping out of the incorrect responses through trial and error. In trying for the correct solution the cat made many vain attempts, committed error after error before gaining success in subsequent trials, tried to avoid the erroneous ways and repeated the right way of manipulating the latch.

- From the above experiments, Thorndike concluded that the following components

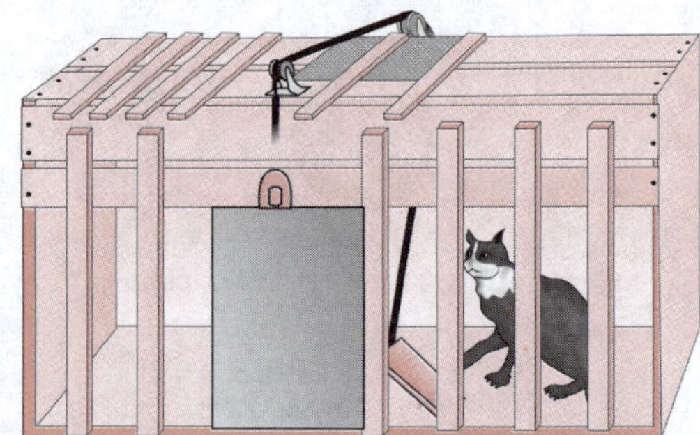

Figure 6.13: Edward Lee Thorndike devised this puzzle box to study trial and error learning

or elements are involved in the process of learning:
  - Drive
  - Goal
  - Barriers or blocks which prevent the individual from reaching the goal
  - Random attempts to overcome the barriers
  - Chance success
  - Selection of the correct response
  - Fixation of the correct response in neuromuscular system of the individual
- Major theoretical principles which form the basis of Thorndike theory of learning are:
  - Learning involves trial and error or selection and connection
  - Learning is a result of formation of connections
  - Learning is improvement in performance not insightful
  - Learning is direct and not mediated by ideas
- Based on his theory, Thorndike put forward the following laws of learning:
  - The law of readiness
  - The law of effect of satisfaction/dissatisfaction
  - The law of exercise or practice
  - The law of multiple responses or varied reactions
  - The law of attitude
  - The law of analogy
  - The law of associative shifting

Educational Implications of Trial and Error Theory

- According to Thorndike, when a child is ready to learn he learns more quickly and effectively. He warns that the child should not be forced to learn when he is not ready and also not to miss any opportunity of providing the right learning experience when the child is prepared to learn. The task of the teacher is to motivate the students by arousing their attention, interest and curiosity, and make them want to learn (law of readiness).
- The teacher must try to strengthen the bonds or connections between stimuli and responses through repetition, drill and practice. Otherwise the bonds get weakened through disuse and learning does not happen (law of practice).
- The child must be provided with a learning experience which gives him a sense of satisfaction. The child must also be suitably rewarded so as to make learning effective (law of effect).
- The learner should try to see similarities and dissimilarities between different kinds of responses to stimuli and by comparison and contrast try to apply the learning from one situation to other similar situations.
- The learner should be encouraged to perform his task independently. He must attempt various solutions to the problem before arriving at the correct one.

In general, Thorndike theory and laws of learning have contributed towards making learning purposeful and goal-oriented and brought out the importance of motivation, rewards and practice in the process of teaching and learning.

2. Theory of Classical Conditioning (or) Type 'S' Conditioning (or) Respondent Learning

The theory of classical conditioning was proposed by Ivan Pavlov (1849-1936), a Russian physiologist. Pavlov while studying the physiology of digestion found that behavior can be classically conditioned. He experimented on a dog and found that food placed in the mouth of a hungry dog automatically causes salivation. In this case salivation is an unlearned response or an unconditioned response and food the unconditioned stimulus (natural). Later a bell was rung each time before the food was served. Pavlov now found that the dog started to salivate at the very sound of the bell. He termed this phenomenon as conditioned response. Here the bell is the conditioned stimulus (artificial stimulus).

In later studies Pavlov noticed that if he did not provide food after the bell was rung, the dog eventually stopped salivating called 'extinction' and demonstrated that reinforcement is essential both to acquire and maintain respondent learning. Pavlov also found that if the dog is given a prolonged rest period during extinction it will once again salivate when the bell is rung. This phenomenon was termed as spontaneous recovery.

- Prior to conditioning the ringing of a bell does not bring about salivation making the bell a neutral stimulus. On the other hand, food naturally brings about salivation making it an unconditioned stimulus and salivation an unconditioned response **(Figures 6.14A and B)**.
- During conditioning the bell is rung just before the food is served **(Figure 6.14C)**.
- After conditioning the ringing of the bell alone brings about salivation. The bell which was earlier considered a neutral stimulus is now considered a conditional stimulus bringing about conditioned response of salivation **(Figure 6.14D)**.

Classical conditioning is a type of learning in which a neutral stimulus brings about a response after it is paired with a stimulus that naturally brings about that response.

Neutral Stimulus

A stimulus which initially produces no specific response other than focusing attention. In other words it is a stimulus that does not produce an automatic response.

Unconditioned Stimulus

A response that is natural and needs no training (e.g., salivation at the smell of food).

Conditioned Stimulus

A neutral stimulus that has been paired with an unconditioned stimulus (UCS) to bring about a response earlier caused only by the UCS.

Conditioned Response

A response which after conditioning follows a previously neutral stimulus (e.g., salivation at the ringing of a bell).

Extinction

The decrease in frequency and eventual disappearance of a previously conditioned response; one of the basic phenomena of learning.

Spontaneous Recovery

The re-emergence of an extinguished conditioned response after a period of rest.

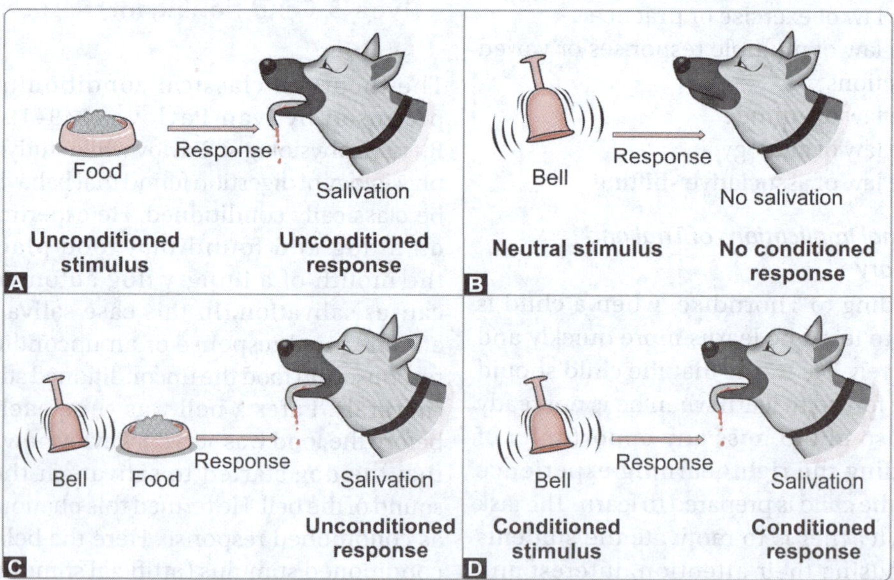

Figures 6.14 A to D: The basic process of classical conditioning: (A and B) Before conditioning; (C) During conditioning; (D) After conditioning

Stimulus Generalization

A response to a stimulus that is similar to but different from a conditioned stimulus. More similar are the two stimuli, more likely the generalization will occur.

Pavlov theory is also termed as type-S conditioning to stress the significance of stimulus that comes before and elicits the response. The theory of conditioning as advocated by Pavlov thus considers learning as habit formation and is based on the principle of association and substitution. It is simply a stimulus-response type of learning where in place of a natural stimulus like food, water, sexual contact, etc., an artificial stimulus like the sound of the bell, sight of light of a definite color, etc., can evoke a natural response. When both the artificial stimulus (ringing of the bell) and the natural stimulus (food) are brought together several times, the dog becomes conditioned to respond to this situation as a perfect association occurs between the types of stimuli presented together. As a result the natural stimulus can later be substituted or replaced with an artificial stimulus capable of evoking a natural stimulus.

Educational Implications of Classical Conditioning Theory

- Fear, love or hatred towards a particular subject is created through conditioning. A teacher with his defective methods of teaching or harsh treatment of students may create a strong dislike among them towards the subject.
- On the other hand interesting and effective methodology in teaching along with sympathetic treatment can have a desirable impact on the students through the process of conditioning. They develop a positive attitude towards the subject as well as the teacher who has imparted the knowledge to them.
- The theory of classical conditioning emphasizes that students should be exposed to positive stimuli in order to develop desirable habits, interests and attitudes in them.
- Conditioning can also be used to remove unhealthy attitudes, superstitions and fears from the minds of students by exposing them to positive stimuli (reconditioning).

3. Theory of Operant Conditioning (or) Type 'R' Conditioning (or) Instrumental Conditioning

The theory of learning by operant conditioning was given by BF Skinner (1904–1990). Basically Skinner revolted against the concept of classical conditioning. He said that man is an active organism and not a victim of his environment. He does not wait for the stimulus; instead he acts or operates on the environment so as to change it in some way. Thus he called it operant behavior.

According to Skinner, operant behavior is determined by events or consequences that follow the response. If the consequences are favorable the individual will repeat the same behavior. In this case the consequences are said to have provided positive reinforcement and caused repetition of behavior. Alternatively, if the consequences are unfavorable they reduce the chances of same behavior from getting repeated. In such a case the consequences are said to have provided negative reinforcement and reduced the chances of behavior from recurring again.

To emphasize the effect of response on future behavior, operant conditioning is also termed as type-R conditioning. Skinner thus proposed that learning is shaped and maintained by its consequences. Following is one of the experiments carried out by Skinner to support his concept of operant conditioning. A hungry rat was placed in a box designed by Skinner which was called the Skinner box or operant chamber. The chamber contained a lever which would drop food pellets into the chamber if pressed. In the beginning the experimenter himself dropped the food pellets into the box and later stopped. The rat being hungry began to explore the box and pressed the lever accidentally. The food pellet was released into the box which the rat ate up. After a while it pressed the lever again and ate the food pellet which got released.

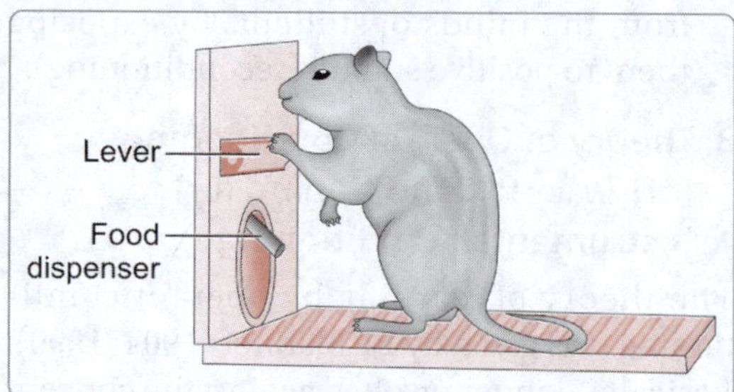

Figure 6.15: A Skinner box used to study operant conditioning

A few attempts later, the rat began to press the lever more rapidly. Food is thus said to have provided positive reinforcement to the rat thereby establishing operant behavior, i.e., the rat continued to press the lever in order to obtain food pellets **(Figure 6.15)**. Based on the findings of his experiments he concluded that behavior is shaped and maintained by its consequences. It is operated by the organism and maintained by its results.

Reinforcement

The process by which a stimulus increases the probability that a preceding behavior will be repeated **(Table 6.6)**.

Reinforcer

Any stimulus that increases the probability that a preceding behavior will occur again.

Positive reinforcer

A stimulus added to the environment that brings about an increase in the preceding response.

Negative reinforcer

An unpleasant stimulus whose removal leads to an increase in the probability that a preceding response will occur again in future.

Punishment

A stimulus that decreases the probability that a previous behavior will occur again.

Schedules of Reinforcement

Objects or events which provide reinforcement are called reinforcers. There are two types of reinforcers: primary and secondary.

1. Primary reinforcers are those which possess inherent reinforcing properties. Examples include food, water, physical comfort, etc.
2. Secondary or conditioned reinforcers are those which acquire their reinforcing qualities through close association with a primary reinforcer. Examples include money, attention, affection and good grades.

Skinner put forward the idea of planning the schedules of reinforcement in order to condition the operant behavior of the individual. The important schedules are as follows **(Table 6.7):**

1. Continuous reinforcement schedule

Continuous reinforcement (CR) schedule is 100% reinforcement schedule where every correct response of the individual is rewarded or reinforced. The learner is rewarded for every correct answer he gives for the questions posed by his teacher.

Table 6.6: Types of reinforcement and punishment

	Effect on behavior	
Procedure	**Increases**	**Decreases**
Presentation of stimulus	**Positive reinforcement** *Example*: Giving a raise for good performance *Result*: Increase in frequency of response (good performance)	**Positive punishment** *Example*: Giving a punishment following misbehavior *Result*: Decrease in frequency of response (misbehavior)
Removal of stimulus	**Negative reinforcement** *Example*: Terminating a headache by taking aspirin *Result*: Increase in frequency of response (taking aspirin)	**Negative punishment** *Example*: Removal of favorite toy after misbehavior *Result*: Decrease in frequency of response (misbehavior)

Table 6.7: Schedules of reinforcement

Schedule of reinforcement	Definitions	Examples	Response pattern
Continuous	Reinforcement after every response	A student is rewarded for every correct answer	Rapid learning of response
Fixed-interval	Reinforcement after a set period of time	A student receives a reward after a fixed period of time during which he performs the desired behavior (for example, a reward for working hard for 10 minutes)	Response rate increases as time for reinforcement approaches, then drops after reinforcement
Fixed-ratio	Reinforcement after a set number of responses	A student receives a reward after he performs a desired behavior for a fixed number of times (for example, a reward every time he attempts an additional question)	Rapid response rate; pause after reinforcement
Variable-ratio	Reinforcement is intermittent and irregular	A student receives a reward after he performs a desired behavior for a variable number of times	Very high response rate; little pause after reinforcement
Variable-interval	Reinforcement after varying lengths of time	A student receives a reward after a variable period of time during which he performs the desired behavior	Slow, steady rate of response; very little pause after reinforcement

2. Fixed-interval reinforcement schedule

In fixed-interval (FI) reinforcement schedule the individual is rewarded for a response only after a set interval of time. What is important here is the fixed responses during this interval. For example:

- Paying salaries for the work done on a weekly or monthly basis.
- Conducting examinations periodically for the students.
- Giving a person a periodic allowance, etc.

3. Fixed-ratio reinforcement schedule

in fixed-ratio (FR) reinforcement schedule the individual is reinforced following a 'fixed' number of correct responses. This schedule usually generated extremely high operant levels in the individuals because the more they respond the more reinforcement they receive. Example: Paying or compensating employees depending on the number of units they produce or sell.

4. Variable-ratio reinforcement schedule

In variable-ratio (VR) reinforcement schedule reinforcement is intermittent and irregular. The individual does not know when he is going to be rewarded and so remains motivated throughout the learning process. The most common example of this schedule is human behavior in gambling. Here rewards are unpredictable and keep the players motivated though the returns are occasional.

5. Variable-interval reinforcement schedule

In variable-interval (VI) reinforcement schedule reinforcement is given to a response after an unpredictable amount of time has passed. However this amount of time is on a changing/variable schedule. This is almost identical to a FI schedule but the reinforcements are given on a variable or changing schedule. Example, checking email at random intervals across the day rather than checking every time a message is delivered. In most cases it is not known when the message will be received, i.e., emails roll in at completely unpredictable times. When we check and see that a message has been received, it acts as a reinforcer for checking the email.

Educational implications of Operant Conditioning Theory

- The key concept in Skinner's theory is reinforcement. For an individual to learn, correct responses must be suitably rewarded or positively reinforced. Thus to provide proper reinforcement the learning process and environment must be designed so as to create minimum frustration and maximum satisfaction to the learner.

  The principle of operant conditioning may be successfully applied in behavior modification. We have to find something that is rewarding for the individual whose behavior we wish to modify, wait until the desired behavior occurs and immediately reward him when it does. When this is done the frequency with which the desired response occurs goes up. When the behavior next occurs it is again rewarded and the rate of response goes up even further. Proceeding in this manner the individual can be induced to learn the desired behavior.
- Operant conditioning emphasizes the importance of schedules in the process of reinforcement of behavior. In trying to impart or teach a particular behavior great care should be taken for the proper planning of the schedules of reinforcement.
- This theory advocated the avoidance of punishment for unlearning the undesirable behavior and shaping the desirable behavior. Punishment proves ineffective in the long run. It appears that punishment simply suppresses behavior and when the threat of punishment is removed the rate with which the behavior occurs returns to its original level. Therefore, operant conditioning experiments suggested appropriate alternatives to punishment in the form of rewarding appropriate behavior and ignoring inappropriate behavior for its gradual extinction.
- The theory of operant conditioning has shown that learning proceeds most effectively if:
  - The learning material is so designed that it produces fewer chances for failure and more opportunities for success.
  - The learner is given rapid feedback concerning the accuracy of his learning.
  - The learner is able to learn at his own pace.

4. Theory of Insightful Learning (Gestalt Psychology)

Gestalt psychology was founded in Germany in 1912 by Max Wertheimer (1880–1943) and his colleagues. The word 'Gestalt' means 'form or shape or a particular arrangement of elements'. The basic idea behind Gestalt learning is that 'the whole is more than the sum of its parts'. Everything cannot be understood by a study of its constituent parts but can be done so by viewing it in totality. The learner while learning always perceives the situation as a whole. After studying and evaluating the different relationships in the situation he takes the proper decision in an intelligent way rather than simply reacting to the specific stimuli.

Gestalt psychologists used the term 'insight' to describe the perception of the whole situation by the learner and his intelligence in responding to the proper relationships. Insight is often referred to as the end process of observational activity. Learning activities are said to be insightful for desired learning. This reinforcement may be provided through verbal praise, positive facial expressions of the teacher, scores, grades, prizes, medals, etc.

In a nutshell, Gestalt psychologists tried to interpret learning as a purposive, exploratory and creative process rather than a mere trial and error or even conditioning. Learning is restructuring the field of perception through insight.

The following are some of the experiments carried out by Gestalt psychologists to support their view on learning:

Kohler put a chimpanzee in a cage and a banana was hung from the roof of the cage. A box was placed inside the cage. The chimpanzee tried to reach the banana by jumping but could not succeed. Suddenly he got an idea and used the box as a jumping platform by placing it just below the bananas **(Figure 6.16)**.

In another experiment the problem was made more difficult and the chimpanzee had to use two or three boxes to reach the bananas. Moreover, the placing of one box over the other required different specific arrangements. In a more complicated arrangement the bananas were placed outside the cage. Two sticks, one longer than the other were placed in the cage.

One stick was hollow at one end so that the other stick could be thrust into forming a longer stick. The bananas were kept at such a distance that they could not be picked up by anyone of the sticks. The chimpanzee first tried these sticks one after the other but could not succeed. Suddenly it got an idea of joining the two sticks together and finally reached the bananas **(Figure 6.17)**.

Based on their experiments, Gestalt psychologists concluded that insight depends on following factors:

- Past experiences which help in the insightful solution.

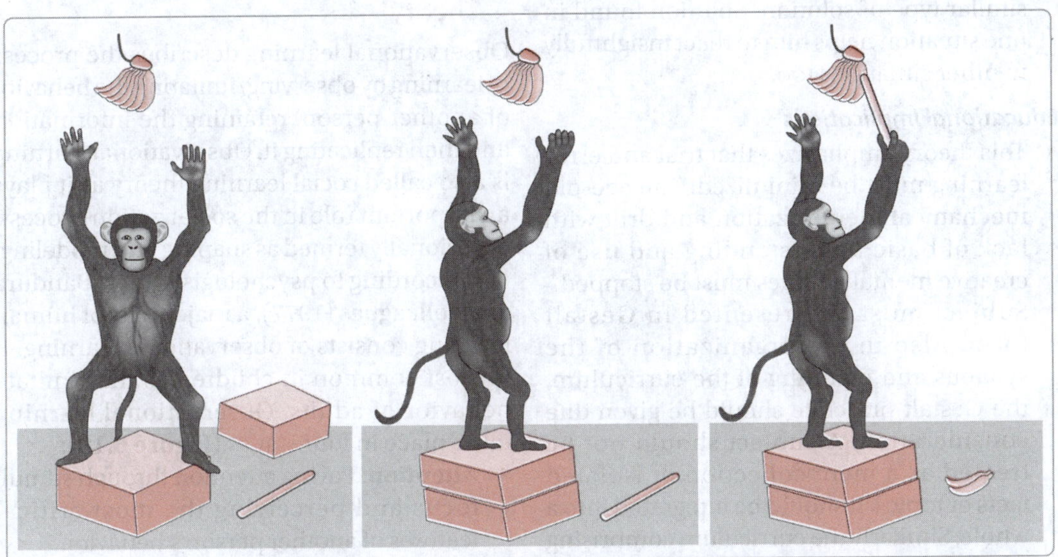

Figure 6.16: Kohler's chimpanzee learns to reach the bananas

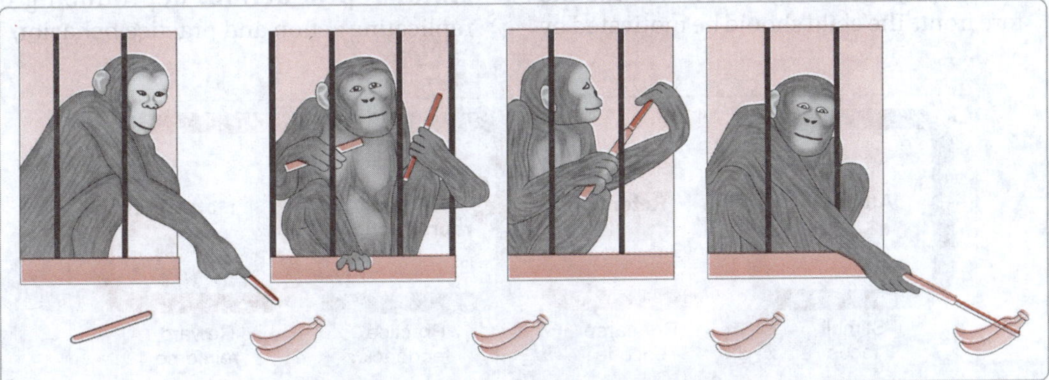

Figure 6.17: Kohler chimpanzee learns to assemble a long stick from two shorter ones

- Insightful solutions depend upon the basic intelligence of the learner. Greater the intelligence, more is the insight.
- Insight recurs when the learning situation is so arranged that all the necessary aspects are open for observation.
- Insightful learning may initially pass through the process of trial and error. But this stage does not last long. These initial efforts in the form of simple trial and error open the way for insightful learning.
- Repetition and generalization.
- After reaching an insightful solution to a particular problem the individual tries to repeat it in another situation demanding similar type of solution. Solution found in one situation helps him to react insightfully in other situations too.

Educational Implications

- This theory emphasizes that trial and error learning must be minimized. The age-old mechanical memorization and drill with lack of basic understanding and use of creative mental abilities must be stopped.
- Subject must be presented in Gestalt form. Also in the organization of the syllabus and planning of the curriculum, the Gestalt principle should be given due consideration. A subject should not be treated as a mere collection of isolated facts or topics. It should be integrated into a whole. Similarly the curriculum comprising of different subjects and activities should reflect unity and integration.
- This theory has brought motivation to the fore front. The child should be motivated by arousing his interest and curiosity so as to make learning goal-oriented and effective.
- The learner must be given plenty of opportunities to use his mental abilities. Neither is classroom or environment in which the child is learning just a body of discrete (separate) stimuli nor are the child's responses to the environment just a trial and error. The world is organized and has a meaning. The child can react with understanding as he has insight. Thus learning should be made meaningful.

5. Observational Learning (or) Learning Through Imitation (Social Learning Theory)

Observational learning describes the process of learning by observing/imitating the behavior of another person, retaining the information and then replicating it. Observational learning is also called social learning theory as it plays an important role in the socialization process, occasionally termed as shaping and modeling.

According to psychologist Albert Bandura and colleagues (1977), a major part of human learning consists of observational learning. It is most common in children as they imitate behavior of adults. Observational learning takes place in four stages **(Figure 6.18)**:

- **Attention**: Paying attention through stimuli focus and perceiving the most critical features of another person's behavior.
- **Retention:** Remembering the behavior through rehearse encode.
- **Motor reproduction**: Reproducing or replicating action and practice behavior.

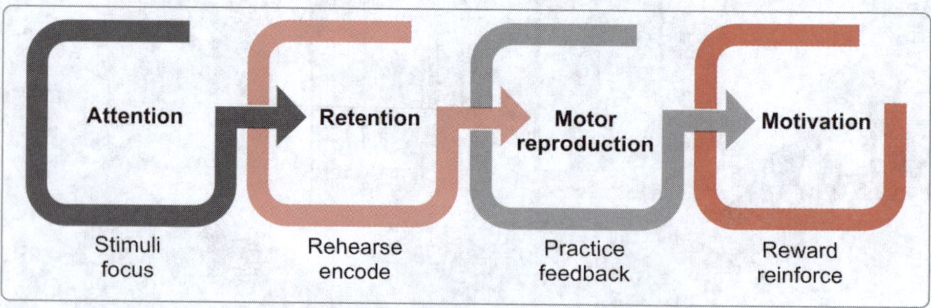

Figure 6.18: Albert Bandura's social learning theory

- **Motivation**: Being motivated to learn and carry out the behavior through reward reinforcement.

For example, a girl is watching a TV program on preparation of some new dishes. First she observes the demonstration on preparation of the new dish on TV screen and tries to memorize it. She then enters her kitchen to convert the stored observation into action. Her learning of the preparation of new dishes may then be reinforced by the response she gets from the members of her family who taste the new dishes.

Summary of Various Theories of Learning

Trial and error theory of learning, classical conditioning and operant conditioning theories interpret learning in terms of connection or association between stimulus and response. Insightful learning and observational learning theories emphasize the role of purpose, insight, understanding, reasoning, memory and other cognitive factors in the process of learning **(Table 6.8)**.

Table 6.8: Summary of various theories of learning

Theory	Theorist	Description
Trial and error theory of learning	Edward Lee Thorndike (1874–1949)	Learning is nothing but the stamping in of the correct responses and stamping out of the incorrect responses through trial and error. It is also called 'learning by selection of the successful variant'.
Theory of classical conditioning	Ivan Pavlov (1849–1936)	Learning occurs from associations between an unconditioned stimulus and a neutral stimulus. It is a type of unconscious or automatic learning process which creates a conditioned response.
Theory of operant conditioning	BF Skinner (1904–1990)	Learning is shaped and maintained by its consequences. Learning is a voluntary response which is strengthened or weakened depending on its favorable or unfavorable consequences
Theory of insightful learning	Wolfgang Kohler (1887–1967)	Learning is a purposive, exploratory and creative process rather than mere trial and error or even conditioning. Learning is restructuring the field of perception through insight
Observational learning	Albert Bandura (1925–2021)	Learning occurs through observational process. It advocates that most of what we learn is acquired through simply observing and imitating the behavior of others who are taken as models

MEMORY

Memory plays a very important role in our learning and psychological growth. Through memory of our past experiences we handle new situations. It helps us in our re-learning, problem solving and thinking. Memory is regarded as the special ability of our mind to conserve or store what has been previously learned or experienced and recollect or reproduce it after sometime.

DEFINITIONS

- Memory consists in remembering what has previously been learned.
  —Wood Worth and Marquis (1948)
- The power that we have to 'store' our experiences and to bring them into the field of consciousness sometime after experiences have occurred is termed memory. **—Ryburn (1956)**

Memory and remembering carry the same meaning. While differentiating between memory and remembering, Levin (1978) says 'Memory can be compared to a giant filing cabinet in the brain with data stored, classified and cross-filed for future reference. Remembering depends upon how the brain goes about coding its input'.

TYPES OF MEMORY/STAGES OF MEMORY

There are three different types of memory: Immediate (sensory memory), short-term memory and long-term memory **(Flowcharts 6.3 and 6.4)**.

Immediate or Sensory Memory

Immediate memory or sensory memory is that memory which helps an individual to recall something a split second after having perceived it. In this type of memory retentive time is extremely brief, generally from a fraction of a second to several seconds.

Immediate memory is needed when we need to remember something for a short time and then forget it. It helps us to learn immediately with speed and accuracy. For example, we look up a telephone number from the directory and remember it but after making the call we usually forget it.

Short-term Memory

Short-term memory (STM) holds a relatively small amount of information, about seven items for a short period of time (20–30 seconds) though not nearly as short-lived as the immediate memory. For example,

Flowchart 6.3: Types of memory

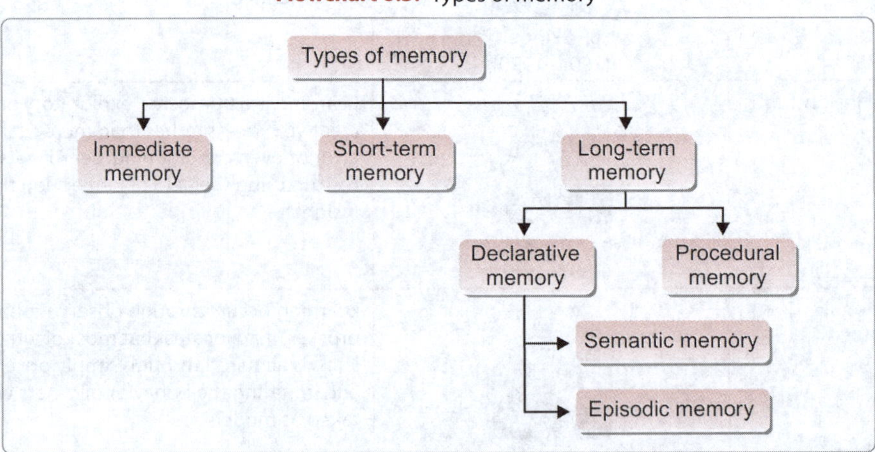

Flowchart 6.4: Three stage model of memory

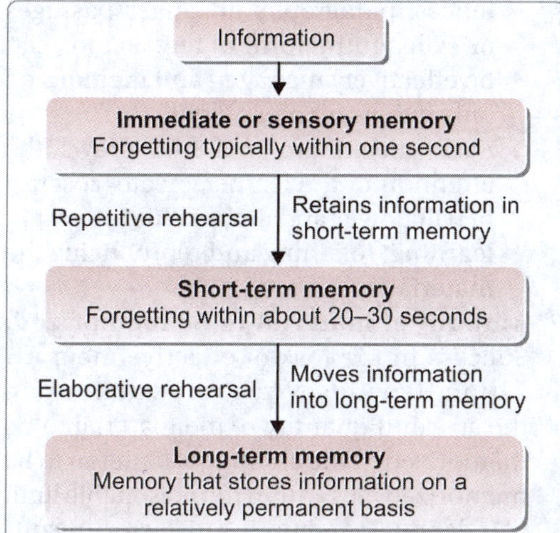

Flowchart 6.5: Classifications of long-term memory

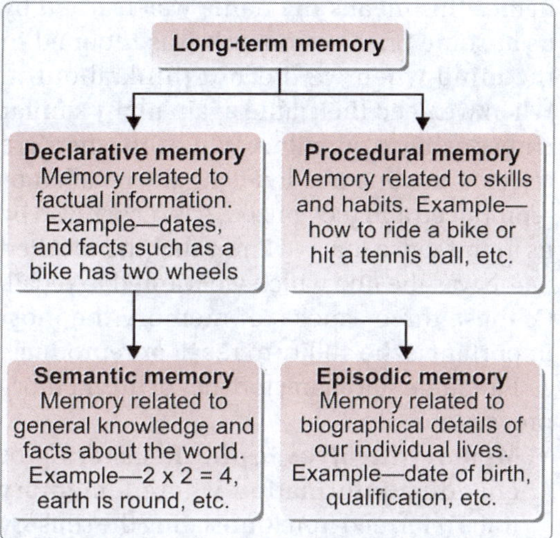

where one parked his vehicle in the morning or what he had for dinner the previous day.

Long-term Memory

Long-term memory (LTM) deals with continuous storage and an unlimited capacity to store information for days, months, years and even a lifetime. LTM codes information according to meaning, pattern and other characteristics. LTM helps in storage, retention and remembrance of life events at record notice making things quite easy.

Long-term memory can be categorized into declarative and procedural memory. Declarative memory also termed as explicit memory is based on recall and retrieval. It deals with the memory of facts, data and events. For example, a student knows that the library is open only till 2.00 pm on Sundays. This fact is stored as declarative memory which can consciously be recalled. Declarative memory can further be subdivided into semantic memory and episodic memory **(Flowchart 6.5)**. Procedural memory on the other hand deals with different actions and skills. For example, riding a scooter, wearing a pair of shoes, cooking, etc.

NATURE OF MEMORY

Memory is a complex process which involves learning, retention, recall and recognition.

Learning or Registration

Our mind has a special ability by virtue of which every experience or learning leaves behind traces. These are conserved in the form of 'engrains.' This is known as learning.

Retention

These engrains or memory traces are preserved in our brain with the help of our nervous system. This process is known as retention.

Recall

Recall means perfect revival of the past experiences.

Recognition

Recognition means that the recalled experience at the conscious level is the same from which the individual wanted to recall and had experienced earlier. Recall and recognition are closely related. Recall provides the material in memory while recognition is the process of accepting or rejecting it. Recall is an active process while recognition is more a passive behavior.

For example, remembering a person's name. This means the name was learned by us at some previous time. It was retained in the mind when we did not think about it. When we need this name again many similar names come to our mind. While the others are rejected the one needed is finally recalled or reproduced and recognized. It is recognized by us in the sense that we knew that the recalled name was the one which we wanted to recall. Of these three aspects of memory the most important is the ability to recall or reproduce.

Fundamental characteristics of the memory process are:

- **Memory involves input:** Registering or encoding information where a memory trace is formed from translating the sensory data.
- **Storage:** It is either temporary or permanent.
- **Output:** It involves retrieval. Memory would be useless unless there is a mechanism to retrieve the information.

FACTORS INFLUENCING MEMORY

Memory refers to the process of remembering. The factors which influence memory are divided into extrinsic factors and intrinsic factors **(Table 6.9)**.

Extrinsic Factors

1. **Meaningfulness of material to be memorized:**
   - Useful and meaningful material which suits the needs, motives and purposes of an individual can be learned properly, retained for a long time and be reproduced easily when needed.
   - Similarly material in the form of sentences, paragraphs or longer passages or skills in the form of any actions can be effectively managed and memorized only if they are meaningful.
   - Such meaningful material draws the attention of the learner, creates a sense of will power and arouses his interest in learning, retaining and reproducing the material.
2. **Amount of material to be memorized:** Success in the task of effective memorization depends to a great extent upon the size and quantity of the material to be memorized. If the amount of material to be memorized falls within the reasonable limit of individual's memory, satisfactory results can be achieved. However, if it crosses one's reasonable limit no such result is likely to be achieved.
   Greater the amount of material and greater the effort in memorization it needs, greater is the possibility of failure in terms of learning, retention and reproduction. Therefore, it is always safer to have a convenient amount of material for memorization at a particular sitting.
3. **Time required to vocalize responses:** Memory span is consistently higher for short words than for long words. This increase in span is due to the lesser duration of time needed to pronounce the shorter words.
4. **Distraction:** Greater the distraction present in the situation, poorer would be the performance of the individual. Alternately, either a calm and quite atmosphere or a stimulating environment proves to be an effective aid to learning.

Table 6.9: Factors influencing memory

Extrinsic factors	Intrinsic factors
◆ Meaningfulness of material ◆ Amount of material ◆ Time required to vocalize response ◆ Distraction	◆ Age ◆ Maturity ◆ Will to learn ◆ Interest and attention ◆ Intelligence ◆ Rest and sleep ◆ Medical conditions

Intrinsic Factors

1. **Age of the individual:** This is a factor which definitely affects memory span. Investigators claim that memory span increases between the age of 16 and 26 years. Youngsters can remember better than the aged.
2. **Maturity:** Very young children cannot retain and remember complex material.

3. **Will to learn:** Material read, heard or seen without genuine interest or inclination is difficult to be remembered or recalled at a later time.
4. **Interest and attention:** Interest as well as attention is essential for learning and memorization. A person who has no interest in what he learns will not give due attention to it and consequently will not be able to learn it.
5. **Intelligence:** A more intelligent person will exhibit better memory than a less intelligent person.
6. **Rest and sleep:** Adequate sleep and rest helps to relieve fatigue and monotony. A mind which is fresh is naturally able to learn more and retain it for a longer period than a mind which is dull and fatigued.
7. **Medical conditions:** Major causes for memory loss are contributed by medical conditions and eating habits.
   - **High blood pressure:** This condition leads to the hardening of the arteries. It does not aid the flow of blood to various parts of the body as it is supposed to. The circulation problem thus caused can lead to memory loss as the blood that carries oxygen and other nutrition to the brain does not reach it. Such effects on the circulation system can also lead to a stroke, a major cause for dementia. Dementia can leave a person with severe memory impairment.
   - **Hypothyroidism:** This is a condition caused when not enough thyroid hormone is produced. The most common symptom of memory loss is hypothyroidism.
   - **Brain tumors:** This is a disease that causes the patients to forget people's names they interact with every day or places that they go to everyday.
   - **Alzheimer's disease:** This is the most common cause of memory loss. Nerve cells are degenerated in this disease.
   - **Attention deficit disorder (ADD) and attention deficit hyperactive disorder (ADHD):** These are conditions that affect a person's ability to learn and remember.
   - **Certain nutritional deficiency** problems can cause memory loss or weak memory. Deficiency of certain minerals, vitamins and other nutrients can cause cognitive problems and also contribute to the beginning of dementia. A deficiency of minerals and vitamins including iron, zinc, vitamins—B_{12}, B_6, folate, selenium, vitamin E and iodine can cause difficulties in concentrating, recalling, risk of developing dementia and low level of oxygen in the brain.
   - **Alcohol** acts as a depressant by slowing down reaction time and thought processes. Short-term memory is affected by excessive drinking.
   - Some **drugs like benzodiazepines** can cause temporary memory disturbance.
   - Patients with a **psychological problem** like anxiety and depression suffer with memory impairment.
   - **Head injury** condition can lead to cognitive problems.

THEORIES OF MEMORY

Theories of memory provide abstract representations of how memory is believed to work. Below are the theories proposed over past years by various psychologists.

1. Theory of General Memory Functions

Theory of general memory functions focuses on three distinct processes of memory—encoding, storage and retrieval **(Figure 6.19)**.

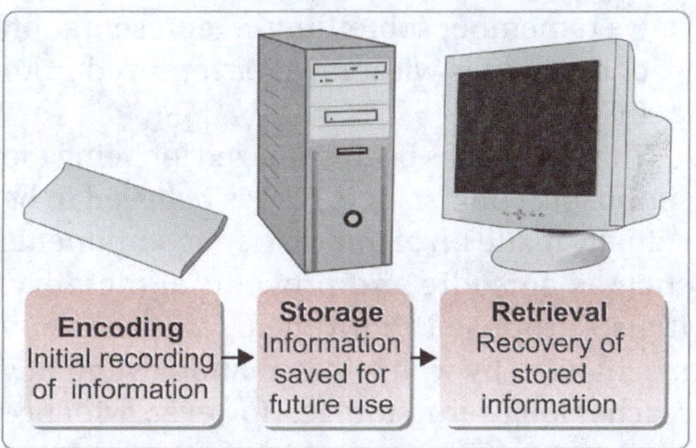

Figure 6.19: Stages of memory

1. *Encoding* is the process of receiving sensory input and transforming it into a code which can be stored.
2. *Storage* is a process of actually putting coded information into memory.
3. *Retrieval* is the process of gaining access to stored coded information when needed. Memory is seldom an accurate record of what was experienced.

2. Information Processing Theory

- Information processing theory was developed by Richard Atkinson and Richard Shiffrin (1968). According to this theory memory starts with a memory input from the environment.
- This input is held for a very brief time-several seconds at most in a sensory register associated with the sensory channels (hearing, taste, touch, smell and vision).
- Information that is attended to and recognized in the sensory register may be passed on to STM where it is held for 20 to 30 seconds.
- Some of the information reaching STM is processed by being rehearsed, i.e., by having attention focused on it perhaps by being repeated over and over or being processed in some other way that will link it up with other information already stored in the memory.
- Information that is rehearsed by then is passed along to LTM. Information not so processed is lost.
- Information placed in LTM is organized into categories where it may reside for days, months, years or for a lifetime. When we remember something, a representation of the item is withdrawn or retrieved from LTM.

This theory has been criticized for being too simplistic. For instance, LTM is believed to be actually made up of multiple subcomponents such as episodic and procedural memory. It also proposed that rehearsal is the only mechanism by which information eventually reaches long-term storage. However, evidence shows that LTM is capable of remembering things even without a rehearsal **(Figure 6.20)**.

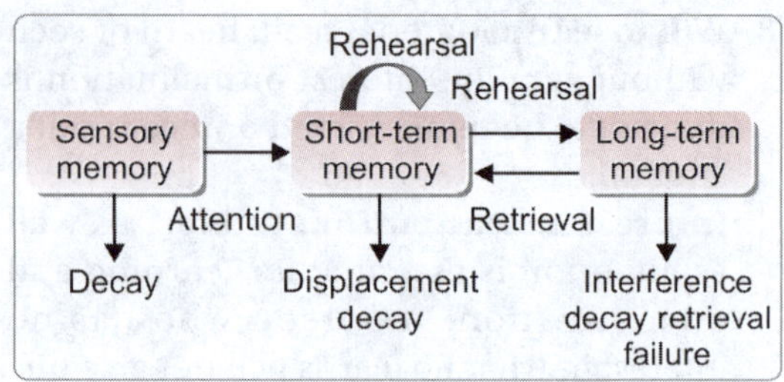

Figure 6.20: Information processing theory

3. Levels of Processing Theory

- Craik and Lockhart (1972) proposed that memory occurs on a continuum from shallow to deep with no limit on the number of different levels.
- The shallow or superficial levels store information about identity of phenomena including numerous attributes. These may be associated with a word or an image. The shallow levels involve analysis in terms of physical or sensory characteristics such as brightness or pitch.
- The intermediate level of memory relates to recognition and labeling.
- Deep level relates to storage of meaning and networks of association. Deeper processing results in more elaborate, long-lasting and stronger memory traces. When the learner analyzes for meaning he may think of other related associations, images and past experiences related to the stimulus.
- Factors which influence the depth of perceptual processing include the amount of attention devoted to the stimulus, its compatibility with existing memory structures in the learner's brain and the amount of processing time available. In addition, the 'self-reference effect' in which new information is related to the learner himself takes learning to deeper levels and therefore promotes LTM.

Craik and Lockhart also discussed rehearsal, the process of cycling information through memory. Craik and Lockhart proposed two kinds of rehearsal. Maintenance rehearsal merely repeats the kind of analysis that has already been carried out. In contrast, elaborate rehearsal involves a deeper, more meaningful

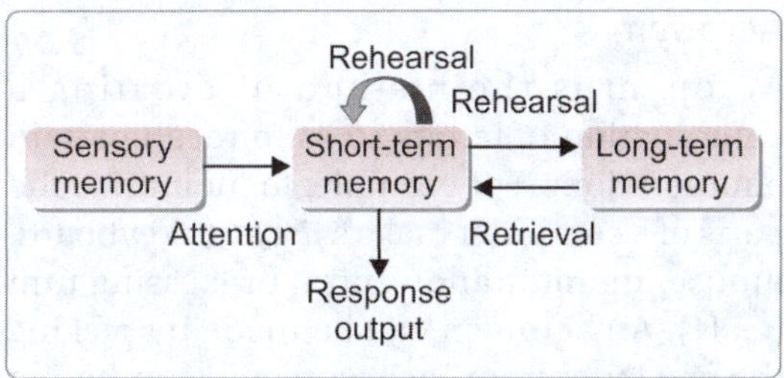

Figure 6.21: Levels of processing theory

analysis of the stimulus. Elaboration is the process of adding more extensive information into the memory system. This serves to make existing information and incoming information more distinctive and unique **(Figure 6.21)**.

Craik and Lockhart suggested three levels in processing of verbal information:

1. **Structural**: This is shallow processing—looking at what the words only look like.
2. **Phonetic**: Processing the sound of the word.
3. **Semantic**: This is deep processing—considering the meaning of the word.

METHODS TO IMPROVE MEMORY

Success in the process of memorization depends much on the methods of learning or memorization adopted by the learner. The choice of a particular method for bringing better results depends upon many factors like the nature of the learner, the learning material and the learning situations, etc. The list of various methods of memorizing is given in **Box 6.1**.

Box 6.1: Methods of memorizing

- Whole and part method
- Space and unspaced method
- Repetition and practice
- Making use of the principles of association
- Grouping and rhythm
- Recitation
- Utilizing as many senses as possible
- Pulling at all together
- Funnel approach
- Acronym
- Acrostic
- Mnemonics

Whole and Part Method

There are two methods of memorizing. For example, a poem can be read again and again from the beginning till the end as a whole or divided into parts with each part memorized separately. The whole method is found to be better than the part method in case of a short poem while the part method proves more advantageous if the poem is a larger one.

Space and Unspaced Method

In the spaced or distributed practice method of memorization the principle of 'work and rest' is followed. For example, if one has to memorize a piece of poetry by this method he will be advised to go on repeating it for sometime before resting. On the other hand, in unspaced or massed practice method of memorization the subject has to memorize the assigned material in one sitting without any rest.

It has been observed that instead of working continuously without taking any rest it is better to distribute the hours of work in these sittings by introducing periods of rest in between. This helps in removing the monotony caused by long periods of study. It also allows the individual to get a fresh start after a period of rest thus continuing to maintain interest in the task.

Repetition and Practice

An intelligent repetition with full understanding always helps in achieving better results in the process of memorization. Things repeated and practiced frequently are remembered for a longer time in comparison to those for which little or no time is spent for repetition and practice.

Making Use of the Principle of Association

It is always good to follow the principle of association in learning or memorization. Always attempts should be made to connect it with one's previous learning on the one hand and with so many related things on the other. Sometimes for association of ideas special techniques and devices are used for recall. For example, 'CAUTION' for cancer symptoms.

Grouping and Rhythm

Grouping facilitates learning. For example, a telephone number 567345234 can be easily memorized and recalled if we try to group it as 567 345 234.

Similarly rhythm also proves as an aid in learning and memorizing. Children learn multiplication tables in sing song fashion effectively. Arrangement of material in the form of a verse with rhyme and rhythm is found very useful in this direction.

Recitation

After reading a lesson a few times the student must try to review it completely without the help of a book. This method is referred to as self-recitation. Several studies have shown that self-recitation is a more economical use of one's study time than mere re-reading. This method not only economizes the energy to be applied but also helps towards permanent retention.

Utilizing as Many Senses as Possible

Things are better learnt and remembered when they are presented through more senses than one. Therefore an attempt should be made to take the help of audiovisual aid material and receive impressions through as many senses as possible.

Pulling at All Together

Organizing and ordering information can significantly improve memory. Learning a large amount of unconnected and unorganized information from various classes can be very challenging. By organizing and adding meaning to the material prior to learning facilitates both storage and retrieval.

Funnel Approach

The funnel approach means learning general concepts before moving onto specific details. When we understand the general concepts first, the details make more sense.

Acronym

Acronym is the method of creating a combination of letters so as to recall certain enumerations. For example, to memorize the parts of a computer make a list, e.g., keyboard, mouse, monitor and central processing unit (CPU). An acronym can be made by picking the first letter from each word and combining it to get KMMC.

Acrostic

It is an invented sentence where the first letter of each word is a clue to an idea that needs to be remembered. Acrostics are useful especially for long list of things whose names do not begin with vowels. For example, to remember the bones of the skull the acrostic sentence can be—'Old People From Texas Eat Spiders–Occipital, Parietal, Frontal, Temporal, Ethmoid and Sphenoid.'

Mnemonics

Mnemonics is another word for memory tool. Mnemonics are techniques for remembering information that is otherwise quite difficult to recall. The idea behind using mnemonics is to encode difficult to remember information in a way that is much easier to remember. These are even more effective when the individual chooses images and links on his own and tries to visualize and organize the information in ways that are particularly meaningful and memorable to him.

- **Mnemonic link system**: It is an age-old memory technique of remembering lists based on creating an association between the elements of that list. It works by turning information into vivid images, then linking those images together in memorable ways. For example, if one wished to remember the list (cat, milk, beehive, apple, glass), one could create a link system such as a story about 'a brown cat jumping from a beehive falling into a large glass of milk balanced on a tiny apple.' This story would be easier to remember than the list itself.
- **Story method:** This method takes the link system a step further by using a story to

connect all the items on the list. Here the individual is required to invent a story that features each item on the list, in the right order. The flow of the story and the strength of the images helps the individual to recall the original information. A funny, strange and exciting story can make it easier to remember the original information. However, if a word on the list does not trigger images, it is preferred to look for another word that looks or sounds similar to it.

- **Songs and rhymes:** Songs and rhymes are very effective as mnemonic devices too. Most young children are taught to remember the entire English alphabet consisting of 26 random letters in a row by reciting it in a simple rhyming tune. Songs and rhymes work for adults as well. A good example is how one can easily sing along when an old song comes on the television or radio. A study has also indicated that singing may improve memory and well-being in people with dementia.
- **Memory peg system**: It is a technique for memorizing lists. The main idea is to establish long-term memory with the help of a well-organized set of images to which the list of items to be remembered can be linked. In number systems one can form an image with each number. For instance, a rhyming system can be used for the numbers 1 through 10. Words that rhyme with the numbers can be thought out—1 is bun, 2 is a shoe, 3 is a tree, 4 is a door and so on. Now when there is a list to remember it can be associated with the items on the list with images of numbers. If the first item on a grocery list is coffee, a steaming cup of coffee next to a plate of buns can be imagined; if the second item is bread, a giant shoe squashing the bread into a paste can be seen and so on through the list associating the number images with what is to be remembered.
- **Method of loci**: 'Loci' is otherwise known as locations. The method of loci is also commonly called the mental walk. It is a method of memory enhancement which uses visualization to organize and recall information. In this technique the subject memorizes the layout of some building or the arrangement of shops on a street or any geographical entity which is composed of a number of discrete loci. When desiring to remember a set of items the individual literally 'walks' through these loci and commits an item to each one by forming an image between the items and any distinguishing feature of that locus. Retrieval of items is achieved by 'walking' through the 'loci' allowing the latter to activate the desired items.
- **Chunking**: This is a technique generally used when remembering numbers. It is based on the idea that STM is limited in the number of things that can be contained. A common rule is that a person can remember 7 (plus or minus 2) 'items' in STM. In other words, people can remember between 5 and 9 things at one given time. When using 'chunking' to remember, the number of items held in the memory is reduced by increasing the size of each item. In remembering the number string 64831996, one could remember each of the 8 numbers individually or think of stringing them as 64 83 19 96 (by creating 'chunks' of numbers). This breaks the group into a smaller number of 'chunks.' Instead of remembering 8 individual numbers it is sufficient to remember 4 larger numbers. This is particularly helpful when 'chunks' that are meaningful or familiar are formed (in this case, the last four numbers in the series are '1996' which can easily be remembered as one chunk of information).

Some of the advantages of using mnemonic devices are:

- It aids active learning as the person is able to sort the information in a way he/she can better remember.
- Mnemonic tools allow recalling large amounts of information that would be incredibly difficult to remember.

- The learner is able to quickly retrieve information from his/her long-term memory.

FORGETTING

Forgetting means a failure to recall a fact, an idea, or a group of ideas. It is the weakening of the bonds that were formed in learning.

Definitions

- Forgetting is the loss, permanent or temporary, of the ability to recall or recognize something learned earlier.

  —Munn (1967)

- Forgetting means failure at any time to recall an experience when attempting to do so or to perform an action previously learned. **—Drever (1952)**

Types of Forgetting

Forgetting is just the opposite of remembering and essentially a failure in the ability to reproduce. It can be classified into natural forgetting and morbid forgetting (abnormal).

1. **Natural forgetting:** Forgetting occurs with lapse of time in a quite normal way without any intention of forgetting on the part of the individual.
2. **Morbid forgetting (abnormal):** Person deliberately tries to forget something (repression).

According to a certain view forgetting may be classified into:

- **General forgetfulness**: One suffers a total loss in one's recalling some previous learning.
- **Specific forgetfulness:** The individual forgets only one or a specific part of his earlier learning.

According to another classification:

- **Physical forgetfulness:** One loses his memory on account of factors like age, disease, biological malfunctioning of the brain and nervous system, accidents, consumption of liquor or other intoxicating materials, etc.
- **Psychological forgetfulness:** One loses his memory on account of factors like stress, anxiety, conflicts, temper provocation, lack of interest, apathy, repression or similar other emotional and psychic difficulties.

Causes of Forgetting

Some of the common physical and psychological factors responsible for forgetfulness are given in **Figure 6.22.**

- **Inadequate impression while learning:** Inadequate or improper learning is likely to be forgotten. Intention or will is the most important factor in remembering. Forced learning either results in no learning or has a very temporary effect.
- **Lapse of time:** Time is said to be a great healing factor. What is learned or experienced is forgotten with lapse of time.
- **Interference of association:** We forget something because what has been learned earlier interferes with the remembering of what has been learnt later on. We also forget because we tend to learn new things all the time and new learning interferes with the retention of old learning.
- **Rise of emotions:** Emotions play a key role in learning as well as in forgetting. Sudden rise of emotions in excess blocks the process of recall.

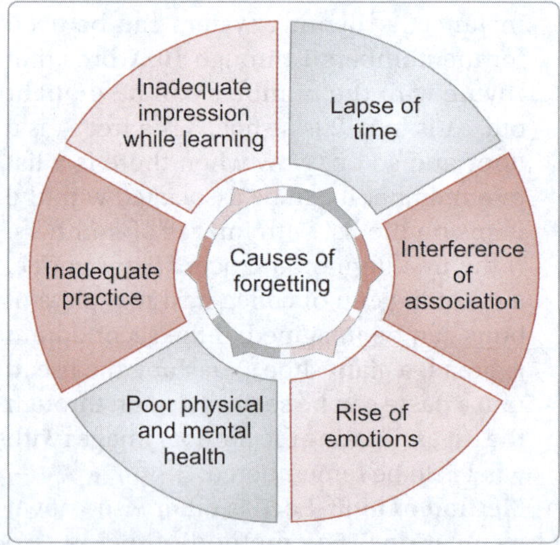

Figure 6.22: Causes of forgetting

- **Poor physical and mental health:** Deterioration in health makes an individual less confident and more perturbed. The individual remains under a state of tension and thus is unable to concentrate upon a thing at a particular time. Neither is he able to learn it effectively nor is he able to recall it easily after sometime. People having lower intelligence quotient (IQ) or suffering from mental defects have generally been found to have poor retention and recall abilities. In some cases a brain injury may also become the sole cause for loss of memory. In such cases people are found to forget all their previous experiences and happenings.
- **Inadequate practice:** We forget facts which we do not subsequently make use of. We forget because of inadequate repetition or practice of learning material that has been over learned with long hours of studying. Studying without proper spacing strains our nerves and results in fatigue.

In addition to factors mentioned above there are many others which result in forgetfulness. They include fatigue, long illness, forces of distraction, lack of interest and purpose, lack of willingness or intention to learn or recall, unfavorable situations or conditions at the time of learning and reproduction. These factors make the material easily slip out of the mind.

Theories of Forgetting

Forgetting is caused by an inability to access information that is represented in memory. Forgetting can be explained by following theories:

1. Trace Decay Theory

According to many psychologists time is the cause of much forgetting. What is learnt or experienced is forgotten with lapse of time. The cause of such natural forgetting can be explained through a process known as decay of the memory trace. It says that learning results in neurological changes leaving certain types of memory traces or engrams in the brain. With the passage of time these memory traces of learning impressions get weaker and weaker and finally fade away through disuse. It leads us to conclude that the older an experience the weaker its memory and as time passes the amount of forgetting goes on increasing.

This theory has proved a failure in many instances of forgetting. In LTM such as learning to ride a bicycle forgetting does not occur even after years of neglect. However, this theory has provided good results in explaining forgetfulness in the case of STM. Drill, practice, rehearsal or repetition of learning always results in preventing decay.

2. Interference Theory

Mechanism of interference is responsible for forgetting. Interference is caused on account of the negative inhibiting effects of one learning experience on another. We forget things because of such interference. The interfering effects of things previously learnt and retained in our memory with the things of our recent memory can work both ways, backward and forward. The psychological term used for these types of interference is retroactive inhibition and proactive inhibition.

- In retroactive inhibition, acquisition of new learning works backward to impair the retention of previously learned material. For example, a second list of words, formulations or equations may impair the retention of a first list.
- Proactive inhibition is just the reverse of retroactive inhibition. Here the old learning or experiences retained in our memory works forward to disrupt the memory of what we acquire or learn afterwards. For example, learning a new formula may be hampered on account of the previously learned formulae in one's memory.

In both the types of inhibitions it can easily be seen that similar experiences when follow each other produce more interference than dissimilar experiences. This is because all experiences are so intermingled that a state of utter confusion prevails in the mind of the individual and consequently he is faced with the difficulty in retention and recall **(Figure 6.23)**.

Interference theory as a whole has proved to be quite successful in providing adequate

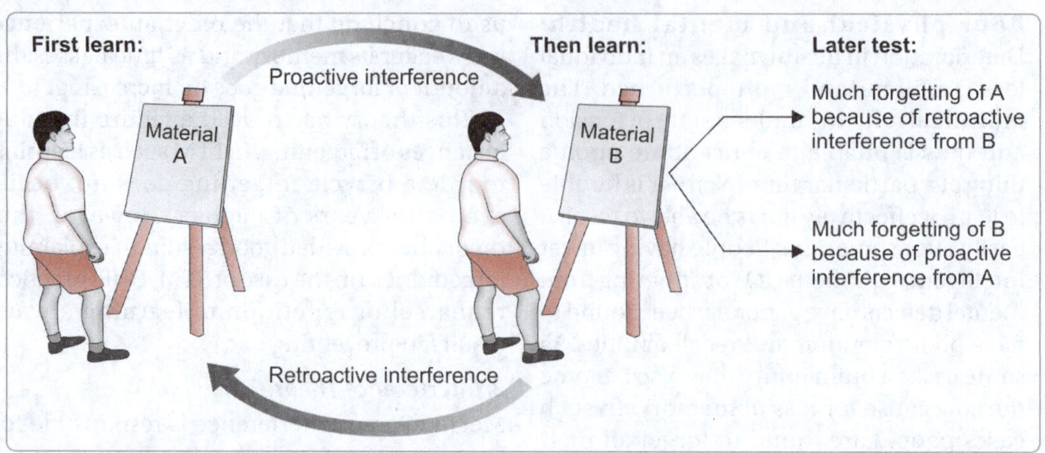

Figure 6.23: Interference theory

Table 6.10: Summary of decay and interference theories

Decay theory	Interference theory
Forgetting occurs as time passes because memory traces gradually fade away with passage of time. A name we once knew is no longer available for recall because the physiological basis for the memory has been eroded	**Proactive interference:** Material learned initially prevents us from recalling the material learned later on (for example, Spanish words learned earlier interfere with the memory of French words learned later on) **Retroactive interference:** Material learned later on prevents from recalling the previously learned material (for example, one cannot remember someone's phone number given at the beginning of a party as subsequent activities block the memory)

explanation for natural and normal forgetting for both STM and LTM **(Table 6.10)**.

3. Repression Theory

The 'repression theory' was put forward by Freud's psychoanalytic school of psychology. Repression according to this school is a mental function that safeguards the mind from the impact of painful experiences. As a result of this function we actually push the unpleasant and painful memories into the unconscious and thus try to avoid at least consciously the conflicts that bother us. This leads to forgetting things which we do not want to remember.

People under a heavy emotional shock are seen to forget even their names, homes, wives and children. Apart from causing abnormal forgetting the impaired emotional behavior of an individual also plays its part in disrupting the normal memory process.

For example, a sudden rise of emotions in excess may completely block the process of recall. When one is taken over by emotions like fear, anger or love, one may forget all he has experienced, learned or thought beforehand. During these emotions one becomes so self-conscious that his thinking is paralyzed. That is why a child fails to recall the answer to a question in the presence of a teacher whom he fears very much.

THINKING

Thinking is a complex mental activity. It is symbolic in character, initiated by a problem which the individual is facing, involves the response of the individual to this problem.

DEFINITIONS

- Thinking is behavior which is often implicit and hidden and in which symbols (images, ideas and concepts) are ordinarily employed. —**Garrett (1968)**

- Thinking is a problem-solving process in which we use ideas or symbols in places of overt activity. —**Gilmer (1970)**

TYPES OF THINKING

Thinking as a mental process is usually classified into the following types **(Figure 6.24)**:

Perceptual or Concrete Thinking

Perceptual thinking is the simplest form of thinking. The basis of this type of thinking is perception, i.e., interpretation of sensation according to one's experience. It is also named as concrete thinking as it is carried by the perception of actual or concrete objects and events. It is thinking of a lower order. Such type of thinking is present in animals and children.

Conceptual or Abstract Thinking

Like perceptual thinking it does not require the perception of actual objects or events. It is a form of abstract thinking where one makes use of concepts, generalized ideas and language. It is regarded superior to perceptual form of thinking as it economizes efforts in understanding and problem solving.

Reflective or Logical Thinking

Reflective thinking aims at solving complex problems rather than simple problems. It requires reorganization of all the relevant experiences and finding new ways of reacting to a situation. Mental activity in reflective thinking does not undergo any mechanical trial and error type of effort. There is an insightful cognitive approach in reflective thinking. It takes logic into account in which all the relevant facts are arranged in a logical order so as to arrive at a solution to the problem on hand.

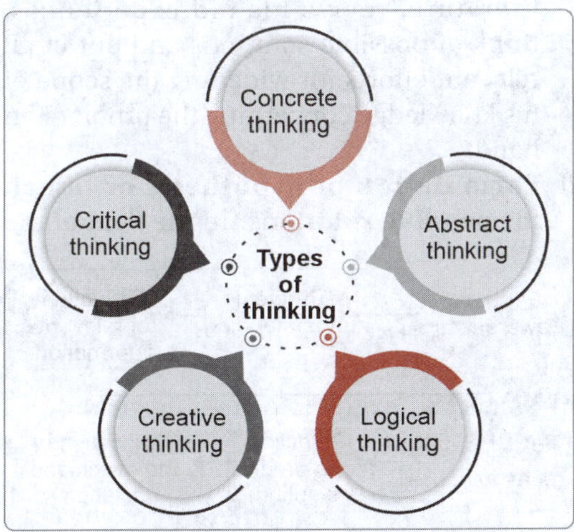

Figure 6.24: Types of thinking

Creative Thinking

Creative thinking is chiefly aimed at creating something new. It is in search of new relationships and associations to describe and interpret the nature of things, events and situations. It is not bound by any pre-established rules. Usually the individual himself formulates the problem and is free to collect evidence and invent tools for its solution. Thinking of scientists or inventors is an example of creative thinking.

Critical Thinking

Critical thinking is a higher order well-disciplined thought process which involves the use of cognitive skills like conceptualization, interpretation, analysis, synthesis and evaluation for arriving at an unbiased, valid and reliable judgment of the gathered or communicated information or data as a guide to one's belief and action.

Two Main Types of Thinking

The two main types of thinking are: controlled thinking and free thinking **(Figure 6.25)**.

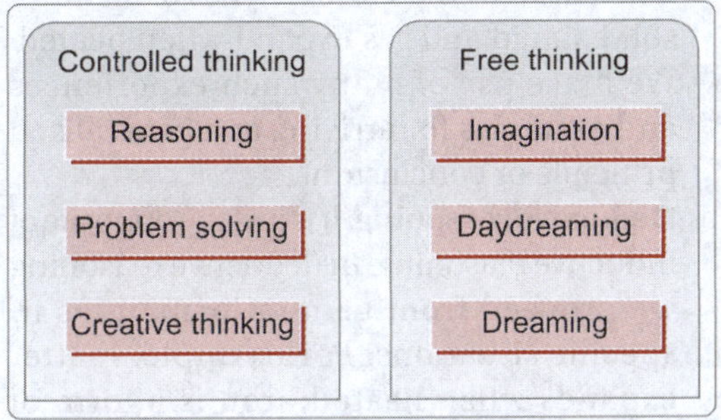

Figure 6.25: Two main types of thinking

Controlled Thinking

In controlled thinking the process of thinking is controlled and regulated. Thoughts keep in close touch with reality and are directed towards the achievement of a specific goal. Reasoning, problem solving and creative thinking are examples of controlled thinking.

1. Reasoning

It is one of the methods of finding solution to a problem. It is referred to as a highly specialized thinking involving some well-organized systematic steps for the mental exploration of a cause and effect relationship or solution of a problem.

Definitions

- Reasoning is stepwise thinking with a purpose or goal in mind.
  —Garrett (1968)
- Reasoning is combining past experience in order to solve a problem which cannot be solved by mere reproduction of earlier solutions. **—Mann (1967)**

Reasoning may be classified into two broad types:

a. **Inductive reasoning**: This type of reasoning involves proceeding from specific facts or observations to general principles. Induction is a way of providing a statement or generalizing a rule or principle that if a statement or a rule is true in one particular case it will be true for cases that appear in the same serial order. Thus it may generally be applied to all such cases. For example, iron expands when heated; water also expands when heated; air also expands when heated. Therefore all types of matter—solid, liquid and gas expand when heated. We make use of many such experiences and examples for arriving at a generalized principle or conclusion.
b. **Deductive reasoning**: It is just the opposite of inductive reasoning. In deductive reasoning we proceed from general principles to specific situations. For example, matter expands when heated; iron is a form of matter and thus expands when heated.

2. Problem Solving

Problem solving as a deliberate and serious act involves the use of some novel methods, higher thinking and systematic scientific steps for the realization of set goals.

Definition

It is a process of overcoming difficulties that appear to interfere with the attainment of a goal. It is a procedure of making adjustments in spite of interferences. **—Skinner (1968)**

Steps in problem solving process (**Figure 6.26**):

a. **Problem awareness:** The first step in problem-solving behavior of an individual concerns his awareness of the difficulty or problem that needs a solution.
b. **Problem understanding:** The difficulty or problem experienced by the individual should be properly identified by a careful analysis. He should be clear about his problem. The problem should then be pinpointed in terms of specific goals and objectives. Thus, all the difficulties and obstacles in the path of the solution must be properly named and identified and what is to be got through the problem-solving efforts should then be properly analyzed.
c. **Collection of relevant information:** In this step the individual is required to collect all the relevant information about the problem through all possible sources. He may consult experienced people, read available literature, revive his old experiences, think of possible solutions and put in all relevant efforts for widening the scope of his knowledge concerning the problem on hand.
d. **Formulation of hypothesis or hunch for possible solutions:** In the light of the

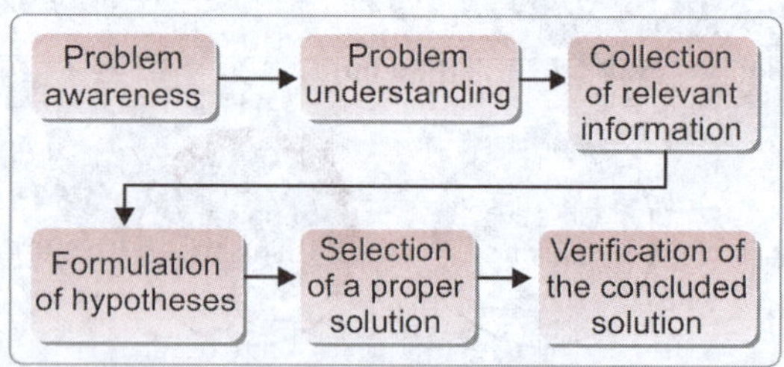

Figure 6.26: Steps in problem solving process

collected relevant information and nature of his problem one may then engage in some serious cognitive activities to explore various possibilities for solving one's problem. As a result he may start with a few possible solutions for his problem.

e. **Selection of a proper solution:** In this step all the possible solutions thought of in the previous step are closely analyzed and evaluated. Gates and others (1946) have suggested the following activities in evaluation of assumed hypothesis or solution:
   - One should determine the conclusion that completely satisfies the demands of the problem.
   - One should find out whether the solution is consistent with other facts and principles which have been well-established.
   - One should make a deliberate search for negative instances which might cast doubts on the conclusion.

   The above suggestions can help the individual to consider a suitable solution for his problem out of the many possible solutions.

f. **Verification of the concluded solution or hypothesis:** The solution arrived at or conclusion drawn must further be verified by applying it in the solution of various similar problems and only if the derived solution helps in the solution of these problems should the same be applied.

John Bransford and Barry Stein (1984) advocated five steps that are basically associated with the task of problem solving. They referred to these steps as 'IDEAL' thinking and arranged them in the following order:

I—Identifying the problem
D—Defining and representing the problem
E—Exploring possible strategies
A—Acting on the strategies
L—Looking back and evaluating the effects of one's activities

3. Creative Thinking

Creative thinking is a process in which the individual generates an original, unusual and productive solution to a problem. It is defined as personal, imaginative thinking which produces a new, novel and useful solution.

Unlike ordinary solution to problems, creative solutions are new ones that other people have not thought of before. The outcome of creative thinking may be a new and unique way of conceptualizing the world around us.

Stages of creative thinking

The five stages of creative thinking are **(Figure 6.27)**:

Stage I–Preparation: Creative thinker formulates the problem and collects facts and materials necessary for arriving at the new solution. Very frequently he finds that the problem cannot be solved despite days, weeks or months of concentrated effort. Failing to solve the problem the thinker turns away from it either deliberately or involuntarily.

Stage II–Incubation: This stage is initiated when the creative thinker turns away from the problem. During this stage the ideas that were interfering with the solution of the problem begin to fade. The unconscious thought processes involved in creative thinking are also at work during this stage. All this leads to the third stage.

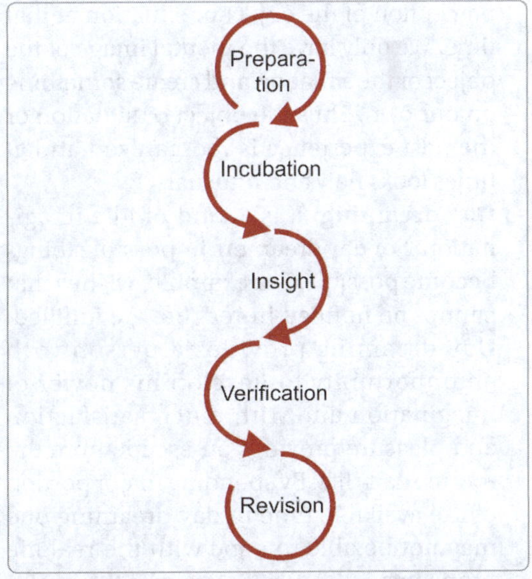

Figure 6.27: Stages of creative thinking

Stage III–Insight (illumination): During this stage the creative thinker experiences sudden appearance of the solution to his problems which is termed as 'insight'.

Stage IV–Verification (evaluation): During this stage the insight is tested to see if it satisfactorily solves the problem. If not satisfactory the thinker is back at the beginning of the creative process. On the other hand if the solution is satisfactory stage V is reached.

Stage V–Revision: During this stage any modifications needed are made. The creative thinker never considers his solution as perfect or final. It is open for modification or revision at any essential time.

Free Thinking

In free thinking thought processes are allowed much greater freedom of action. Neither is there any restriction of reality in terms of time and space nor any desire on the part of the thinker to achieve a certain goal which is realistic. Examples of free thinking are imagination, day dreaming and dreaming.

- **Imagination**: It is a mental activity in which we make use of images and also go beyond them. When we are imagining an object or situation we do not have any sense perception of the object or situation at that time. We only have the mental image of the object or the situation and create something on our own. Thus the object or situation or the past experience is reorganized and at times looks new and unusual.
- **Day dreaming**: It is a kind of idle imagination. For day dreamers impossible things become possible. For example, wishes that cannot be fulfilled in real life are fulfilled. Day dreaming provides a person with an opportunity to develop his power of imagination and with much satisfaction and pleasure provides an escape from the routine daily life. By spending major portion of the available time in day dreaming one may not be able to cope with the real life problems.
- **Dreaming**: Dreams are mental activities of lighter sleep. It is not subject to the personal and environmental controls that operate when we are awake. They emerge in response to some stimulus either internal or external. In some of our dreams we solve the problems which were perplexing us during our waking hours. Some dreams may be simple reminiscences or reproductions of what happened during the day.

LEVELS OF THINKING (BASED ON 'BLOOM'S TAXONOMY)

Bloom's Taxonomy was created by Dr Benjamin Bloom in 1956 to promote higher forms of thinking in education such as analyzing and evaluating concepts, processes, procedures, and principles rather than just remembering facts (rote learning). This process of thinking involves six levels. While infants and toddlers mostly use the first two levels, by the age of 3 years children can use all six **(Figure 6.28)**.

Bloom's Revised Taxonomy

However, in 2001, a group of cognitive psychologists, curriculum theorists and researchers published a revision of Bloom's Taxonomy with the title "A Taxonomy for Teaching and Assessment". The authors revised taxonomy using verbs to label their categories and subcategories. These action words describe the cognitive processes. The revised Bloom's Taxonomy involves following six levels.

1. Remember

This level helps us to recall foundational or factual information—names, dates, formulas, definitions, components or methods. Appropriate learning outcome verbs for this level include—cite, define, describe, label, list match, name, outline, quote, recall, report, reproduce, retrieve, show, state, and tell.

2. Understand

This level helps us to explain main ideas and concepts and make meaning by interpreting,

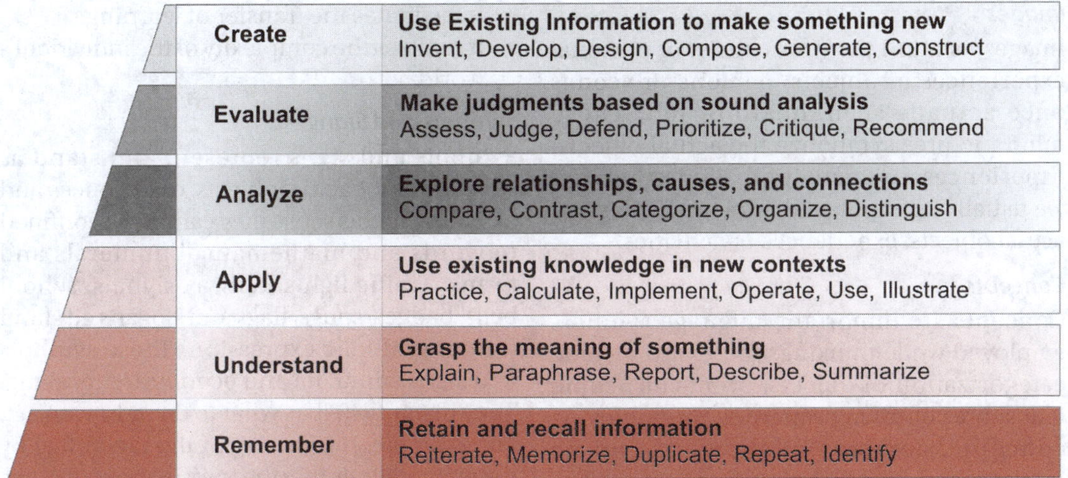

Figure 6.28: Bloom's levels of thinking

classifying, summarizing, inferring, comparing and explaining. Appropriate learning outcome verbs for this level are abstract, arrange, articulate, categorize, clarify, compare, compute, conclude, contrast, differentiate, discuss, distinguish, estimate, explain, give examples of, illustrate, interpret, match, outline, predict, rearrange, rephrase, restate, summarize, and translate.

3. Apply

This level helps us to recognize or use concepts in real world situations and address when, where or how to employ methods and ideas. Appropriate learning outcome verbs for this level include—apply, calculate, carry out, classify, compute, demonstrate, employ, examine, experiment, generalize, illustrate, implement, infer, interpret, manipulate, modify, outline, predict and use.

4. Analyze

Analyze means breaking a topic or idea into components or examining a subject from various perspectives. It helps us to see, how the whole is created from the parts. Appropriate learning outcome verbs for this level include—analyze, arrange, breakdown, categorize, classify, compare, connect, contrast, detect, differentiate, distinguish, identify, organize, separate and structure.

5. Evaluate

It means making judgments about something based on criteria and standards. This requires checking and critiquing an argument or concept to form an opinion about its value. Appropriate learning outcome verbs for this level include—appraise, assess, compare, conclude, consider, criticize, critique, decide, determine, evaluate, judge, justify, rate, recommend, review, score, select, test and validate.

6. Create

It involves putting elements together to form a coherent or functional whole. Creating includes reorganizing elements into a new pattern or structure through planning. This is the highest and most advanced level of Bloom's taxonomy. Appropriate learning outcome verbs for this level include—arrange, assemble, build, collect, construct, design, develop, devise, reorganize, revise, rewrite, specify, synthesize and write.

Elements in Development of Thought (Tools of Thinking)

Thinking is one of the most important aspects in a learning process. The ability to learn and solve problems depends upon our ability to think correctly which in turn helps in adjustment for a successful living. The various elements involved in development of thought process are:

Images

Images as mind pictures consist of personal experiences of objects, persons or scenes once actually seen, heard or felt. These mind pictures symbolize the actual objects, experiences and activities. While thinking we usually manipulate the images instead of actual objects, experiences or activities.

Concepts

Concepts are important language symbols employed while thinking. These also include categorization of objects, events or people that share common properties. By employing concepts, complex phenomena can be reorganized into simple phenomena. For example, with the concept of 'soft' we sort out objects into soft and hard. The features we select define the concept and form the basis for making classifications. When a classification has been made we tend to behave accordingly and think about the members of the class in similar ways. Therefore, concepts being the means of classifying diverse elements in the world around us they are the most convenient tools for solving problems and thinking about the world around us.

Steps in concept development

1. First step in the development of a concept is the awareness of a variety of connected experiences revealed to the individual through perception.
2. Second step deals with comparison of these experiences highlighting the essential attributes commonly found in all these experiences.
3. Third step involves abstraction of these common characteristics. Here abstraction refers to the mental step of conceiving qualities apart from the things in which they are present. The abstracted common traits are verified and a name/tag coined to represent the unity. Thus the said name is tagged for the concept.
4. Language plays a significant role in the development and stability of concepts.

Uses of concepts

- It is a time and labor saving device.
- It facilitates the transfer of learning.
- It reduces the complexity of the individual's world.

Symbols and Signs

Symbols and signs represent and stand as substitutes for actual objects, experiences and activities. In this sense they cannot be confined to words and mathematical numerals and terms. Traffic lights, railway signals, school bells, badges, songs, flags and slogans all stand for the symbolic expression. These symbols and signs stimulate and economize thinking. They instantly tell us what to do or how to act. For example, the waving of the green flag by the guard tells us that the train is about to move and we should get into the train.

Languages

Language is the most efficient and developed vehicle for carrying out the thinking process. It broadens our thinking. When one listens, reads or writes words, phrases or sentences or observes gestures in any language, one is stimulated to think. Reading and writing of the written documents and literature also helps in stimulating and promoting our thinking process.

Brain Functions

Our mind or brain is said to be the chief instrument or reservoir for carrying out the process of thinking. Whatever is experienced through our sense organs carries no meaning and thus cannot serve as a stimulating agent unless the same is received by our brain cells and properly interpreted for driving some meaning. The mental pictures or images can be stored, formed, reconstructed or put to some use only through the functioning of the brain.

Errors in Thinking

Our response to stimuli is determined entirely by the information present in our brain at that time. When our information about the stimulus is complete and correct we respond appropriately and achieve our objective. However when information about the stimulus is incomplete and/or incorrect our response is inappropriate. Such an inappropriate response is called an error. All errors in thinking occur because of incomplete or incorrect information on how to deal with the stimuli detected.

It is necessary that we are aware of the errors in thinking. Various errors in thinking are:

- **Partialism**: This error occurs when the thinker observes the problem through one perspective only, i.e., the thinker examines only one or two factors of the problem and arrives at a premature solution.
- **Adversary thinking**: This is like 'You are wrong. So, I should be right.' type of reasoning. Politicians are masters in this type of thinking and use it to their advantage.
- **Time scale error**: This is a kind of partialism in thinking wherein the thinker sees the problem from a limited time frame. It is similar to short-sightedness.
- **Initial judgment**: Here the thinker becomes very subjective. Instead of considering the issue or problem objectively the thinker approaches it with prejudice or bias.
- **Arrogance and conceit**: This error is sometimes called the 'Village Venus Effect'. It is a phenomenon wherein the villagers think that the prettiest girl in the village is the most beautiful girl in the world. Simply stated, the thinker has his own perception and believes that there is no other better solution than the one he has already found. This blocks creativity.
- **Black and white thinking**: Thinking of things in absolute terms, like 'always', 'every' or 'never'. For example, if your performance falls short of perfect you see yourself as a total failure.
- **Overgeneralization**: Taking isolated cases and using them to make wide generalizations. For example, you see a single negative event as a never-ending pattern of defeat: 'She yelled at me. She is always yelling at me. She does not like me.'
- **Mental filter**: Focusing exclusively on negative or upsetting aspects of something while ignoring the rest. For example, you selectively hear the one tiny negative thing surrounded by all the huge positive stuff.
- **Jumping to conclusions:** Assuming something negative when there is actually no evidence to support it.
- **Magnification and minimization**: Exaggerating negatives and understating positives.
- **Emotional reasoning**: Making decisions and arguments based on how you feel rather than objective reality.

STAGES IN DEVELOPMENT OF THINKING

Jean Piaget (1896–1980), a Swiss philosopher and psychologist dedicated his life to observing and interacting with children so as to determine how their thinking processes differed from adults **(Figure 6.29)**. He formulated theory of children's thinking that helped shape current ideas about developmental psychology. According to Piaget, development is influenced by biological maturation, social experiences and experiences with the physical environment. During cognitive development the individual strives to find an equilibrium between the self and environment.

Cognitive theory explains how thought processes are structured and developed, and their influence on behavior. Structuring of thought processes occurs through the development of schema (i.e., mental

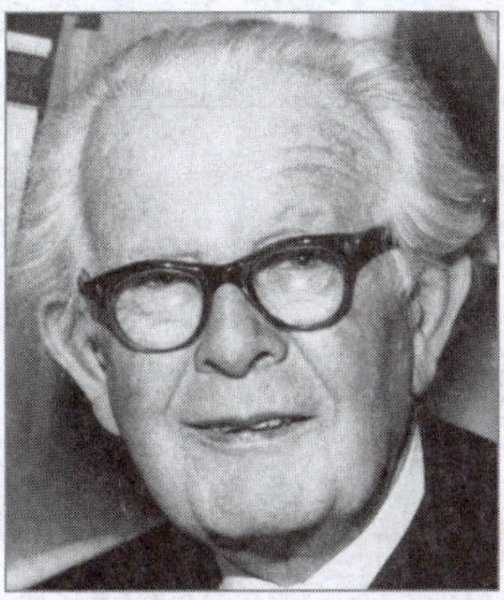

Figure 6.29: Jean Piaget

images or cognitive structures). Thought processes develop through assimilation and accommodation. When a child encounters new information that is recognized and understood within the existing schema, assimilation of that new information occurs. If new information cannot be linked to existing schema, the child must learn to develop new mental images or patterns through the process of accommodation. As long as the child is able to assimilate or accommodate adequately to the new knowledge it is able to achieve equilibrium or mental balance. When schemas are inadequate to facilitate learning disequilibrium may creep in.

According to Piaget's theory of cognitive development the developing child passes through four main discrete stages: (i) sensorimotor stage (ii) preoperational stage (iii) stage of concrete operations and (iv) stage of formal operations. Each stage reflects a range of organizational patterns that occur in definite sequence and within an approximate age span **(Figure 6.30 and Table 6.11)**.

Sensorimotor (Birth to 2 Years)

During this stage the child learns about himself and his environment through motor and reflex actions. Thought derives from sensation and movement. The child learns that he is separate from his environment and that aspects of his environment—his parents or favorite toy continue to exist even though they may be outside the reach of his senses.

Preoperational (2–7 Years)

During this stage sensory motor operations are replaced by words and the child learns the language. Applying his new knowledge of language, the child begins to use symbols to represent objects. He is now better able to think about things and events that are not immediately present. His thought process at this stage usually displays a high degree of egocentricism, i.e., an inability to take the point of view of another person. His thinking is influenced by fantasy—the way he would like things to be and he assumes that others see situations from his viewpoint. He gathers information and then modifies it in his mind to fit in his ideas. Children in this stage do not understand cause-effect relationships.

Concrete Operational (7–11 Years)

During this stage accommodation increases. The child develops an ability to think abstractly and make rational judgments about concrete or observable phenomena which in the past he needed to manipulate physically to understand. During this stage children use logic and begin to grasp such important principles of nature such as number, classification and conservation of mass and length. Their thought processes are limited to

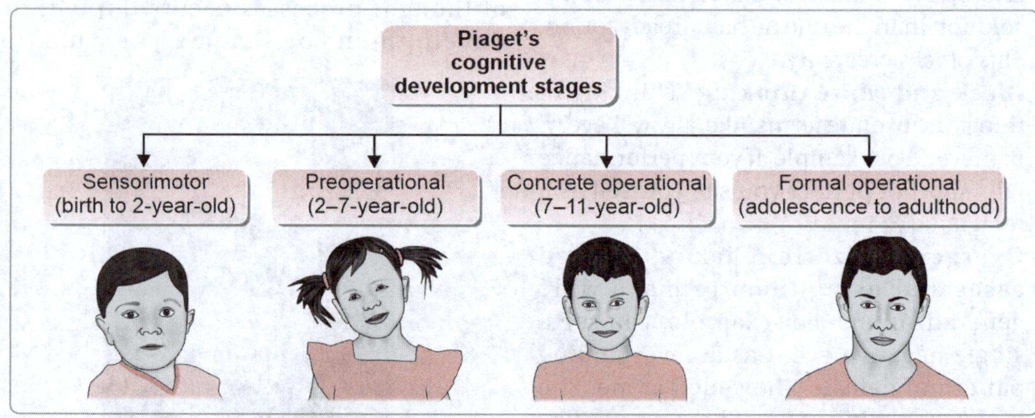

Figure 6.30: Piaget's four stages of cognitive development

Table 6.11: Piaget's four stages of cognitive development

Stage and age range	Description
Sensorimotor (Birth to 2 years)	An infant progresses from reflexive, instinctual action at birth to the beginning of symbolic thought. The infant constructs an understanding of the world by coordinating sensory experiences with physical actions
Preoperational (2–7 years)	The child begins to represent the world with words and images. These words and images reflect increased symbolic thinking and go beyond the connection of sensory information and physical action
Concrete operational (7–11 years)	The child can now reason logically about concrete events and classify objects into different sets
Formal operational (11–15 years)	The adolescent reasons in more abstract and logical ways. Thought is more idealistic

concrete objects and events. Due to influence of social environment, school, peers and teachers there is corresponding expansion in their perception of people.

Formal Operational (11–15 Years)

This stage brings cognition to its final form. During this stage the person thinks in terms of abstract concepts that are not physically present in nature. The child develops ability to think on scientific basis and find solutions to problems. At this point he is capable of hypothetical and deductive reasoning.

APTITUDE

Aptitude means quickness in learning and understanding. It may be a natural talent or an acquired ability. It is the special aptness or fitness for a special ability such as mechanical, musical, artistic, scholastic or religious.

People differ in terms of performance and human activity like leadership, music, art, teaching, etc. Individuals possess specific aptitude or ability in addition to intellectual abilities or intelligence which helps them to achieve success in certain occupations or activities. Thus aptitude means specific ability or capacity distinct from general intellectual ability that helps to acquire proficiency or achievement in a given field.

DEFINITIONS

- Aptitude is variously defined as an innate learning ability, the specific ability needed to facilitate learning a job, aptness, knack, suitability, readiness, tendency, natural or acquired disposition or capacity for a particular activity or innate component of a competency.
- Aptitude refers to those qualities characterizing a person's way of behavior which serve to indicate how well he can learn to meet and solve a certain specified kind of problem. **—Bingham (1937)**
- An aptitude is a combination of characteristics indicative of an individual's capacity to acquire (with training) some specific knowledge, skill or set of organized responses such as the ability to speak a language, become a musician or do mechanical work. **—Freeman (1971)**

CONCEPTS

- An aptitude is an innate component of a competency to do a certain kind of work at a certain level. Aptitudes may be physical or mental. Aptitude is not knowledge, understanding, learned or acquired abilities (skills) or attitude. The innate nature of aptitude in contrast to achievement represents knowledge or ability that is gained.
- Aptitudes are latent potentialities. Given the opportunities for development they would result in great achievement.
- Aptitude is derived from general mental ability and predicts one's possible success or failure in a vocation.

- An aptitude is an innate inborn ability to do a certain kind of work. Aptitudes may be physical or mental. Many of them have been identified and are testable.
- Aptitude helps an individual to learn faster and achieve success.
- Aptitude can be very helpful in choosing an activity in which we wish to be successful or enjoy. For example, an individual with good aptitude for dance will not only enjoy it but also be successful in dance training. However, the lack of such aptitude will result in the individual developing a dislike for it. He would neither enjoy nor progress in dance despite a great deal of training. Doing things in which one has an aptitude protects them from frustrations and failures. It also helps to adjust and be successful much more quickly.
- To predict an achievement in a particular job or a training course, more needs to be known about the individual's aptitudes rather than his intelligence or general ability.
- Aptitude is a special ability whereas intelligence is a general ability. With the knowledge of an individual's level of intelligence we can predict his success in a number of situations involving mental function or activity. The knowledge of aptitude on the other hand acquaints us with the specific abilities and capabilities of an individual to succeed in a particular field of activity.
- Aptitude differs from ability and achievement in that it is forward looking in nature. While aptitude gives an indication of the future success of an individual, ability limits itself to the present performance of an individual. Achievement with its past oriented nature merely indicates what an individual has learned or acquired.
- Aptitude should not be confused with interest. One may show interest in a particular act or job but may or may not have the aptitude for it. The opposite is also true. However to achieve the desired success in a given task one must have both interest as well as aptitude. Interest usually grows with knowledge. For example, if one has an interest in something he will learn more about it. With a greater amount of learning the interest and zeal will also grow. Likewise an interest in nursing will grow with progress in nursing education.
- Aptitude is different from skill and proficiency. Skill is the ability to perform a given act with ease and precision. For example, we may say that a person is skilled in carpentry or playing a piano.

Skill refers to psychomotor ability. Proficiency has much the same meaning except that it is more comprehensive. It includes not only skills in certain types of motor and manual activities but also in other types of activities as shown by the extent of one's competence in language, book-keeping, etc.

TYPES

Various types of aptitude are:

Manual aptitude: It indicates motor abilities or skills required for semi-skilled occupations.

Mechanical aptitude: It involves the ability to understand and solve problems involving mechanical relationships and arrangements such as those which occur in the adjustment, repair and assembly of machinery.

Clerical aptitude: It indicates perceptual and intellectual abilities, mental and motor skills.

Other types of aptitude: These include musical, graphic, scholastic/professional aptitudes.

Commonly recognized aptitudes that are testable include:

- General learning ability
- Verbal aptitude
- Numerical aptitude
- Inductive reasoning aptitude (differentiation or inductive learning ability)
- Finger dexterity aptitude
- Number series aptitude
- Language learning aptitude
- Mechanical comprehension
- Symbolic reasoning aptitude (analytical reasoning)
- Visual memory
- Visual pursuit (line tracing)

INDIVIDUAL DIFFERENCES AND VARIABILITY IN APTITUDE

Suppose two persons of equal intelligence have the same opportunities to learn a job or develop a skill, attend the same on the job training or classes, study the same material and practice the same length of time, while one of them acquires the knowledge or skill easily, the other has difficulty and takes more time if at all he masters the skill. These two people differ in aptitude for this type of work or skill acquisition.

Aptitudes are highly individualized and specialized apart from one's general level of intelligence. For example, two individuals may have the same level of intelligence but not do well in the same kind of education or training due to differences in their aptitude. It is these differences in aptitude that will decide the area in which they will practice successfully. One nurse may have an aptitude for handling surgical instruments and do well in the operation theater; another may have an aptitude for problem-solving in research and enjoy research and teaching. Aptitudes are very important in determining success in professional practices.

An aptitude is a composite of different component abilities that together make for success in performance in a particular field. Higher the aptitude, higher are the chances of success and lower the aptitude, lower is the probability of achievement. Higher the aptitude, lesser is the time required for learning and mastery. Lower the aptitude, greater is the time required for learning.

PSYCHOMETRIC ASSESSMENT OF COGNITIVE PROCESSES

Neuropsychological testing is a procedure that measures and identifies cognitive impairment and functioning in individuals. Neuropsychological testing provides diagnostic clarification and grading of clinical severity for patients with subtle or obvious cognitive disorders. These include:

- Children who are not achieving appropriate developmental milestones
- Fetus exposed to drugs, alcohol or illness
- Patients with head injuries
- Patients with Parkinson disease or other neurological diseases
- Patients exposed to chemicals or toxins
- Substance abusing patients
- Stroke victims
- Patients with dementia

Neurological tests for assessing various cognitive processes are shown in **Table 6.12**.

Measurement of Aptitude

Aptitude assessments are used to predict success or failure in an activity. For vocational/career guidance and planning they are used to measure different aptitudes such as general learning ability, numerical ability, verbal ability, spatial perception and clerical perception. Objective aptitude tests are based on timed subtests. Results are compared to age-group norms or other criteria as opposed to self-report inventories of abilities often found in computerized career exploration systems. For helping a person find and pursue a career, course of study or work experience program, aptitude assessment should logically precede achievement testing or skills assessment.

Aptitude tests measure the degree or level of one's special flair. They are chiefly used to estimate the extent to which an individual would benefit from a specific course or training or predict the quality of his or her achievement in a given situation.

For example, mechanical aptitude test measures a person's aptitude for mechanical work; clerical aptitude tests are employed for measuring the aptitude for clerical work; musical aptitude tests measure the musical talent, etc.

Types of Aptitude Test

Aptitude tests can be classified as follows:

- **Verbal reasoning:** A verbal reasoning test is an aptitude test which measures the ability to comprehend complex written materials and deduct relevant information

Table 6.12: Neurological tests for assessing various cognitive processes

Domain	Neurological tests
Intellectual functioning	• Wechsler Scales • Wechsler Adult Intelligence Scale-Revised (WAIS-R) • Wechsler Adult Intelligence Scale-III (WAIS-III) • Wechsler Intelligence Scale for Children-IV (WISC-IV) • Stanford-Binet Intelligence Scale-IV
Academic achievement	• Wechsler Individual Achievement Test (WIAT) • Woodcock–Johnson Achievement Test
Language processing	• Multilingual Aphasia Examination • Boston Diagnostic Aphasia Examination • Token Test
Visuospatial processing	• WAIS Block Design Subtest • Judgment of Line Orientation • Hooper Visual Organization Test
Attention/ concentration	• Digit Span Forward and Reversed • Cancellation Tasks (letter and symbol)
Verbal learning and memory	• Wechsler Memory Scale (WMS) • Logical Memory I and II: Contextualized prose • Verbal Paired: Associates • WMS-III Verbal Memory Index
Visual learning and memory	• Visual Reproduction I and II • Non-verbal Selective Reminding Test • Continuous Recognition Memory Test • Visuo-Motor Integration Test-Block Design
Executive functions	• Wisconsin Card Sorting Test • WAIS Subtests of Similarities and Block Design
Speed of processing	• Simple and Choice Reaction Time • Symbol Digit Modalities Test: Written and oral
Sensory-perceptual functions	• Halstead–Reitan Neuropsychological Battery (HRNB) • Actual Performance Test and Sensory Perceptual Examination
Motor speed and strength	Index Finger Tapping
Motivation	• Rey 15 Item Test • Dot Counting • Forced-Choice Symptom Validity Testing
Personality assessment	• Minnesota Multiphasic Personality Inventory (MMPI) • Beck Depression Inventory (BDI) • Rorschach Test • Thematic Apperception Test for Children or Adults

and conclusions. Verbal reasoning tests also include spelling, grammar, logic and vocabulary tests. Aptitude tests administered to candidates vary greatly depending upon the profession they are trying to get into.

- **Numerical reasoning**: A numerical reasoning test includes a wide range of aptitude tests varying from 'basic arithmetic tests' through 'estimation tests' that measure the speed in making educated mathematical estimations to 'advanced numerical reasoning tests' that measure the ability to interpret complex data presented in various graphic forms, deduce information and make conclusions.
- **Abstract/inductive/diagrammatic reasoning**: These aptitude tests measure logical reasoning and perceptual reasoning skills. These aptitude tests do not rely on acquired linguistic or numeric abilities but on innate abilities and are thus termed non-verbal reasoning tests.
- **Logical reasoning:** A logical reasoning test is an aptitude test meant to assess the ability to understand and make comprehensive conclusions from the provided data. It is one of the most common aptitude tests and though may seem as one of the most difficult, becomes much simpler with practice than it initially seems to be.
- **Specialty/technical/information technology (IT) tests:** Certain sectors and positions require an aptitude test that

measures specific skills related to certain positions. For example, there are a wide variety of niche aptitude tests for IT personnel and clerical positions. These tests are administered in addition to the main aptitude test.

Other Types of Aptitude Tests

Other types of aptitude tests are mechanical aptitude test, musical aptitude test, art judgment test, professional aptitude test, scholastic aptitude test, clerical aptitude test.

- **Manual aptitude:** It indicates motor abilities or skills required for semi-skilled occupations. Two tests that measure manual aptitude are O'Connor Finger Dexterity and Tweezer Dexterity tests.
- **Mechanical aptitude:** It covers a variety of factors such as spatial visualization, perceptual speed, mechanical information and manual dexterity. This aptitude involves the ability to understand and solve problems involving mechanical relationships and arrangements such as those which occur in the adjustment, repair and assembly of machinery. Some of the well-known mechanical aptitude tests are Minnesota mechanical assembly test, Minnesota spatial relations test, Battery of mechanical aptitude tests and Bennett tests of mechanical comprehension.
- **Clerical aptitude:** This aptitude indicates different abilities like perceptual, intellectual abilities, mental skills and motor skills. Some of the popular clerical aptitude tests are Detroit clerical aptitude examination and Minnesota vocational test for clerical workers.

Standardized aptitude tests are also available for the measurement of scholastic and professional aptitudes [scholastic aptitude tests (SAT)] of individuals for the specific courses or professions like engineering, medicine, law, business management, teaching, etc.

Instead of employing specialized aptitude tests for measuring specific aptitudes the present trend is to use multiple aptitude test batteries to assess the suitability of persons for different professions on the basis of scores in the relevant aptitude tests. Like intelligence tests, multiple aptitude test batteries measure a number of abilities. For example, while General Aptitude Test Battery (GATB) measures the verbal aptitude, numerical aptitude, spatial aptitude, clerical perception and mortar co-ordination, Differential Aptitude Test (DAT) measures verbal reasoning, numerical ability, abstract reasoning, spatial relation, mechanical reasoning, clerical ability and linguistic ability.

Aptitude tests have a wide range of application. They have proven to be the backbone of all kinds of guidance services and selection programs as they are very useful for predicting the suitability of individuals for specific jobs and lines of work.

ALTERATIONS IN COGNITIVE PROCESSES

Cognitive alterations can be defined as changes or disruptions in cognitive process which alter and distort the pre-existing mental function. Six important alterations in cognitive processes are presented in **Figure 6.31:** (1) Sensation, (2) Perception, (3) Learning, (4) Memory, (5) Thinking and (6) Intelligence.

Alterations in Attention

Normal people typically pay selective attention to a single message while screening out the stream of other distracting stimuli and thoughts. For example, when one is reading he can ignore the noise and the visual clutter that could divert him from the goal of completing the sentence. However, people with schizophrenia and attention deficit hyperactivity disorder (ADHD) are easily distracted.

ADHD is a disorder marked by inattention, impulsiveness, a low tolerance for frustration and generally a great deal of inappropriate activity.

ADHD children have difficulty in sustaining attention, are distractible and often fail to follow instructions.

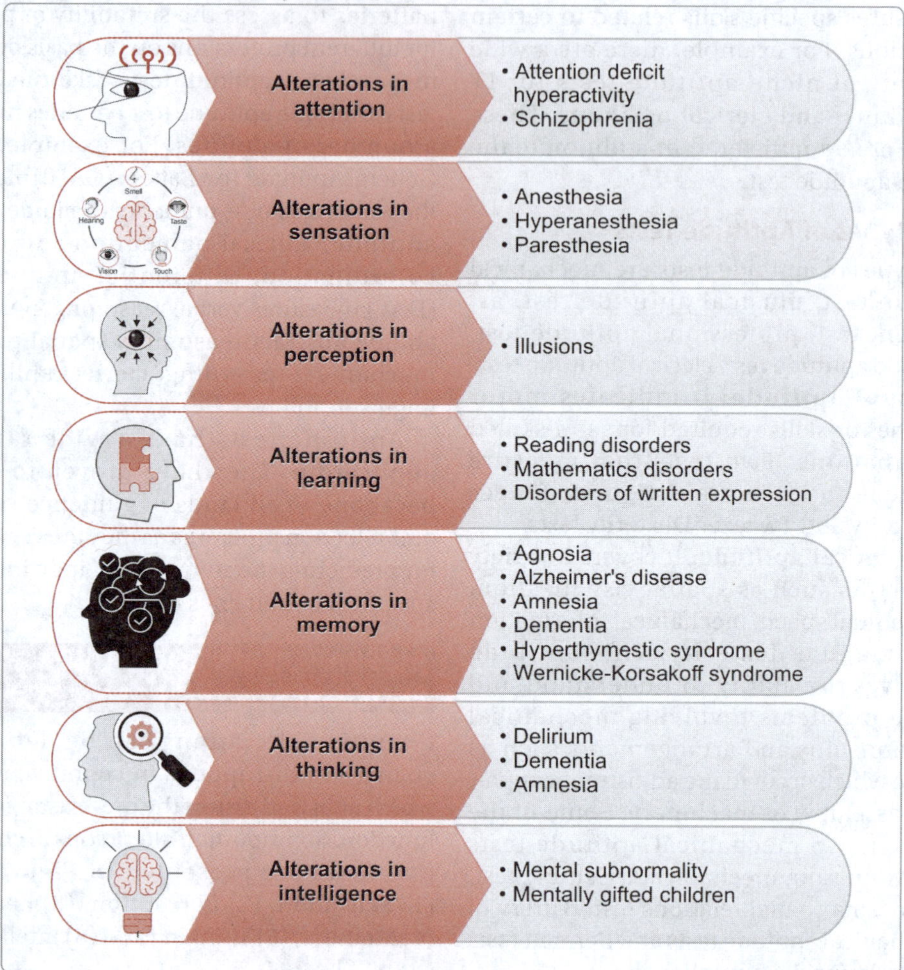

Figure 6.31: Alterations in cognitive processes

Alterations in Sensation

The three common sensory abnormalities are:

1. **Anesthesia**: It means a loss or absence of sensitivity. It implies complete inability to respond to sensory stimuli. It may be caused by defective sense organs, effects of drugs or also by some emotional or functional factors.
2. **Hyperesthesia**: It means excessive response to stimuli. When patients are extremely ill they often exhibit this in their behavior. A slight wrinkle in the sheet may be very irritating, a soft sound may seem very harsh or dim light may seem to be very bright and glaring.
3. **Paresthesia**: It is an abnormal touch sensation such as burning or prickling that occurs without an outside stimulus. This may occur due to poor blood supply to the nerve or nerve injury or dysfunction. For example, numbness or tingling sensation in the hand or feet when they are in one position for too long.

Alterations in Perception

Sensory information received by our sensory receptors is interpreted and given some meaning through the process of perception. Sometimes this interpretation goes wrong resulting in the failure of the perception to

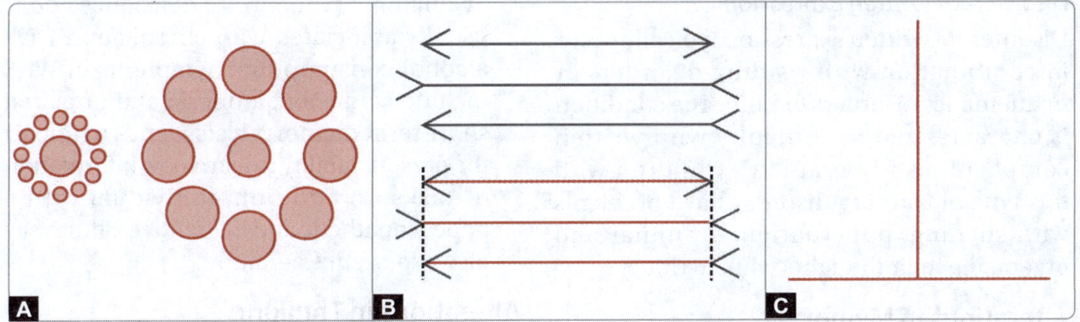

Figures 6.32A to C: (A) Illusion of size; (B) Illusion of length; (C) Horizontal vertical illusion

correspond with reality. Such false perceptions are called perceptual illusions.

Types of Illusions

- **Illusion of size:** This type of illusion provides false perception of the size of objects. A larger background always makes the objects look smaller in comparison to a smaller background where they will be perceived as larger. For example, in Ebbinghaus illusion, two circles of the same size are perceived to be of different sizes because of the size of the surrounding objects **(Figure 6.32A)**.
- **Illusion of length**: In Muller–Lyer illusion, line segments of the same size appear to be of different lengths based on the shapes placed at their ends **(Figure 6.32B)**.
- **Horizontal vertical illusion:** This type of illusion involves two straight lines, a horizontal line and a vertical line. Though both are invariably of the same length, the vertical one is perceived to be longer than the horizontal one **(Figure 6.32C)**.

All these are good examples of optical illusions. Illusions arise either because of the ambiguous qualities of what is perceived or the state of the perceiving person or both.

Alterations in Learning

Learning disorders are academic difficulties experienced by children and adults of average to above average intelligence. People with learning disorders have difficulty with reading, writing, mathematics or a combination of the three. These difficulties significantly interfere with academic achievement or daily living.

Learning disorders are thought to be caused by neurological abnormalities that trigger impairments in the regions of the brain that control visual and language processing, attention and planning. These traits maybe genetically linked. Children from families with a history of learning disorders are more likely to develop disorders themselves. Learning difficulties may also be caused by such medical conditions as a traumatic brain injury or brain infections such as encephalitis or meningitis. The three main types of learning disorders are—reading disorders, mathematics disorders and disorders of written expression.

Reading Disorders

Children with reading disorders have difficulty in recognizing and interpreting letters and words (dyslexia). They are unable to recognize and decode the sounds and syllables (phonetic structure) behind written words and language in general. This condition lowers accuracy and comprehension in reading.

Mathematics Disorders

Children with mathematics disorders (dyscalculia) have problems recognizing and counting numbers correctly. The child's math ability is far below the normal for their age, intelligence and education level. They have difficulty using numbers in everyday settings. Mathematics disorders are typically diagnosed in the first few years of elementary school when formal teaching of numbers and basic mathematical concepts begins.

Disorders of Written Expression

Disorders of written expression typically occur in combination with reading disorders or mathematics disorders or both. The condition is characterized by difficulty with written compositions (dysgraphia). Children with this type of learning disorder have problems with spelling, punctuation, grammar and organizing their thoughts while writing.

Alterations in Memory

Memory can be defined as an organism's ability to encode, retain and recall information. Alterations in memory though can range from mild to severe, are all a result of damage to neuroanatomical structures either in part or full. This damage hinders the storage, retention and recollection of memories. The common memory disorders are listed below:

1. **Agnosia** is the inability to recognize certain objects, persons or sounds. Examples of specific types of agnosia include—visual agnosia, auditory agnosia, prosopagnosia, somatosensory agnosia, apraxia, associative agnosia, etc.
2. **Alzheimer's disease** is a progressive, degenerative and fatal brain disease in which cell to cell connections in the brain are lost. As a result the death of brain cells occurs leading to severe cognitive impairment.
3. **Amnesia** is an abnormal mental state in which memory and learning are affected out of all proportion to other cognitive functions. The two forms of amnesia are—anterograde amnesia and retrograde amnesia.
4. **Dementia** refers to a large class of disorders characterized by the progressive deterioration of thinking ability and memory as the brain becomes damaged.
5. **Hyperthymestic syndrome** causes an individual to have an extremely detailed autobiographical memory. Patients with this disorder are able to recall events from each day of their lives. This disorder is very rare with only a few confirmed cases.
6. **Wernicke-Korsakoff syndrome (WKS)** is a severe neurological disorder caused by thiamine (vitamin B_1) deficiency and is usually associated with chronic excessive alcohol consumption. Symptoms of WKS include confusion, amnesia and impaired short-term memory. It also tends to impair the person's ability to learn new information or tasks. In addition, individuals often appear apathetic and inattentive. Some may also experience agitation.

Alterations in Thinking

Cognitive disorders are mental conditions that cause people to have difficulty thinking clearly and precisely. Although symptoms of cognitive disorders vary they are generally marked by impaired awareness, perception, reasoning, memory and judgment. A wide variety of factors can lead to cognitive disorders including general medical conditions, brain infections and head injury. The four major categories of cognitive disorders are:

1. **Delirium**: A change in consciousness that develops over a short period of time in which people have a reduced awareness of their environment.
2. **Dementia**: A progressive deterioration of brain function that is marked by impairment of memory, confusion and inability to concentrate.
3. **Amnesia**: A significant loss of memory despite no loss of other cognitive functions like in dementia.
4. **Cognitive disorders not otherwise specified**: Cognitive impairment presumed to be due to a general medical condition or substance use and that which does not fit into other categories.

Alterations in Intelligence

People differ in intellectual ability and capacities like reasoning and thinking, power of imagination, creative expression, concentration, etc. Intelligence level differs from individual to individual. Individuals can be classified between super normal (IQ above 120) and idiots (IQ from 0 to 50) on the basis of their intelligence level. *(Refer Chapter 6 - Page Nos. 122 and 123 for details on mental deficiency and mentally gifted children)*.

APPLICATIONS IN NURSING PROFESSION

Nursing Implications of Attention

- Attention helps in bringing mental alertness and preparedness. As a result the nurse becomes mentally alert and tries to exercise one's mental powers as effectively as possible for providing care.
- Attention helps the nurse to concentrate by focusing consciousness on one object at a time rather than two.
- Attention helps the nurse for better organization of the perceptual field for maximum clarity and understanding of the patient condition.
- Attention provides strength and ability to continue the task of cognitive functioning despite the obstacles laid by the distractions.
- The nurse can use psychology of attention for invoking not only voluntary but also involuntary attention to her job.

Nursing Implications of Sensory Process

- The nurse should always be alert to malfunctioning of sense organs and abnormal sensations in patients. A sick person reacts to colors. During illness even moderate lighting may irritate and cause discomfort. For patients who need rest and sleep, lights can be subdued. For stimulation and encouragement warm bright lights can be used. An ageing patient may need a great deal of help than younger patients to comprehend the visual details.
- A sick person is very much averse to loud noises. Loud noises increase the patient's irritability. The nurse must avoid loud noises in the ward. Patients with hearing loss require special effort by the nurse to be sure that the instructions are given clearly and questions answered and understood.
- Patients with loss of skin sensation require special attention to prevent further injuries to the skin while treating or using treatments or applications of any kind. Bandages, adhesive tapes, plaster casts, heat or cold, even wrinkled linens may be very irritating to a patient. Gentle skin care is necessary to prevent irritation. Patients always should be handled gently and smoothly to avoid pain and discomfort.
- In healthcare environment the possible sources for bad odor are—body eliminations, treatment procedures, dressings, drainages and medications. These must be controlled to the maximum possible extent by proper ventilation and prompt disposal of waste.
- A sick person may not relish his food. Taste can be improved with good mouth care and well prepared, clean and fresh food served in an appetizing way. Those having dizziness may need help in walking and protection from accidents and injury. Rough, fast or jerky movements cause discomfort and irritation to the patient. Patients should always be handled gently and smoothly to avoid discomfort.
- A nurse can use the knowledge of sense organs for training her senses. This will enable the trained senses to observe her functions.

Nursing Implications of Perception

- Accurate perception and observation are very important for a nurse to provide quality patient care. All nursing activities require accurate observation and perception. For example, checking vital signs, assessing patient, administering medications, etc.
- If the nurse is not a keen observer she will not be able to note some very critical or important symptoms resulting in premature patient death.
- Accurate perception and observation will help the nurse to gather accurate information and knowledge which in turn will help her to learn more easily and adjust more quickly to new situations. It also prevents accidents and incidents harmful to the patient.
- With accurate perception there is an improvement not only in nurse's memory but also the recording and reporting is more accurate. This makes her more resourceful for the patient and the healthcare team.

- All types of false perceptions and illusions should be scrupulously avoided by the nurse.

Nursing Implications of Learning

- Learning is fundamental to the development and modification of behavior. Thus knowledge of the learning process may be successfully applied to academic work and many clinical situations.
- Many of our subjective feelings, emotions and attitudes are probably conditioned responses. Through generalization it becomes difficult to identify the origin of our emotional responses. Both our adaptive emotional responses as well as maladaptive responses are learned and can be unlearned through principle of learning.
- Learning methods have wide applications in educational settings. In programed learning the material to be learned is broken up into small easy steps so that the learner can accomplish without any frustration. While programed learning enables the learner to master the task at his own pace, versatile and flexible learning enables the improvement in learning style.
- Application of reinforcement principles can often increase productivity both at studies and vocation.
- A nurse should understand the nature of learning so also the factors affecting learning. As learning modifies our behavior it is necessary for the nurse to gather only correct and factual knowledge. It ensures modification in the right direction.
- A nurse must have a well-defined purpose and goal in all learning situations.
- A nurse should always connect the new material with the old material.
- Repeated practice is very important for effective learning. Modern nursing requires skills in many complicated techniques. In order that these skills are learned proficiently the nurse will need repeated day-to-day practice. Besides practice the nurse needs to observe the demonstrated techniques attentively so as to understand the instructions given by the teacher and make use of her intelligence, thinking and memory.

Nursing Implications of Memory

The following tips aid in improving memory retention:

- Learning needs a desire, a receptive mood and an interest in the learning task before any success can be anticipated.
- Things are better remembered when presented through more than one sense. Materials when seen and heard are better retained than the ones which are only seen or heard. Use imagery to visualize the material and give auditory stimulation by reading aloud. For example, while studying nervous system—visualize the structure of the nervous system and also read loudly.
- As many associations as possible should be developed between the material presented and the one already learnt. A child for example learns the alphabets easily through associations such as: A for 'apple', etc.
- Rhythm is an aid to learning. Children learn nursery rhymes easily because of the rhythm.
- Learning must be distributed as much as possible. Studying in smaller units but over a longer period ensures greater retention than crammed up material.
- Rehearsal and recitation are useful in memorizing. Recitation gives us a chance for self-evaluation and builds confidence in oneself. Elaborative rehearsal is more effective than maintenance rehearsal.
- Retention occurs better if an attempt is made at having a general look at the entire material even before the intensive study is taken up. Going over the whole unit gives the general picture before it is broken into units.
- Since forgetting is much faster during the period immediately following learning the obvious thing to do is to review early and often. Periodical review will help retention of the material learnt.

- Meaningful material is not only more easily learnt than nonsense material but also remembered longer and more fully.
- Short pauses may be given between study times. It would help to consolidate the learned material. Periods of rest and preferably sleep help retention.
- Over learning aids retention.
- Very often forgetting may occur due to interference. Teachers should normally avoid presenting ideas which might easily be confused in close succession.
- Review before examination is desirable.

Nursing Interventions for Impaired Memory

- Encourage the patient to use written cues such as calendar lists or a note book. These cues will soon reduce the patients need to recall appointments and activities without much assistance.
- Provide single step instructions to patients as those with memory impairment cannot recall multistep instructions.
- Keep environmental changes to a bare minimum.
- It is important to maximize independent functioning and assist the patient unobtrusively when memory function has deteriorated further.
- It is important to preserve the patient's dignity and minimize his frustration with progressive memory loss.

Nursing Implications of Thinking

Correct thinking is one of the greatest assets for a nurse. Certain recommendations for student nurses to think correctly and reason out properly are as under:

- The nurse should confront the problems directly instead of evading them or shifting responsibility to another person. She should look for the central problem.
- The job of a nurse requires a lot of thinking. The knowledge of psychology of thinking as well as the technique is therefore very helpful for a nurse. The nurse uses her thinking to understand the rationale behind each procedure. In order to think correctly a nurse should have adequate knowledge and experience. She should be able to distinguish between facts and opinion.
- Logical thinking helps to think correctly. Hence she should develop the habit of thinking scientifically.
- The nurse should be able to size up the whole situation. A nurse should try to think on definite lines with a definite purpose. Unless there is a definite aim or purpose thinking cannot proceed on the right track.
- Nurses with past experiences or habitual methods may at time find it difficult to resolve problems. She should thus strive for new associations, relationships and possibilities for arriving at satisfactory results.
- She should form a habit of looking for relationships and generalizing from facts.
- She should cultivate the right habits of observation and attention for collection of factual data on which the thinking can be based.
- A nurse should also adopt a flexible attitude towards patient's problems.
- Nurse's emotions should not influence the reasoning ability. Also moods, attitudes or behavior of the patients should not interfere with her scientific thoughts and ideas related to treatment. Nurse should avoid prejudice and look for a new meaning.
- Muscular responses should be recognized as an important part of thinking. It is possible to recognize muscular tensions in oneself and others when thinking deeply. Some muscle tension may be exhibited by the patient using body language which needs to be observed and understood by the nurse.
- It is an error to assume that a person cannot think when paralyzed or seriously ill.
- In the midst of all the superstitions and contrary beliefs of patients, the nurse must always insist upon what is factual, rational and helpful to the patient.

Nursing Implications of Intelligence

- Knowledge about the nature of intelligence and its measurement is useful to the nurse in understanding herself, colleagues and patients.

- Nurse's explanations or guidance to the patient would be according to the patient's intellectual level.
- As a student and later as a teacher, the knowledge of intellectual function is useful for a nurse. Teaching method, content of the subject matter and expectations from students should be based on student's intellectual functioning.
- Knowledge regarding intelligence helps the nurse in diagnosing a patient with mental subnormality or with very superior intelligence.
- In diseases related to neuropsychiatric disorders, epilepsy, psychiatric disorders and some of the endocrinal disorders, assessment of intelligence is of great assistance in their management.
- Knowledge about abnormalities in newborns and development of their intelligence helps the nurse in providing suitable care.
- Aging patients though physically slow, retain their levels of intelligence. Respect and encouragement with combined nursing care has to be ensured.

Every individual is unique especially when intelligence is the judging factor. A nurse in the course of discharging her duties has to heavily rely on verbal and non-verbal communication patterns. Nurses may have to interact with the patient, patient's family members, explain and clarify procedures and medications. The intelligence level of the patient and family members decides how effectively the nurse is able to communicate and discharge her duties. Lower the levels of intelligence, more the time and patience the nurse will have to invest in caring for the patient. The instructions may have to be simple and repeated more often. However, where the patient is more intelligent he can be expected to take an active part in his own health care in the future.

Nursing Implications of Aptitude

- Knowledge of aptitudes, their measurements and conditions will be helpful to the nurse to develop a proper aptitude for her profession and guide those around her entering professions according to their aptitudes.
- The knowledge of aptitude will also give her optimism in her own future success.
- If nurse has an aptitude for her profession she is bound to be a successful nurse whatever the impediments she might face in her path.

SYNOPSIS

- Attention is the focus of conscious on a particular object at a particular time.
- There are two types of attention—voluntary and involuntary.
- Maximum amount of material that can be attended to in one period of attention is called span of attention.
- Maximum amount of time one can attend to an object without a break is called duration of attention.
- Any stimulus whose presence interferes with the process of attention is called distraction.
- Perception is the interpretation of sensory stimuli reaching the sense organs and the brain.
- There are individual differences in perceptual abilities.
- When errors creep into the process of perception it leads to impaired perception.
- Intelligence is the general capacity for comprehension and reasoning that manifests itself in various ways.
- Both nurture and nature play an important role in the development of heredity.
- Learning is the acquisition of habits, knowledge and attitudes.
- The learning process includes three elements: learner, type of experience, resources.
- According to trial and error theory learning consists of making bonds or connections between stimuli and responses.
- Classical conditioning is a type of learning in which a neutral stimulus comes to bring about a response after it is paired with a stimulus.
- According to operant conditioning behavior is shaped and manifested by it consequences.

- According to theory of insightfulness learning is restructuring the field of perception through insight.
- According to observational theory learning is acquired through imitation and observation.
- A habit is the tendency of the individual to behave in the same way as he has behaved earlier.
- Memory is the special ability of our mind to store what has been learned and reproduce it after sometime.
- The three different types of memory are: immediate, short-term and long-term.
- Failure to recollect a fact or idea is called forgetting.
- Thinking is a problem solving process in which we use ideas or symbols.
- Attitude is the special aptness for a special ability.
- Neuropsychological testing is used to measure cognitive impairment and cognitive ability in individuals.

Review Questions

ATTENTION AND PERCEPTION

Long Essays

1. Define perception. Discuss organization of perception.
2. What are the factors influencing perception? Describe the relationship between sensation and perception.

Short Essays

1. Explain factors influencing attention.
2. Varieties of attention.
3. Can attention be divided? Explain.
4. Describe factors that control and direct attention.
5. Briefly discuss objective conditions of attention.
6. Enumerate and explain determinants of attention.
7. Define perception. Discuss salient features of perception.
8. Organization of perception.
9. Characteristics of perception.
10. Errors in perception.
11. Factors influencing perception.
12. Describe principles of perceptual organization.

Short Notes

1. Attention
2. Determinants of attention
3. Division of attention
4. Span of attention
5. Varieties of attention
6. Distraction of attention
7. Fluctuation of attention
8. Perception
9. Extrasensory perception
10. Common errors in perception
11. Illusions
12. Law of proximity

Multiple Choice Questions

1. Stimulus operating on our nervous system is termed as:

a. Sensation
b. Observation
c. Attention
d. Perception

2. Which of the following factors influence an individual's perception?

a. Motives and needs
b. Learning
c. Person's mental set up
d. All of the above

3. According to which of the principles do items close together in space of time tend to be perceived as belonging together or forming an organized group?

a. Similarity
b. Proximity
c. Good figure
d. Closure

4. A common type of perceptual error found in a psychotic patient is:
a. Illusion
b. Hallucination
c. Delusion
d. Thought disorder

5. Concentration of consciousness upon one object rather than upon another is called:
a. Observation
b. Sensation
c. Attention
d. Perception

6. What is voluntary attention?
a. It does not demand conscious effort on the subject
b. It demands conscious effort on the subject
c. It demands single act of will
d. It demands repeated acts of will

7. Certain situations neither demand any conscious effort nor strike to catch our attention but we still attend to it. It is:
a. Voluntary attention
b. Involuntary attention
c. Habitual attention
d. None of the above

8. A person busy writing an assignment hears a loud sound and immediately attends to it. It is an example of:
a. Involuntary attention
b. Voluntary attention
c. Habitual attention
d. Partial voluntary attention

9. Solving a mathematical problem is an example of:
a. Voluntary attention
b. Involuntary attention
c. Habitual attention
d. All of the above

10. Maximum amount of material that can be attended to in one period of attention is called:
a. Variety of attention
b. Span of attention
c. Division of attention
d. None of the above

11. Time range for visual span of attention is:
a. 1/100 to1/5 of a second
b. 1/200 to1/10 of a second
c. 1/300 to1/15 of a second
d. 1/400 to1/20 of a second

12. Number of units that can be perceived at a brief glance in visual span of attention is:
a. 4 or 5 units
b. 6 or 7 units
c. 7 or 8 units
d. 8 or 9 units

13. Attending to two or more tasks simultaneously is termed as:
a. Visual span of attention
b. Auditory span of attention
c. Division of attention
d. Variety of attention

14. When we travel in a train we attend to the scenery as well as to the talks of our companions. This is called:
a. Variety of attention
b. Subjective factor of attention
c. Objective factor of attention
d. Division of attention

15. To achieve our goal we make deliberate effort and focus our conscious upon an object. It is termed as:
a. Involuntary attention
b. Voluntary attention
c. Habitual attention
d. Partially voluntary and partially involuntary attention

16. Leakage of LPG gas in your house catches your attention. It is an example of:
a. Involuntary attention
b. Habitual attention
c. Voluntary attention
d. None of the above

17. Attention which makes you wish every time you see the teacher is an example of:
   a. Voluntary attention
   b. Involuntary attention
   c. Habitual attention
   d. None of the above

18. A skillful knitter who can knit and read at the same time has learnt to knit quite automatically. This is an example of:
   a. Visual span of attention
   b. Auditory span of attention
   c. Division of attention
   d. Variety of attention

19. The term absolute threshold refers to the ______ intensity of a stimulus that must be present for the stimulus to be detected.

20. When a car passes you on the road and appears to shrink as it gets farther away the phenomenon of ____ permits you to realize that the car is not in fact getting smaller.

LEARNING

Long Essays

1. Define learning. Explain operant conditioning given by Skinner.
2. Define learning. Explain classical conditioning theory.
3. Discuss the laws of learning. Explain the role of motivation and anxiety in learning process.
4. Define learning. Describe learning by conditioning and its educational implication in nursing.
5. Explain laws of learning. Describe factors influencing our memory.
6. Define learning. What are the laws of learning? Explain the different types of learning quoting examples wherever necessary.

Short Essays

1. Explain various types of learning.
2. Classical conditioning.
3. Techniques of learning.
4. Describe the laws of learning and their educational implications.
5. Explain part vs whole and massed vs spaced method of learning.
6. What is learning? Explain trial and error method of learning.
7. Enumerate the differences between learning by classical conditioning and operant conditioning.
8. Explain classical conditioning with special reference to Pavlov.
9. Describe operant conditioning by Skinner.
10. Discuss different methods of learning with suitable examples.
11. Steps in learning.
12. Characteristics of habits.

Short Notes

1. Reinforcement
2. Insightful learning
3. Learning
4. Extinction and spontaneous recovery
5. Trial and error
6. Maturation and learning
7. List any four factors affecting learning
8. 'Aha! Effect' in insight learning

Multiple Choice Questions

1. A relatively enduring behavioral change brought about by an experience is called:
   a. Learning
   b. Habituation
   c. Growth
   d. All of the above

2. The process of learning:
   a. Improves adjustment

b. Improves efficiency
c. Is continuous
d. All of the above

3. Which of the following factors is not conducive to learning?
a. Intelligence
b. Motivation
c. Distracting conditions
d. Good physical health

4. Learning results in:
a. A more or less permanent change in behavior
b. Poor control of one's emotions
c. Frequent motivational conflicts
d. All of the above

5. Ivan Pavlov proposed the concept of:
a. Operant conditioning
b. Classical conditioning
c. Learning by trial and error
d. Learning by insight

6. In Pavlov's original experiment meat was the:
a. Unconditioned stimulus
b. Conditioned stimulus
c. Unconditioned response
d. Conditioned response

7. You begin to salivate at the sight of a pizza hut sign. When this happens the sight of the sign is an example of:
a. Unconditioned stimulus
b. Discriminative stimulus
c. Conditioned stimulus
d. Conditioned response

8. In classical conditioning ______ is capable of eliciting a response previously triggered by the unconditioned stimulus.
a. Aversive stimulus
b. Conditioned stimulus
c. Secondary reinforcer
d. Primary reinforcer

9. Extinction occurs in classical conditioning:
a. After repeated trials wherein conditioned stimulus is presented by itself
b. When the delay between conditioned stimulus and unconditioned stimulus is reduced to approximately half a second
c. When unconditioned stimulus loses its ability to elicit unconditioned response
d. When conditioned stimulus and unconditioned stimulus are paired during every trial

10. According to behavioral view of learning:
a. Human beings can be taught to do anything
b. Human learning cannot be modified
c. Human learning is rigid
d. None of the above

11. BF Skinner proposed the concept of:
a. Operant conditioning
b. Classical conditioning
c. Learning by trial and error
d. Learning by insight

12. Adding something pleasant is ___ and removing something good is ______.
a. Positive reinforcement; negative reinforcement
b. Positive reinforcement; punishment by removal
c. Negative reinforcement; punishment by application
d. Punishment; reinforcement

13. Someone who offers money in a temple every week is doing so according to a ______ reinforcement schedule.
a. Fixed-interval
b. Variable-interval
c. Fixed-ratio
d. Variable-ratio

14. Rewards that satisfy a biological need are called:
a. Negative reinforcers
b. Positive reinforcers
c. Secondary reinforcers
d. Primary reinforcers

15. Prizes in lotteries are given on a:
   a. Variable-interval reinforcement basis
   b. Variable-ratio reinforcement basis
   c. Continuous basis
   d. Fixed-ratio reinforcement basis

16. Trial and error learning was propagated by:
   a. Erikson
   b. Pavlov
   c. Thorndike
   d. Skinner

17. What is a habit?
   a. Acquisition of new skill
   b. Tendency of an individual to behave in a new way compared to previous situation
   c. Tendency of an individual to behave in the same way as he behaved earlier
   d. Continuously practicing the new skill

18. Following habits are risk factors for specific diseases, *except*:
   a. Excessive sunbathing
   b. Excessive eating of certain foods
   c. Poor personal hygiene
   d. Balanced diet

19. While learning involves changes brought about by experience, ________ describes changes due to biological development.

20. In a ______ reinforcement schedule behavior is reinforced some of the time while in a ______ reinforcement schedule behavior is reinforced all the time.

21. Cognitive-social learning theorists are concerned only with overt behavior not with its internal cause. True or False?

22. Bandura's theory of ______ learning states that people learn through watching a ______; another person displaying the behavior of interest.

23. A man wishes to quit smoking. Upon the advice of a psychologist he begins a program in which he sets goals for his withdrawal, carefully records his progress and rewards himself for not smoking during a certain period of time. What type of program is he following?

MEMORY

Long Essays

1. What is memory? Explain techniques to improve memory.
2. What is forgetting? Explain theories of forgetting.
3. Define learning and explain efficient methods of memorizing.

Short Essays

1. List factors influencing forgetting.
2. Differentiate between long-term and short-term memory.
3. Theories of forgetting.
4. What is forgetting? How can it be minimized?
5. Mention the meaning and nature of forgetting.
6. Discuss various economical methods of memorization and their use in education.
7. Explain factors influencing memory.
8. What are the types of memory? How can memory be improved?
9. Elaborate effective ways of memorizing.
10. Explain the causes of forgetting.
11. Define memory. Explain methods to improve memory.
12. What are the organic (biological) causes of forgetting?

Short Notes

1. Chunking
2. Types of memory
3. Amnesia
4. Short-term memory

5. Mnemonics
6. Learning
7. Distributed practice in memorization
8. Forgetting
9. Remembering
10. Proactive and retroactive inhibition

Multiple Choice Questions

1. In psychology which of the following mental processes provides the basis for all cognitive processes?
a. Thinking
b. Learning
c. Memory
d. Motivation

2. The first stage of memory is:
a. Encoding
b. Storage
c. Retrieval
d. Imagination

3. Short-term memory is also known as:
a. Iconic memory
b. Working memory
c. Echoic memory
d. Sensory memory

4. Long-term memories may last for:
a. Days
b. Months
c. Years
d. All of the above

5. Memory images or traces are present in the mind in the form of:
a. Pictures
b. Engrams
c. Signals
d. Diagrams

6. Which of the following types of memory helps an individual to recall something asplit second after having perceived it?
a. Short-term memory
b. Immediate or sensory memory
c. Long-term memory
d. Delayed memory

7. Semantic memory is memory for:
a. Language and knowledge
b. Visuospatial orientation
c. Events occurring in one's life
d. Events occurring in external world

8. Which of the following is a measure of memory?
a. Recall or reproduction
b. Recognition
c. Repetition
d. Registration

9. Which of the following components of a memory system refers to transformation of a physical stimulus into a form acceptable by the human memory?
a. Encoding
b. Storage
c. Retrieval
d. Recognition

10. Which of the following types of long-term memory deals with individual's personal experiences?
a. Semantic memory
b. Episodic memory
c. Procedural memory
d. All of the above

11. Which of the following is a center for recent memory?
a. Temporal lobe
b. Parietal lobe
c. Hippocampus
d. Thalamus

12. Partial or complete loss of memory is called:
a. Agnosia
b. Ataxia
c. Amnesia
d. Forgetting

13. Amnesia associated with total failure of memory for events that occurred before the trauma which resulted in memory impairment is called:
a. Anterograde amnesia
b. Retrograde amnesia
c. Transient amnesia
d. Functional amnesia

14. Most evidence suggests that memory loss in older adults:
   a. Is not an inevitable part of the aging process
   b. Is genetically preprogrammed
   c. Usually affects all memory functions of the individual
   d. Is caused by senility

15. When new memories interfere in the retrieval of old memory it is called:
   a. Proactive interference
   b. Saving
   c. Retroactive interference
   d. Implicit memory

16. A professor forgets the names of students who attended her class two semesters ago because she learned the names of all the students this semester. This is a typical example of a memory problem called:
   a. Alzheimer disease
   b. Decay
   c. Proactive interference
   d. Retroactive interference

17. Memory for a personal anecdote such as, 'How I lost the ring on the morning of my wedding day,' would be stored in________ long-term memory.
   a. Semantic
   b. Episodic
   c. Working
   d. Implicit

18. __________are organized bodies of information stored in memory that bias the way new information is interpreted, stored and recalled.

19. If after learning a poem for a test a year ago you now find yourself unable to recall what you learned, you are experiencing memory ________ caused by non-use.

20. _________ interference occurs when material is difficult to retrieve because of exposure to later material. _________interference refers to the difficulty in retrieving material due to the interference of previous material.

THINKING

Long Essay

1. Define thinking. Describe the process of concept formation.

Short Essays

1. What is reasoning? Explain errors in thinking.
2. Explain Piaget and Bruner's contribution in concept formation.
3. What is concept and how is it developed?
4. Describe the steps involved in scientific problem solving.
5. What are errors in thinking?
6. What is thinking? What are the types of thinking? Explain the influence of language on thought.

Short Notes

1. Problem solving
2. Tools of thinking
3. Define thinking
4. Types of thinking
5. Types of reasoning
6. Errors in thinking
7. Abstract thinking
8. Define concepts
9. Reasoning
10. Inductive reasoning
11. Freethinking

Multiple Choice Questions

1. Thinking is:
   a. Higher mental process
   b. Physical activity
   c. Imagination
   d. None of the above

2. Thinking involves:
   a. Id, ego, superego
   b. Receptors, connectors, effectors
   c. Both a and b
   d. None of the above

3. **In which of the following do we use a system of symbols to communicate with each other?**
   a. Perception
   b. Concepts
   c. Language
   d. Thinking
4. **When a symbol stands for a class of objects or events with common properties, it refers to a:**
   a. Language b. Concept
   c. Emotion d. Experiment
5. **Which cognitive process is characterized by the use of symbols as representations of objects and events?**
   a. Perception b. Learning
   c. Thinking d. Memory
6. **Who among the following psychologists emphasized cognitive approach in his research on development of understanding in a child?**
   a. Edward C Tolman
   b. Jean Piaget
   c. Sigmund Freud
   d. W Kohler
7. **A form of thinking which aims at solving complex problems is:**
   a. Perceptual thinking
   b. Reflective thinking
   c. Abstract thinking
   d. Creative thinking
8. **You are asked the question, 'How many windows are there in your parent's house?' To answer, you visualize the building and take a mental walk around it counting the windows. In achieving the answer you use a(n):**
   a. Mental image
   b. Precursor to perception
   c. Imaginary delusion
   d. Visual nondistractor
9. **Being able to generate unusual but appropriate responses to problems or questions is called:**
   a. Availability heuristic
   b. Divergent thinking
   c. Cognitive complexity
   d. Convergent thinking
10. **Higher type of thinking, being careful, systematic and organized in functioning is termed as:**
    a. Concrete thinking
    b. Perceptual thinking
    c. Critical thinking
    d. Thinking
11. **Divergent thinking involves:**
    a. Logical possibility
    b. Logical recognition
    c. Artistic thinking
    d. Free association
12. **A particular kind of thinking that can point thoughts in the wrong direction is called:**
    a. Functional solution
    b. Functional fixedness
    c. Fixedness
    d. Formal thinking
13. **Reasoning is step wise thinking with:**
    a. Imagination
    b. Purpose or goal
    c. Laws
    d. Both a and b
14. **Which of the following is a cognitive activity that controls as well as affects the total behavior and personality?**
    a. Concept formation
    b. Reasoning
    c. Problem solving
    d. Thinking
15. **During which stage of creative thinking does the thinker feel that he has no sight of solution to his problem?**
    a. Preparation
    b. Incubation
    c. Inspiration or illumination
    d. Verification or revision

16. Awareness, understanding, collection of relevant information, formulation of hypotheses, selection of proper solution, verification of solution are steps in:
   a. Problem solving
   b. Creative thinking
   c. Reasoning
   d. Thinking

17. Following is a method of problem solving in which one is presented with several alternatives among which one must choose
   a. Algorithms
   b. Heuristics
   c. Decision making
   d. Weighing alternatives

18. Problem solving as a deliberate and serious act involves the use of:
   a. Novel methods
   b. Consideration of alternatives
   c. Higher thinking
   d. All of the above

19. _______are categorizations of objects that share common properties.

20. _________ is a term used to describe the sudden 'flash' of revelation that often accompanies the solution to a problem.

21. Thinking of an object only in terms of its typical use is known as _______.

22. A broader, related tendency for old problem-solving patterns to persist is known as a _______.

INTELLIGENCE AND APTITUDE

Long Essays

1. What is intelligence? Explain different tools used for measurement of IQ.
2. Discuss the various intelligence tests and their use in a nursing situation.

Short Essays

1. Measurement of intelligence.
2. Types of intelligence tests.
3. What is IQ? Discuss the present status of intelligence tests and their use in nursing.
4. Discuss the factors influencing intelligence.
5. How is intelligence distributed in the general population?
6. Explain the nature and factors influencing creativity.
7. What is an intelligence test? Elucidate its uses with examples.
8. What is IQ? Write a note on mental retardation and mentally superior.
9. What are aptitudes? Write a note on measurement of aptitudes and skills.
10. Name verbal and performance tests of intelligence.
11. Define mental retardation. Explain various types of MR.
12. Nature and assessment of aptitudes.
13. Bring out the various steps in creative thinking.

Short Notes

1. IQ
2. Creativity
3. Genius
4. Intelligence
5. Steps involved in creative thinking
6. Who proposed the term 'IQ'? How do you calculate IQ?
7. Name two tests each pertaining to intelligence and personality.
8. Aptitudes
9. Aptitude test

Multiple Choice Questions

1. IQ stands for:
   a. International quotient
   b. Intelligence quotient
   c. Intelligent quotient
   d. None of the above

2. Average IQ range is:
   a. 90–110   b. 80–90
   c. 70–80   d. Below 70

3. **When both mental age and chronological age are same, IQ is:**
   a. 95
   b. 98
   c. 110
   d. 100
4. **Intelligence not only helps in career building but also encourages development of better health and relationships in later life. This is called:**
   a. Verbal intelligence
   b. Performance intelligence
   c. Non-verbal intelligence
   d. Emotional intelligence
5. **Intelligence is influenced by:**
   a. Hereditary factors
   b. Environmental factors
   c. Organic factors
   d. Both hereditary and environmental factors
6. **When no language is used in an intelligence test it is called:**
   a. Performance test
   b. Non-performance test
   c. Verbal test
   d. Both a and b
7. **Which measure of intelligence takes into account the individual's chronological age and mental age?**
   a. Triarchic intelligence
   b. Crystallized intelligence
   c. Deviation score
   d. Intelligence quotient
8. **Mental retardation occurs when a person shows:**
   a. Dependency on others for basic living needs such as food, shelter or protection
   b. Preference to live in an institution for special needs
   c. Below average cognition with limitations in related skills
   d. Abnormally excessive fantasizing or day dreaming to an extent that it interferes in daily social interaction with others
9. **The most common biological cause of mental retardation is:**
   a. Brain starvation of oxygen at birth
   b. Severe car accidents or other injuries
   c. Physical abuse during infancy
   d. Down syndrome
10. **Mental retardation is caused due to:**
    a. Physical hazards at birth
    b. Accidental head injury
    c. Infection of the brain
    d. All of the above
11. **Spearman's (1927) G-factor of intelligence**
    a. Is a hypothesized general factor of mental ability that is measured by IQ tests
    b. Represents an array of many independent factors that generate various mental abilities
    c. Is a quantitative measure of degree of cultural bias present in IQ tests
    d. Is calculated as one's level of fluid intelligence minus one's level of crystallized intelligence
12. **During which of the following stages does a creative thinker turn away from the problem?**
    a. Preparation
    b. Incubation
    c. Insight
    d. Verification
13. **Ability to handle words, numbers, formulae and scientific principles is ____________.**
14. **While ____________ tests predict a person's ability in a specific area, ____________ tests determine the specific level of knowledge.**
15. **Some forms of retardation can have a genetic basis and be passed through families. True or False?**

16. People with high intelligence are generally shy and socially withdrawn. True or False?

17. IQ tests can accurately determine the intelligence of an entire group of people. True or False?

18. Intelligence can be seen as a combination of______and______factors.

19. Lower IQ test scores during late adulthood do not necessarily mean a decrease in intelligence. True or False?

ANSWER KEY

ATTENTION AND PERCEPTION					
1. a	2. d	3. b	4. b	5. c	6. b
7. c	8. a	9. a	10. b	11. a	12. a
13. c	14. d	15. b	16. a	17. c	18. c
19. Smallest	20. Perceptual constancy				
LEARNING					
1. a	2. d	3. c	4. a	5. b	6. a
7. a	8. b	9. c	10. a	11. a	12. a
13. a	14. d	15. b	16. c	17. c	18. d
19. Maturation	20. Partial, continuous	21. False, cognitive-social learning theorists are primarily concerned with mental processes	22. Observational, model	23. Behavior modification	
MEMORY					
1. c	2. a	3. b	4. d	5. b	6. b
7. a	8. a	9. a	10. b	11. c	12. c
13. b	14. d	15. c	16. d	17. b	18. Schemas
19. Decay	20. Retroactive, Proactive				
THINKING					
1. a	2. b	3. c	4. b	5. c	6. b
7. b	8. a	9. b	10. c	11. a	12. b
13. b	14. b	15. b	16. a	17. c	18. d
19. Concepts	20. Insight	21. Functional fixedness	22. Mental set		
INTELLIGENCE AND APTITUDE					
1. b	2. a	3. d	4. d	5. d	6. a
7. d	8. c	9. d	10. d	11. b	12. b

13. Abstract intelligence	14. Aptitude, achievement	15. True	16. False, the gifted are generally more socially adept than those with lower IQ	17. False, IQ tests are used to measure individual intelligence. Within any group there are wide variations in individual intelligence
18. Hereditary, environmental	19. True			

CHAPTER

7 Motivation and Emotional Processes

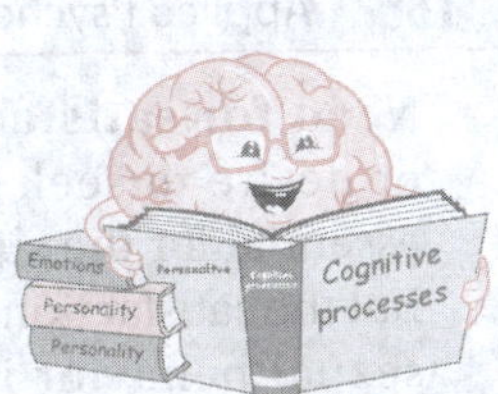

CHAPTER OUTLINE

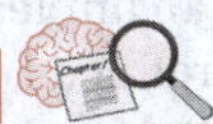

- Needs, drives, incentives, motivation
- Motivation—concepts, types, theories, nursing implications
- Emotions—components, theories, emotional adjustments
- Stress—stress cycle, effects, coping with stress
- Attitude—nature, effects, factors affecting attitudinal change
- Role of attitude in health and sickness
- Psychometric assessment of motivation, emotions and attitudes
- Role of nurse in caring for emotionally sick client

Psychology deals not only with what people do but also why they do so. Why they do and how they behave in a particular fashion at a particular moment can be understood in terms of motivation. Motivation is an organized condition of the individual which serves to direct behavior towards a certain goal. Motives are inferences from observations of behavior. While they serve as powerful tools for explanation of behavior, they also allow us to make predictions about future behavior. In motivation, activating forces such as needs, drives and motives mostly at work.

NEEDS

Needs are general wants or desires that are the very basis of our behavior. They essentially motivate us into action as a stimulated need leads to inner tension driving us into action. Needs can either be objective and physical, such as food and water, or can be subjective and psychological such as the need for self-esteem. Our behavior and feelings about ourselves and others, our values and priorities we set for ourselves all relate to our physiological and psychological needs. Every human being has to strive for the satisfaction of his basic needs if he is to maintain and actualize or enhance himself in this world. They can broadly be classified into biological and psychosocial needs.

Biological Needs

Also called physiological or unlearned needs these are necessary for the survival of an individual. These are generally caused by bodily wants. Biological needs include all our bodily or organic needs like need for oxygen, food, water, temperature, rest, sleep and sex, etc. These needs must be met at least to the minimum for maintaining life.

- **Need for oxygen, water and food** are most fundamental for our survival and existence. Prolonged deprivation of any of these needs may cause death. Oxygen is the most essential of all needs because all body cells require oxygen for survival. Healthy people drink fluids to satisfy thirst and maintain fluid balance. Food is a physiological need. Balance is maintained through digestive and metabolic processes.
- **Temperature, rest and sleep** are essential for survival. The human body functions best at 98.6°F (37°C). Rest and sleep allow time for the body to rejuvenate and be free of stress.

- **Need for satisfaction of the sex urge** or desire to seek sex experiences is not essential for the survival of the individual. But the satisfaction of this need and normal sexual behavior is most essential for a happy domestic life and the continuity and survival of the human species.

Psychosocial Needs

Also called secondary needs these are acquired through social learning and contact with others. These are linked with sociocultural environment and psychological makeup of an individual. These needs transform into dynamic forces underlying behavior.

Needs falling under this category include need for freedom, security, love and affection, recognition and social approval, social company, self-assertion and self-actualization.

- All human beings have an urge to remain free and independent.
- Each one of us needs to feel secure which means being protected from potential or actual harm. Safety and security need also includes trusting others and being free from fear, anxiety and apprehension.
- Love and belonging need includes the understanding and acceptance of others in both giving and receiving love and the feeling of belonging to families, peers, friends, neighborhood and a community. People who believe that their love and belonging needs are unmet, feel lonely and isolated.
- Each one of us has an inherent desire to gain recognition and appreciation from others.
- Man is called a social animal in the sense that he has a strong urge to be with his own kind and maintain social relations with them.
- Each one of us has an inherent desire to get an opportunity to rule or dominate over others. It may vary in intensity from person to person but is exhibited by us all in one or the other situation.
- We all have an inherent craving for the expression of self and actualization of our own potentialities.

DRIVES

A drive is an aroused state resulting from some bodily or tissue need. This aroused condition motivates the individual to initiate behavior to remedy the need. For example, lack of food produces certain chemical changes in the blood indicating a need for food which in turn creates an unpleasant state, a tension that needs to be reduced. The individual seeks out ways to fulfill these biological needs.

Need refers to the physiological state of tissue deprivation while drive refers to the psychological consequences of a need. Drive does not necessarily get stronger as need gets stronger. A starved individual may be so weakened by his great need for food that drive (the motivation to get it) is weakened. People who have fasted for long periods report that their feelings of hunger (drive level) come and go even though their need for food persists. The strength of a drive depends upon the strength of the stimuli involving the related need. Drives of any nature are divided into two categories:

1. Biological or primary drive
2. Socio-psychological or secondary drive

Biological Drive or Primary Drive

Biological needs give birth to biological drives such as hunger, thirst, sex and escape from pain. These drives are basically unlearned in nature. They arise from our biological needs as a result of a biological mechanism called homeostasis.

Homeostasis: Our body system constantly works to maintain optimum level of functioning between input and output. For example, when blood sugar level drops, glands, stomach and other body parts send signals to the brain which activate a hunger drive making one feel hungry. After food has been consumed by the individual's body it returns to a state of balance. This maintenance of an overall physiological balance is called homeostasis. In the event of an imbalance there is a need to restore balance giving rise to a drive which in turn serves as an instigator of behavior.

Socio-psychological or Secondary Drive

It includes fear or anxiety, desire for approval, striving for achievement, aggression and dependence. These drives are not related to our physiological needs and therefore do not arise on account of imbalance in the body's internal functioning. They arise from socio-psychological needs and are said to be acquired through social learning as a result of one's interaction with his socio-cultural environment. These drives move an individual to act for the satisfaction of his socio-psychological needs which in turn act as a reinforcer for such behavior and furthermore its continuity and maintenance. Drives are thus the basic activating force behind a behavior.

INCENTIVES

Anything that incites, rouses or encourages a person is termed as an incentive. Drives are influenced and guided by incentives. Praise, appreciation, regards, bonus etc., are examples of incentives. Incentive works as a reinforcing agent as it adds more strength to a drive like adding fuel to the already ignited fire. A piece of candy, chocolate or a toy may work as an incentive for a child giving more strength to its drive resulting in further motivation to act or behave in a desirable way. Whether primary or secondary, the drive is greatly affected and directed by incentives. These incentives work more forcefully in the case of an individual who remains deprived of them for long.

MOTIVATION

A motive etymologically means that 'which moves'. A motive may be considered as an energetic force or tendency (learned or innate) working within the individual to compel, persuade or inspire him to act for the satisfaction of his basic needs or attainment of some specific purpose. Motives can be seen in the form of various needs, desires and aspirations of an individual.

Definitions

A need gives rise to one or more motives. A motive is a rather specific process which has been learned. It is directed towards a goal.

—Carol (1969)

A motive may be defined as the readiness or disposition to respond in some ways and not others to a variety of situations.

—Rosen, Fox and Gregory (1972)

Motive is an inner state of mind or an aroused feeling generated through basic needs or drives which compel an individual to respond by creating a kind of tension or urge to act.

Motive may thus be considered as an energetic force or a tendency (learned or innate) working within the individual to compel, persuade or inspire him to act either for the satisfaction of his basic needs or the attainment of some specific purpose.

CONCEPTS OF MOTIVATION

- Motivation is generated through basic needs or drives.
- It compels an individual to respond by creating a kind of tension or urge to act.
- It is a goal-directed activity pursued till the attainment of the goal.
- Attainment of a goal helps in the release of tension aroused by a specific motive.
- A change in goal may bring an alteration in the nature and strength of the motive.
- Motivation is an inner state or an aroused feeling.
- We experience motives as feelings of want, need and desire.
- Motive may be considered as a learned response or tendency and also an innate disposition.
- We cannot see motives directly but must infer them from behavior of people.

TYPES OF MOTIVES

Psychologists have divided motives into two main categories: Innate or unlearned and

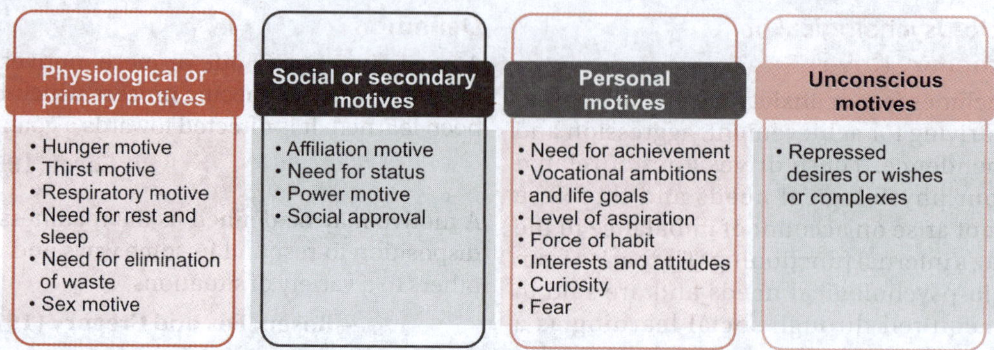

Figure 7.1: Types of motives

acquired or learned. Common types of motives are depicted in **Figure 7.1.**

Physiological or Biological or Primary Motives

Physiological motives are called biological or organic motives. These include hunger, sex, thirst, need for oxygen, rest and sleep, avoid or seek relief from pain, activity and elimination needs.

Hunger Motive

Hunger is seen to be a very dominant motive. If hunger motive is not adequately satisfied behavior of the individual undergoes a series of changes which includes lowering of morale. When food supply to the body is exhausted certain biochemical changes take place in the tissues of the body. This causes the stomach to contract resulting in hunger pains. Hunger must be satisfied so as to help the body return to a physiological balance or homeostasis.

Thirst Motive

When deprived of water over a long period the individual becomes excessively restless thereby creating an urgency for intake of water. Tissues of the body lose fluid in the absence of fluid intake resulting in the mucous membranes of the throat to become dry and cause sensation of thirst.

Respiratory Motive

It is the drive for air and oxygen. One cannot survive for long without a regular supply of air or oxygen. When an individual suffers from oxygen want, his memory, sensory activity and muscular control are seriously impaired.

Need for Rest and Sleep

Need for sleep is another physiological motive. When the body continues to perform activities for a long time without adequate rest or sleep it is possible that confusion, fatigue or discomfort are experienced.

Need for Elimination of Waste

When the bladder or intestine becomes distended with waste material they cause pressure and discomfort. The person becomes restless until the waste material is disposed off and the pressure relieved.

Sex Motive

With the onset of puberty the sex glands start functioning and as a result the sex drive is stimulated. Though it is a physiological drive it is regulated by customs, traditions and religious conventions. A number of taboos are associated with the satisfaction of sex drive. This motive within certain limits influences man's behavior a great deal. Its adequate satisfaction is desirable for the maintenance of normal mental health. It is considered a biological drive since it is dependent on physiological conditions. Unlike hunger and thirst, sex is not essential for survival of the individual but is necessary for the survival of the species. The initial drive for sex activity comes from nerves tensions within the body set up by sex hormones. Its expression is subject to moral codes and civil law. We have to sublimate this sex drive by engaging ourselves with art and painting, creative writing, dramatics, etc.

The nurse has to recognize all these basic needs and drives in her patients. She has to remember that due to illness many of these drives become weak and abnormal in their expression. She should strive to satisfy as many basic needs of the patient as possible.

Social or Secondary Motives

Human beings are not only biological but also social beings. Therefore human behavior is activated by social motives such as affiliation motives, need for status, power motives and social approval. These motives develop through relationship with people.

Affiliation Motives

In general, human beings love company and resent loneliness as pleasures of life cannot be enjoyed alone. Even the simple routine activities of eating and drinking cannot be enjoyed without company. The need to be with other people is referred to as the affiliation need. It is revealed by a need to be attached to others through friendship, sociability or group membership. Need to rely on others also called the dependency motive is one form of the need for affiliation. The motive of affiliation is universally seen in all human cultures.

Need for Status

Most individuals have a desire to demonstrate some standing or position among the people of their society or group. Nobody likes to be considered inferior.

Power Motive

The desire to be in a position of control, to be the boss, to give orders, to command respect and obedience is called the power motive. Power motive directs the behavior of dictators, gang leaders and the builders of fraudulent financial empires.

Social Approval

We try our best to avoid doing anything that may evoke social disapproval. We often show an almost compulsive tendency to conform to the norms set by our social group.

A nurse has to remember that all such social motives are at work in the life of her patients, colleagues and in her own daily relationships. She has to note the manifestations of these motives in her patients carefully because some of them adopt peculiar means to satisfy them.

Personal Motives

Though allied with physiological needs and common social motives, personal motives are no longer common as they are so much individualized. They are our wants and aspirations which are not shared commonly by others. Need for achievement, vocational ambitions and life goals, specific interests, habits and attitudes, levels of aspiration, curiosity and fear are our personal motives.

Need for Achievement

Achievement motivation refers to a drive towards some standard of excellence. People with high need for achievement prefer tasks which would promise success and are moderately difficult. David C McClelland has found that while high achievers tend to succeed, low achievers tend to avoid failures. High achievers challenge failures and work harder while low achievers accept failure and settle for less difficult tasks. High achievers prefer personal responsibility and like to get feedback about their works.

Vocational Ambitions and Life Goals

These desires though common to all, there is something unique about each one's desires. These are powerful determinants of our behavior.

Levels of Aspiration

Levels of aspiration imply the degrees of expectation which a person has i.e., how much he expects to accomplish or achieve. We may have the same ambition or life goal but may have different levels of aspiration. In general, people tend to set their goals slightly higher than the level they are sure of attaining. This is a healthy tendency for progress. However, there are a few who set their level of aspiration much higher or lower in comparison to their actual level of performance leading to frustrations and disappointments. Repeated failure may lower the level of aspiration.

Force of Habit

A habit which has been formed acts as a drive and compels us to continue with the accustomed ways of doing things. In other words, habits once formed persist and influence our behavior greatly.

Interests and Attitudes

The interests we have developed and the attitudes we have formed color our everyday behavior in many ways.

Curiosity

This is a motive which is close to exploration. Exploration is a drive that aids the satisfaction of curiosity. The extent of man's knowledge and experience widens as a result of this drive. Curiosity thus adds to our competency.

Fear

Fear is a learned motive. It motivates individuals to escape from fear producing situations. Fear may also interfere with the satisfaction of other motives.

A nurse should understand that personal motives are no longer common. They are our wants and aspirations which are not shared commonly by others. She has to put extra-attention to understand the personal motives.

Unconscious Motives

Unconscious motives are those of which we are not aware of. They may be in the form of our repressed desires or wishes or complexes. They determine our irrational fears or phobias, eccentric likes and dislikes, chronic headaches and gastric troubles (for which we have no organic causes) and also neuroses and insanities.

According to Freud, it is the unconscious mind that guides, directs and motivates dreams. The root cause of mental diseases is traced to the unconscious mind.

THEORIES OF MOTIVATION

Theories of motivation try to provide general sets of principles to guide our understanding of the urges, wants, needs, desires and goals which fall under the category of motivation **(Table 7.1)**.

Table 7.1: Major approaches to motivation

Theory	Main points
Instinct	◆ Innate biological instincts guide behavior
Drive reduction	◆ Behavior is guided by biological needs and learned ways of reducing drives arising from those needs
Arousal	◆ People seek to maintain an optimal level of physiological arousal which differs from person-to-person ◆ Maximum performance occurs at optimal level of arousal
Incentive	◆ External stimuli direct and energize behavior
Hierarchy of needs	◆ Needs form a hierarchy ◆ Lower order needs must be fulfilled before higher-order needs are met

1. Instinct Theory of Motivation

According to instinct theories people are motivated to behave in certain ways because they are evolutionarily programmed to do so. An example of this in the animal world is seasonal migration. These animals do not learn to do this; it is instead an inborn pattern of behavior.

William James created a list of human instincts that included such things as attachment, play, shame, anger, fear, shyness, modesty and love. The main problem with this theory is that it did not really explain behavior, it just described it. By the1920s, though instinct theories were pushed aside in favor of other motivational theories, contemporary evolutionary psychologists still continued to study the influence of genetics and heredity on human behavior.

According to William McDougall all behavioral acts are essentially instinctive and this instinctive behavior is found to have three aspects:

1. Cognitive (knowing)

2. Affective (feeling)
3. Conative (acting or doing)

For example, when a child sees a monkey coming towards him, he first sees the monkey, secondly experiences an emotion of fear and finally tries to run away. Thus all human behaviors could be explained in terms of some instinct.

2. Drive Theory (Push Theory of Motivation)

Drive theory was developed by Clark Leonard Hull in 1943. According to drive theory of motivation people are motivated to take certain actions so as to reduce the internal tension caused by unmet needs. For example, a person might be motivated to consume food to reduce the internal state of hunger **(Figure 7.2)**. Humans and other animals are motivated by four drives: hunger, thirst, sex and avoidance of pain. This theory is useful in explaining behaviors that have a strong biological component such as hunger or thirst. The problem with the drive theory of motivation is that these behaviors are not always motivated purely by physiological needs. For example, people often eat even when they are not really hungry.

Drive theories might be described as the 'push theories of motivation'. This is because behavior is 'pushed' towards the goals by driving states within the person. Drive theories say—when an internal drive state is aroused the individual is pushed to engage in a behavior that will lead to the goal thus reducing the intensity of the drive state. Motivation consists of:

- A drive state
- Goal-directed behavior initiated by the drive state
- Attainment of an appropriate goal
- Relief on reaching the goal leading to subjective satisfaction and reduction in the drive state

The sequence of events can be depicted using a motivational cycle **(Figure 7.3)**.

Drive theory includes the influence of learning in secondary drives. Primary drives are those which arise from basic biological needs such as hunger, thirst and elimination, etc. However, through the process of conditioning and learning people can acquire other drives. These learned drives are known as secondary drives. People are said to have learned drives for power, aggression or achievement, etc. Such learned driving states become enduring characteristics of the particular person and push him towards appropriate goals.

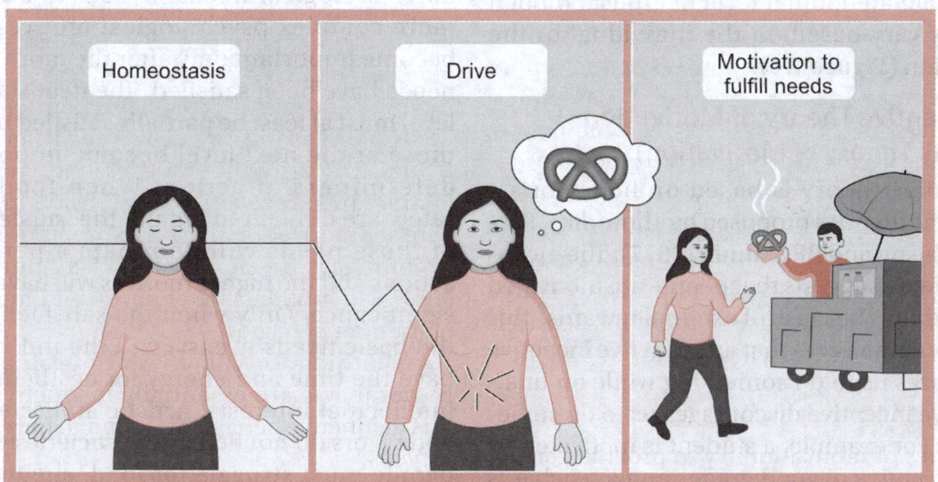

Figure 7.2: Drive theory

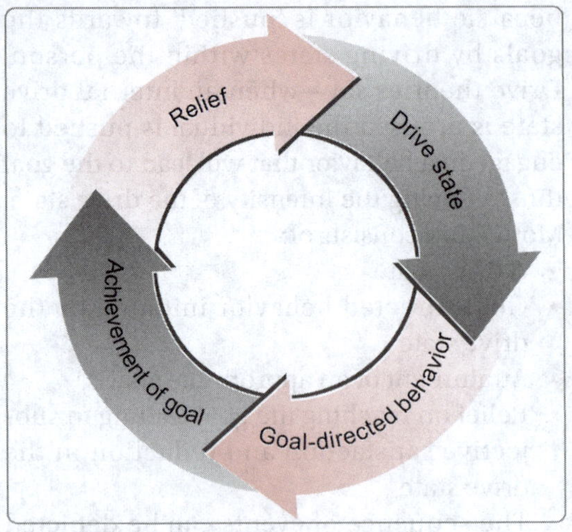

Figure 7.3: Motivational cycle

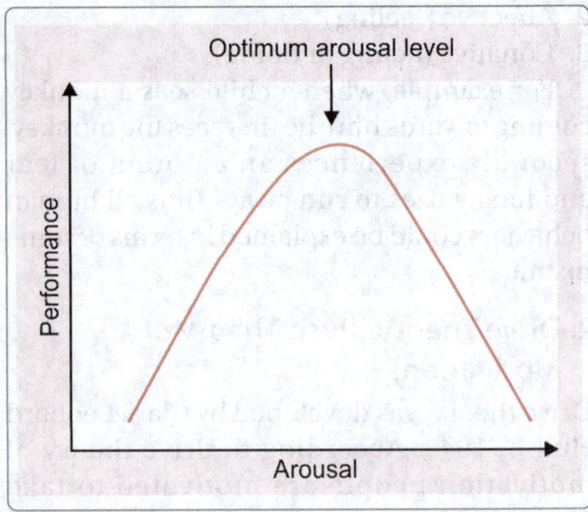

Figure 7.4: Arousal theory of motivation

3. Arousal Theory of Motivation

Arousal is the level of alertness, wakefulness and activation caused by activity in the central nervous system. The optimal level of arousal varies with person and activity. The arousal theory of motivation suggests that people take certain actions to either increase or decrease levels of arousal. For example, when arousal levels get too low a person might go for a jog or watch an exciting movie. On the other hand when the arousal levels get too high the person would probably look for ways to relax either by way of meditation or reading a book. According to this theory, we are motivated to maintain an optimal level of arousal though it may vary based on the individual or the situation **(Figure 7.4)**.

4. Incentive Theory of Motivation (Pull Theory of Motivation)

Incentive theory is based on behaviorists learning theories proposed by Thorndike, Pavlov, Watson and BF Skinner (1977). The incentive theory suggests that people are motivated to do things because of external rewards. This theory emphasizes that an attractive incentive energizes us to do something while an unattractive incentive discourages us to do something. For example, a student is motivated by the incentive of good grades and a teacher is motivated by the incentive of a promotion.

In contrast with the push of drive theories, incentive theories are pull theories of motivation. They stress on the principle that environmental stimuli may motivate behavior by 'pulling' people towards them. We are pushed by our drives and pulled by incentives. While drive is a need, incentive is a reward **(Figure 7.5)**.

5. Maslow's Hierarchy of Needs

Abraham Maslow (1908–1970), a leader in the development of humanistic psychology proposed an interesting way of classifying human motives **(Figure 7.6)**. He assumed a hierarchy of motives ascending from the basic biological needs present at birth to more complex psychological motives that become important only after the more basic needs have been satisfied. The needs at one level must at least be partially satisfied before those at the next level become important determiners of action. When food and safety are difficult to obtain, the satisfaction of these needs will dominate a person's actions and the higher motives will have little significance. Only when the satisfaction of the basic needs is easy, will the individual have the time and energy for aesthetic and intellectual interests. Artistic and scientific endeavors do not flourish in societies where people must struggle for food, shelter and safety.

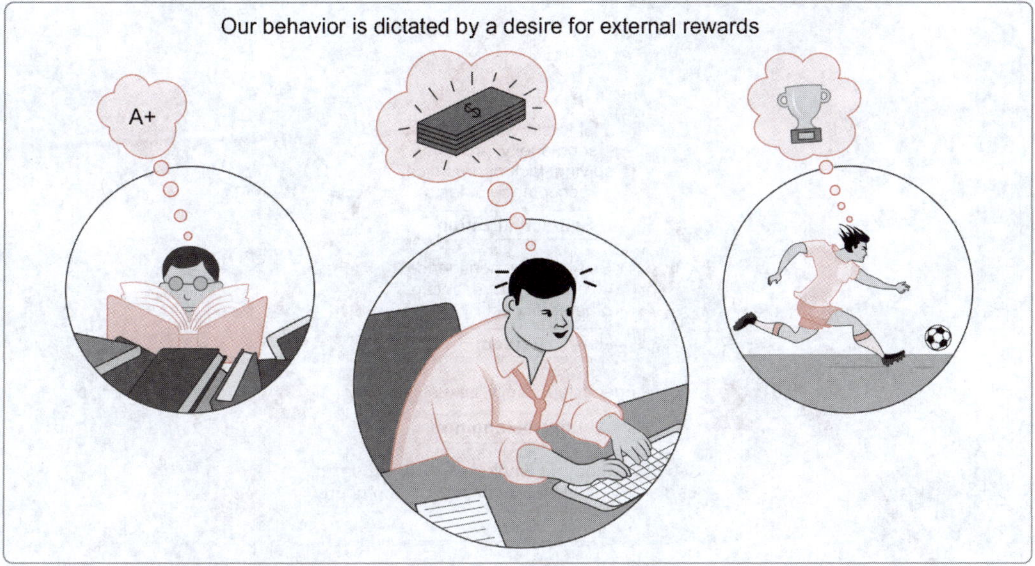

Figure 7.5: Incentive theory of motivation

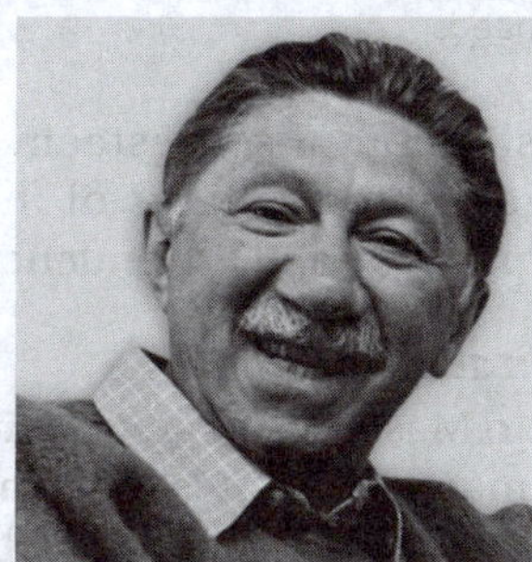

Figure 7.6: Abraham Maslow, leader in the development of humanistic psychology

One of the basic themes underlying Maslow's theory is that motivation affects the person as a whole rather than just a part. Maslow believed that people are motivated to seek personal goals which make their lives rewarding and meaningful.

Abraham Maslow suggested that five basic classes of needs or motives influence human behavior. According to Maslow, needs at the lowest level of hierarchy must be satisfied before people can be motivated by higher-level goals **(Figure 7.7)**. According to Maslow the five levels of motives from bottom to the top of the hierarchy are:

Physiological Needs

Physiological needs are the most basic, powerful and urgent of all human needs that are essential to physical survival. Even if one of these needs remains unsatisfied the individual rapidly becomes dominated by it making all other needs secondary. The needs included in this group are food, water, oxygen, activity, sleep, sex, homeostasis and excretion.

Safety and Security Needs

Once the physiological needs are fairly well-satisfied, safety and security needs predominate. The needs included in this level are the need for security of body, employment, resources, morality, family, health and property. Safety needs are of greater importance in childhood. The failure to satisfy the needs of children may make them fearful and insecure adults unable to cope with the ordinary demands of the environment.

Need for Love and Belongingness

These needs become prominent when the physiological and safety/security needs have been met. A person at this level longs for affectionate relationship with others and for a place in his family and social groups. The

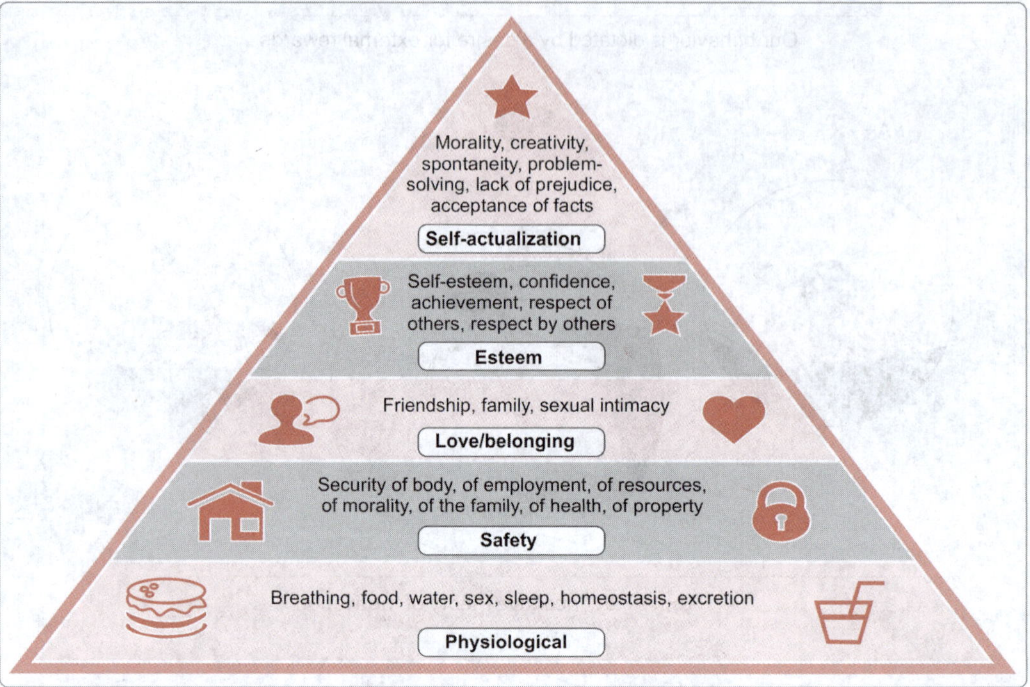

Figure 7.7: Maslow's hierarchy of needs

secure individual will be able to reach out for friends, affiliate with a group and ultimately take on the responsibilities in marriage of being both a spouse and a parent. The needs included in this level are need for friendship, family and sexual intimacy.

Self-esteem Needs

Once people find themselves loved and being members of an accepting circle they then need to think highly of themselves and have others think highly of them. They want self-respect and the respect, confidence and admiration of others. Maslow divided these needs into two types—(1) self-respect and (2) respect from others.

Self-respect includes a person's desire for competence, confidence, achievement and independence. Respect from others includes his desire for prestige, reputation, status, recognition, appreciation and acceptance from others. Satisfaction of self-esteem needs generates feelings of self-confidence, self-worth and a sense of being useful and necessary in the world.

Dissatisfaction of self-esteem needs in contrast generates feelings of inferiority, weakness, passivity and dependency.

Self-actualization

According to Maslow, self-actualization is the highest human motive. It is the need for self-fulfillment, the sense that one is becoming everything that he is capable of being. A person who has achieved this highest-level presses towards the full use of his talents, capacities and potentialities. In short, the self-actualized person is someone who has reached the peak of his potential. Characteristics that distinguish self-actualized people from others are listed in **Box 7.1**.

Maslow's hierarchy provides a framework for nursing assessment and for understanding the needs of the patient at all levels so that interventions to meet the needs become a part of the care plans.

MOTIVES AND BEHAVIOR

- Motives act as an immediate force to energize, direct, sustain and stop a behavior.

Box 7.1: Characteristics of self-actualized individual

- They are realistically oriented
- They accept themselves for what they are
- Their thought is unconventional and spontaneous
- They are problem centered
- They have a need for privacy
- They are independent
- Their appreciation of people is fresh
- They have spiritual experiences
- They identify with people
- They have intimate relationships
- They are democratic
- They have a good sense of humor
- They do not confuse between means and ends
- They are creative and non-confirmist
- They appreciate the environment

- Motives are a powerful tool for explaining behavior.
- Motives help us to make predictions about behavior in many different situations.
- Motives do not tell us exactly what will happen but only give us an idea about the range of things a person will do. A person with a need to achieve will work hard in school, business, work situations, etc.
- Motives are inner forces that control an individual's behavior in a subtle manner.

Nursing Implications of Motives

The nurse should know how behavior is motivated by different needs. The nurse should understand the role of primary, social, personal and unconscious motives in human behavior. She should understand her own motives so that she can better understand patient motives.

- With an insight into the dynamics of motivation she can maintain her mental health and stay cheerful.
- Knowledge about physiological needs such as hunger and sleep help her in the physical care of the patient.
- Knowledge of psychological needs give her an insight into how to use them favorably for patient cure.
- It gives her an insight into the etiology of patient behavior leading to a better understanding.

Understanding motives in a patient helps the nurse in the following ways:

- To recognize motives underlying the behavior of a patient.
- To recognize patient's needs and desires.
- To build a good relationship between the patient and the health team members.
- To provide priority care (i.e., meeting primary needs before meeting other needs).
- To satisfy patient needs.
- To promote healing and health in the patient.

Knowledge of human needs assists nurses in responding therapeutically to patient's behavior and in understanding themselves and their own responses to needs. Human needs serve as a framework for assessing behavior, assigning priorities to desired outcomes and planning nursing interventions.

EMOTIONS

Etymologically the word 'emotion' is derived from the Latin word, 'emovere' which means 'to stir up' or 'to excite'. In common usage emotion is referred to as a subjective feeling.

Feelings are simple experiences of the affective type, pleasant or unpleasant. Emotions are more complex affective experiences in which the whole individual is stirred up. Emotions are feelings or affective experiences characterized by physiological changes that generally lead them to perform some or the other types of behavioral acts.

Definitions

- Emotions are conscious mental reactions, such as anger or fear subjectively experienced as strong feelings usually directed toward a specific object and typically accompanied by physiological and behavioral changes in the body.
- Emotion is an affective experience that accompanies generalized inner adjustment and mental and physiological stirred-up

states in the individual that shows itself in his overt behavior.

—**Crow and Crow (1973)**

COMPONENTS OF EMOTION

Dennis Coon described four components of emotion **(Figure 7.8)**.

Subjective Feeling

Subjective feelings are what you believe and what you are feeling. It is conscious and an intellectual perception of a situation. If the situation is intense enough it may provoke an emotion. Emotional feelings are experienced before expression.

Emotional Expression or Expressive Behavior

There are three ways in which an emotion can be expressed:

- **Facial:** The face is believed to be the most expressive part of the body. Some emotions like guilt, joy, anger, etc., can be perceived fairly accurately through facial expressions.
- **Vocal:** Voice also tells us about an emotional state of an individual. A scream communicates fear, surprise or pain; a trembling voice means sorrow or disappointment; a loud, sharp, high pitched voice means anger, irritability or frustration. Slow monotonous voice usually communicates sadness.
- **Bodily movements or gestures:** Bodily movements or gestures also indicate the emotional state of an individual. In anger, a person clenches his fists and moves forward to attack. In fear a person runs away. In joy the person is excited, holds his head high and chest out.

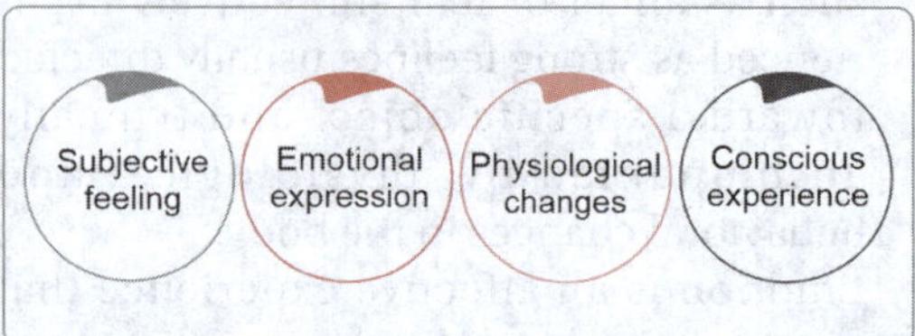

Figure 7.8: Components of emotion

Physiological Changes

Physiological changes occurring during an emotional state are mainly due to the autonomic nervous system and the endocrine gland system. The autonomic nervous system has two sub divisions—*sympathetic division* and *parasympathetic division*. The sympathetic division of the autonomic nervous system prepares the body for emergency action during aroused states. It causes discharge of hormones, epinephrine (adrenaline) and norepinephrine (noradrenaline). Adrenaline gets circulated to different parts of the body through blood and is responsible for the following physical changes:

- Increased blood pressure (BP) and heart rate
- Changes in the rate of respiration
- Dilation of pupils
- Sweating and decreased secretion of saliva
- Increased blood sugar level
- Decreased mobility of the gastrointestinal tract
- Erect hair on the skin
- Muscular tensions and tremors

When a period of intense emotion ends, the physiological response of the body is taken over by the parasympathetic branch of the nervous system. This system slows down the entire metabolism of the body to bring it into balance once again. The parasympathetic system acts much more slowly than the sympathetic system. This is why the body responds very quickly to an intense emotion but recovers its balance very slowly. The physiological changes produced by the parasympathetic nervous system are as follows:

- Reduction of heart rate and BP
- Diversion of blood to the internal organs and digestive tract
- Regulation of salt and water level in the body
- Building up and conservation of body energy

Conscious Experience

An emotion is not only a pattern of bodily changes but also an experience. Emotional experience is generally a conscious feeling. Feelings and emotional experiences are both important indicators to assess an individual's emotion.

TYPES OF EMOTIONS

According to Paul Eckman, 1972 there are six types of emotions—fear, disgust, anger, surprise, happiness and sadness **(Figure 7.9)**. In 1999, Eckman expanded this list of emotions and included embarrassment, shame, excitement, pride, satisfaction and amusement.

Happiness: It is pleasant emotion accompanied by a sense of well-being and satisfaction. It is often expressed by smiling or speaking in a cheerful tone or voice.

Sadness: It is unpleasant emotion accompanied by sadness, grief, disappointment or hopelessness. It is often expressed by crying, being quite or withdrawing from others.

Fear: It is an unpleasant emotion in response to actual or perceived danger or threat. It can increase heart rate, cause racing thoughts or trigger the fight or flight response.

Disgust: It is a strong feeling of aversion towards something offensive. It can be triggered by a physical experience of seeing or smelling. Moral disgust may occur when someone sees another person doing something immoral.

Anger: It is an intense emotional state involving a strong feeling of being annoyed or upset of something wrong or bad. It can be expressed with facial expressions, such as frowning, yelling or violent behavior.

Surprise: It is a feeling which occurs when something unexpected happens. It can be pleasant or unpleasant. When surprised the person might open his mouth or gasp.

CHARACTERISTICS OF EMOTIONS

- Emotions are prevalent in every living organism
- Emotional experiences are associated with some drives
- Emotions are the product of perception
- The core of an emotion is feeling
- Every emotional experience brings physical and psychological changes in the organism

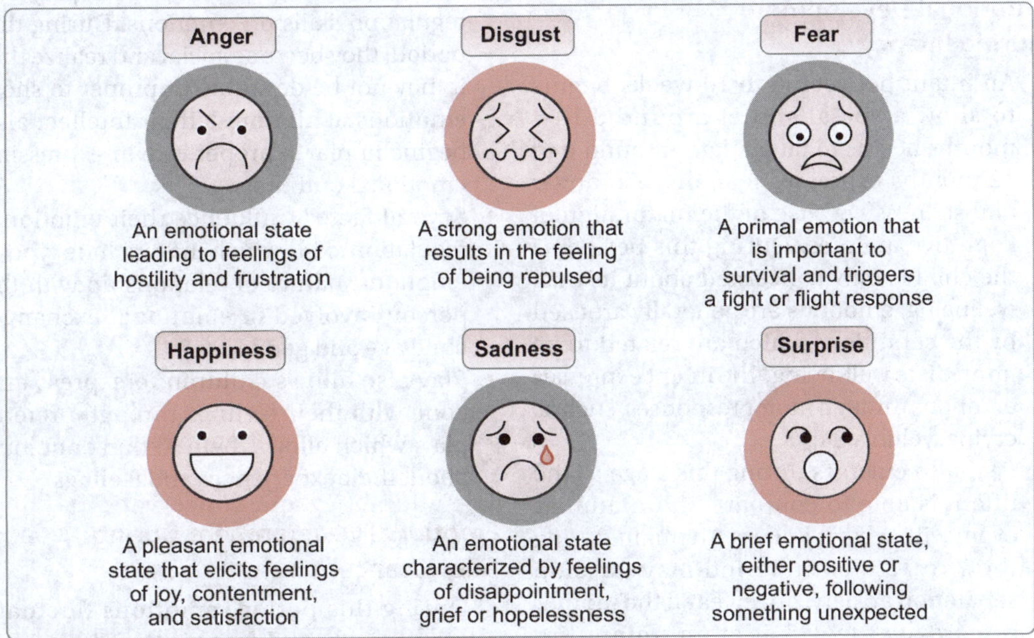

Figure 7.9: Types of emotions.

- Emotions are present at all stages of development
- Emotions differ from person to person and are most individual
- Emotions rise abruptly but die slowly
- An emotion once aroused tends to persist and leaves behind an emotional mood

DEVELOPMENT OF EMOTIONS

Development of emotions is one of the key aspects of human growth and development. Emotions such as happiness, anger, fear and sadness play a greater role in personality development.

- Emotional development refers to an ability to recognize, express and manage feelings at different stages of life and have empathy for the feelings of others.
- Emotional development is the gradual learning process of a person to experience, recognize and express various emotions.
- Emotional development begins during infancy and continues into adulthood. Both positive and negative emotions are largely influenced by the relationship with parents, siblings and peers.

Emotional Development During Infancy

- An infant between 6 to 10 weeks begins to show a social smile, around 3 to 4 months begins to laugh, later around 6 to 12 months expresses fear, disgust, anger and sadness because of the maturation of cognitive abilities. During this period as the child is only concerned about its own wellbeing, emotions are generally aroused by the conditions which are related to its immediate well-being. The infant expresses emotions through motor responses, such as crying, yelling, etc.
- Fear also emerges during this stage as the infant is able to compare an unfamiliar event with what it knows. An infant during the 7 to 12 month period may develop separation anxiety, cry in fear if the mother or caregiver leaves it at an unfamiliar location.
- An infant will respond to its emotions to the degree that their caregivers respond and then from their emotional facial clues.

Emotional Development During Childhood

- During toddler period, the child expresses shame, embarrassment and pride. During this period, it acquires language and learns to express emotions of affection, distress, anger, etc.
- At the age of two, the child begins to acquire complex emotional response of empathy by reading other's emotional cues and understanding their perspectives.
- At the age of 3, the child understands societal rules regarding appropriate expression of emotions.
- At around 4 years, the child acquires the ability to alter its emotional expressions. It can display external expressions that do not match with its internal feelings.
- Parents help the preschooler acquire skills to cope with negative emotional states by teaching, modeling, reasoning and explaining the situation.
- Children during ages 7 to 11 display self regulation skills on emotions. During this period, they become social and realize that it may not be desirable or proper to show emotions at all times. Their intellect also begins to play a proper role in expressing emotional outbursts.
- Several factors influence their emotional regulation skills which may include type of emotions, nature of relationship with the person involved in emotional exchange, child age and gender.
- Play also allows children to express and cope with their feelings through pretend play, which allows them to think out loud about their experiences and feelings.

Emotional Development During Adolescence

- During this period, emotions fluctuate very quickly and frequently. There is so much uncertainty in their emotional states that within a short span of time they move from being extremely happy to being extremely sad and moody. As individuals during this period experience strong emotional energy it is difficult for them to exercise control over their emotions. The sudden functioning of sexual glands and tremendous increase in physical energy makes them restless.

- Another factor that plays a significant role in regulation of emotions is that they are very sensitive to other's evaluation, more self-aware and self conscious.
- Boys are less likely than girls to disclose their fearful emotions during times of distress.

EMOTIONAL DISORDERS

It refers to a mental disorder in which one's thoughts and emotions are disturbed to a great extent and not in a proper state.

According to the American Psychological Association's dictionary of psychology, emotional disorders include psychological disorders where people have mal-adjustive emotional reactions that are inappropriate or disproportionate to their cause. In a clinical setting, emotional disorders are termed as mood disorders. Common mood disorders include:

- Depressive disorder
- Bipolar disorder
- Premenstrual dysphoric disorder
- Anxiety disorder
- Obsessive compulsive disorder

CHANGES IN EMOTIONAL REACTIONS

Emotional reactions affect the autonomic nervous system the most. The following external, internal and psychological changes occur during emotional states **(Figures 7.10 and 7.11)**.

External Changes

Facial expressions: They differ in different emotional reactions. The face is flushed in anger and pale in fear. Mouth turns down in unpleasant emotions and turns up in pleasant emotions.

Bodily movement and gestures: Unexpected fearful situation might cause a startle pattern in which the eyes close, mouth widens, head and neck are thrust forward. In anger one may clench ones fists and move to attack.

Voice disturbances: A tremor or a break in the voice may denote deep sorrow. A loud, sharp high-pitched voice usually denotes anger. Speech is low and monotonous in dejection and sadness and rapid in tension and excitement.

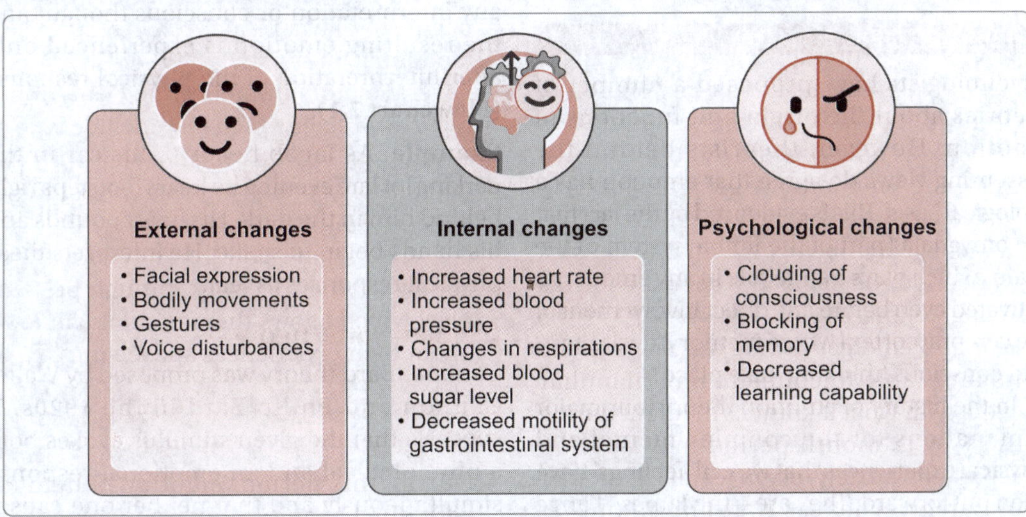

Figure 7.10: Changes in emotional reactions

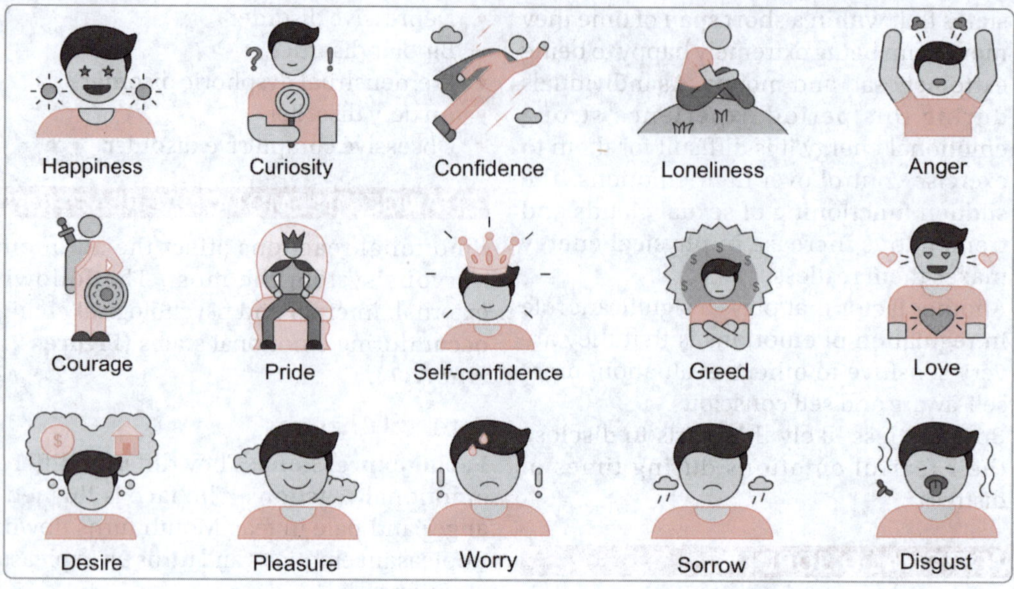

Figure 7.11: Various emotional reactions

Internal Changes

During fear and anger the pulse rate or heart rate increases. Blood pressure increases during emotional excitement. During excitement breathing is in short quick gasps but in depression it is slow.

Psychological Changes

During emotional experiences perception, learning, consciousness and memory are affected.

THEORIES OF EMOTION

Psychologists have proposed a number of theories about the origin and functions of emotion. However, theorists behind the dissenting views do agree that emotion has a biological basis. This is evidenced by the fact that the amygdala (part of the limbic system of the brain) which plays a large role in any emotion is activated even before any direct involvement of the cerebral cortex (where memory, awareness, and conscious 'thinking' take place).

In the history of emotion theory four major explanations for the complex mental and physical experiences that we call 'feelings' have been put forward. They are—the James- Lange theory in the1920s, the Cannon-Bard theory in the 1930s, the Schachter–Singer theory in the 1960s, and most recently the Lazarus theory developed in the 1980s and '90s **(Figure 7.12)**.

James–Lange Theory

In 1880, S William James formulated the first modern theory of emotion at almost the same time a Danish psychologist Carl Lange reached the same conclusion independently. The James–Lange theory proposes that an event or stimulus causes a physiological arousal without any interpretation or conscious thought and the resulting emotion is experienced only after interpretation of the physical response **(Flowchart 7.1)**.

Example: As Jacob heads to his car in the parking lot late evening he hears footsteps right behind him in the dark. His heart pounds and his hands begin to shake. He interprets these physical responses as fear.

Cannon–Bard Theory

Cannon–Bard theory was proposed by Walter Cannon and Philip Bard in the 1920s. It suggests that the given stimulus evokes both a physiological and an emotional response simultaneously and that neither one causes the other. According to Cannon's theory,

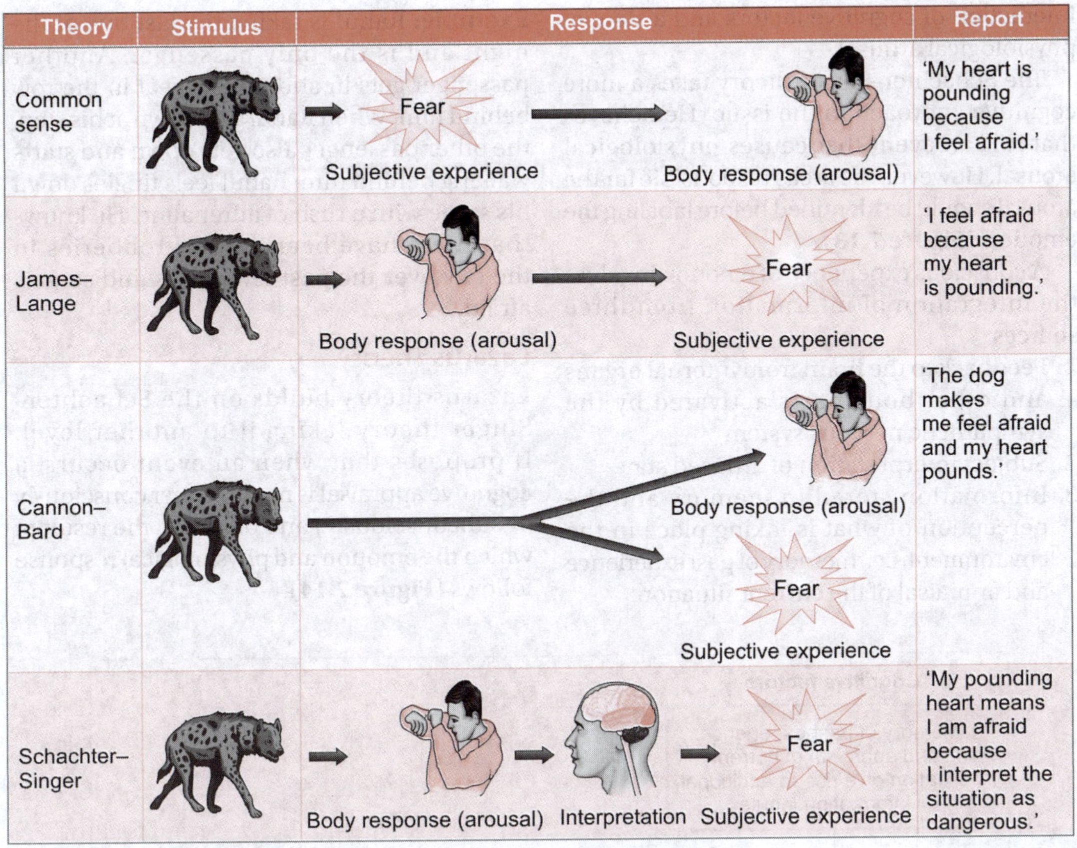

Theory	Stimulus	Response	Report
Common sense		Fear → Subjective experience → Body response (arousal)	'My heart is pounding because I feel afraid.'
James–Lange		Body response (arousal) → Fear → Subjective experience	'I feel afraid because my heart is pounding.'
Cannon–Bard		Body response (arousal); Fear → Subjective experience	'The dog makes me feel afraid and my heart pounds.'
Schachter–Singer		Body response (arousal) → Interpretation → Fear → Subjective experience	'My pounding heart means I am afraid because I interpret the situation as dangerous.'

Figure 7.12: Theories of emotion

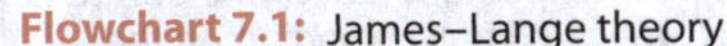

Flowchart 7.1: James–Lange theory

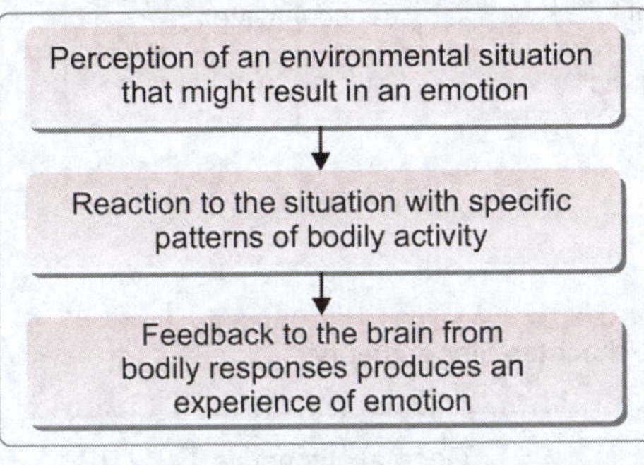

Flowchart 7.2: Cannon–Bard theory

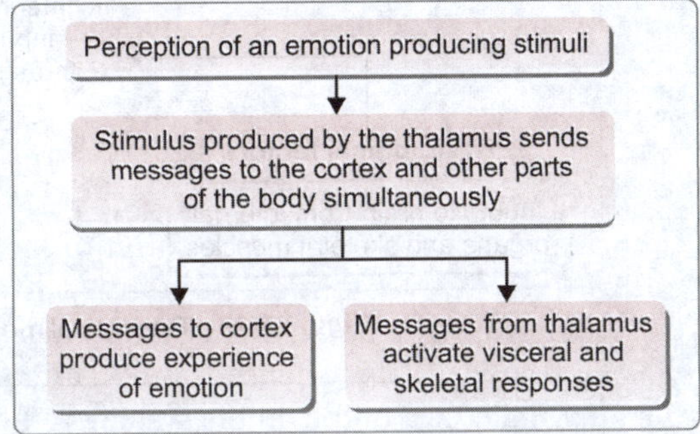

the emotional experience occurs as soon as the cortex receives the message from the thalamus. It does not depend upon the feedback from internal organs and skeletal responses **(Flowchart 7.2).**

Example: Manisha is home alone and hears a creaking sound in the hallway outside her room. She begins to tremble and sweat and feels afraid.

Schachter–Singer Theory (1962)

Schachter-Singer theory is called 'cognitive theory of emotion'. Schachter proposed that emotional states are a function of the interaction of cognitive factors and a state of physiological arousal.

The Schachter–Singer theory takes a more cognitive approach to the issue. He believes that it is an event that causes physiological arousal. However, the areas responsible for the arousal should be identified before labeling the emotion **(Figure 7.13)**.

A conscious experience of emotion involves the integration of information from three sources:

1. Feedback to the brain from internal organs and other body parts activated by the sympathetic nervous system
2. Subject interpretation of aroused state
3. Information stored in memory and the perception of what is taking place in the environment, i.e., memory of past experience and appraisal of the current situation.

Example: Rahul is taking the last bus of the night and is the only passenger. Another passenger gets in and takes a seat in the row behind him. When Rahul gets down at his stop, the other passenger also gets down and starts walking behind him. Rahul feels tingles down his spine with a rush of adrenaline. He knows that there have been several robberies in the city over the past few weeks and so gets afraid.

Lazarus Theory

Lazarus theory builds on the Schachter-Singer theory taking it to another level. It proposes that when an event occurs, a cognitive appraisal is made (either consciously or subconsciously) and based on the result of which the emotion and physiological response follows **(Figure 7.14)**.

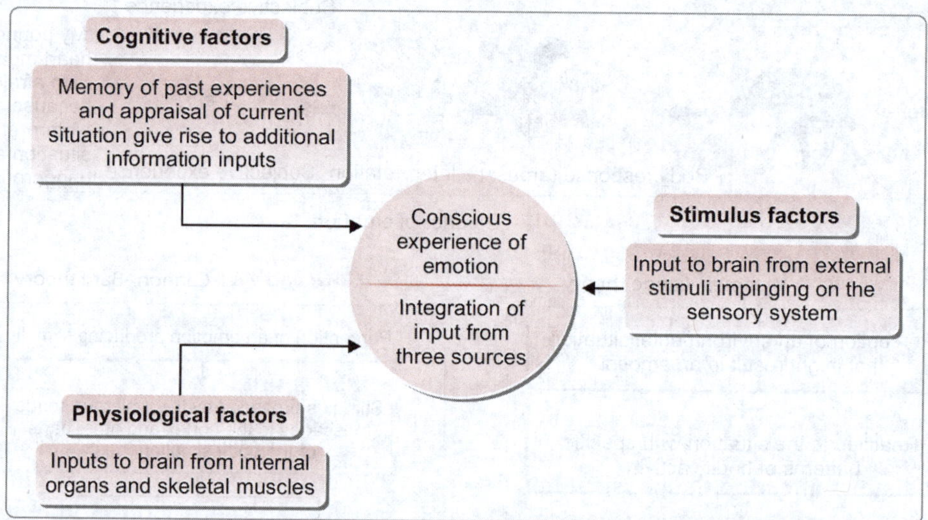

Figure 7.13: Theoretical model of Schachter–Singer theory

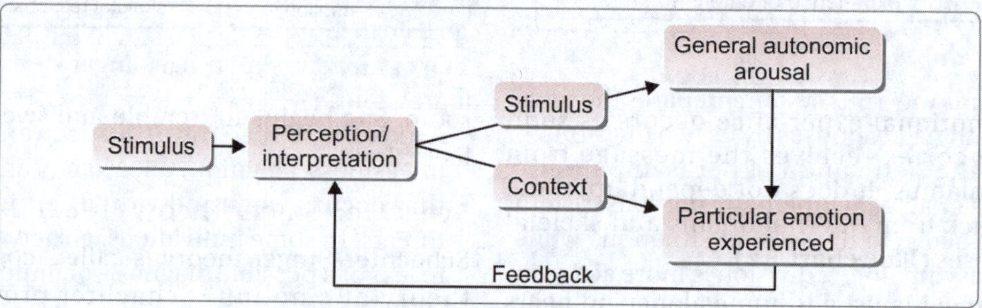

Figure 7.14: Lazarus theory

Example: Rakshit is buying a few items at the super store when two young men in hooded sweatshirts enter the store in a hurry with hands in their jacket pockets. He thinks that they are here to rob the place. He gets scared and feels like he might throw up.

While each of these theories is based on research there is no absolute proof as yet how emotions arise in our bodies and minds or what determines our own individual experiences of them. What we do know is that feelings are a powerful force to be reckoned with and should never be belittled.

EMOTIONAL ADJUSTMENTS

Emotional adjustment (also referred to as emotional equilibrium, emotional stability, neuroticism, personal adjustment or psychological adjustment) is the maintenance of emotional equilibrium in the face of internal and external stressors. This is facilitated by cognitive processes of acceptance and adaptation. An example would be to maintain emotional control and coping behavior in the face of an identity crisis.

Emotions play an important role in human life. Under ordinary circumstances the physiological reactions during an emotion facilitate adjustment in an individual. These physiological reactions last for a little time and do not have any harmful effects on our body. But when an emotion recurs again and again and lingers for a longer time it may lead to distress affecting the physical health adversely. Autonomic nervous system, brain structures and hormones play an important role in emotional adjustment.

Autonomic Nervous System

Autonomic nervous system prepares the body for emotional responses by its two divisions—(1) sympathetic and (2) parasympathetic nervous system. Sympathetic nervous system is more active in unpleasant situations while the parasympathetic division is more active in pleasant situations. Strong emotional reactions like fear, anger, etc., stimulate the sympathetic nervous system that releases hormones from the adrenal gland.

The parasympathetic nervous system makes us calm by inhibiting the release of these hormones.

Brain Structures

Hypothalamus and limbic system are the structures which control emotional systems by signaling the pituitary gland to release epinephrine which is associated with the sympathetic nervous system.

Amygdala is another key player within the limbic system. It receives information from the cortex and thalamus, involves in processing emotions like patterns of attack, defense and flight. Right hemisphere regulates facial expressions while the left hemisphere deciphers emotional tone from the messages we fear.

Hormones

Hormones play an important role in regulation of emotions. During emotional states there is an increase in hormonal level in blood and urine.

EMOTIONS IN SICKNESS

People react differently to illness. Individual's emotional reactions depend on the nature of illness, their attitude towards it, the reaction of others to it, patient's perception of illness, visibility of symptoms, availability of support system, economic variables and patient's coping skills. Short-term, non-life threatening illness evokes few emotional changes. Severe illness, particularly one that is life-threatening can lead to more extensive emotional reactions such as anxiety, shock, fear, anger, denial and depression.

- **Anxiety:** A feeling of apprehension, uneasiness, agitation, uncertainty and fear that occurs when individuals anticipate threats. In some individuals, anxiety is due to fear of a possible diagnosis or impending surgery, etc.

- **Worry:** A mild form of anxiety characterized by preoccupation of a problem. Common anxiety producing factors in a hospital environment are separation from significant others, lack of privacy, lack of understanding of hospital language, strange sights, sounds, odors, etc.
- **Fear:** An emotional state characterized by expected harm or unpleasantness.
- **Shock:** A response when patient or families are informed of a severe or life-threatening illness. They hear what has been said but fail to respond or respond in a totally inappropriate manner.
- **Denial:** A mechanism by which the patient or family avoids emotional conflict and anxiety by refusing to acknowledge difficult facts. For example, a family knowing that their loved one has cancer may deny the diagnosis and attempt to continue as though nothing were wrong. Short-term denial can be an effective way of coping with illness.
- **Anger:** An emotional state characterized by feelings of frustration and struggle with a threatening or unpleasant situation. Anger may have effects on patient's social or spiritual dimensions.
- **Depression:** An emotional state characterized by a dejected mood. It occurs due to the absence of cure or loss of personal control.

Handling Emotions in Self and Other

"Being aware of our internal emotional state and being more mindful and present with how our mind and body respond to situations enables us to manage stress better"

—**Annie Miller**

Emotions are reactions that human beings experience in response to events or situations. These are strongly linked to memory and known to have a strong influence on our daily lives. The type of emotion a person experiences is determined by the circumstance that triggers the emotion. We make decisions based on whether we are happy, angry, sad, bored, or frustrated. We also choose activities and hobbies based on the emotions they incite. Emotions are controlled by the limbic system in the brain.

Understanding emotions can help to improve emotional regulation and emotional resilience and attain lower levels of anxiety thereby navigating life with greater ease and stability. Although, positive emotions such as joy and happiness are easy to deal with, negative emotions are mostly difficult to handle. Negative emotions can be best handled in the following ways:

- **Identify emotions or emotional awareness:** It is the process of recognizing and acknowledging one's own feelings. Generally, emotions are accompanied by physical and mental reactions. Paying attention to one's own physical and mental cues can help the individual to identify what specific emotion he is experiencing.
- **Listen to emotions:** Emotions are expressed in various forms. For example, fears are expressed as rage, sleeplessness, headache or other psychological and physiological symptoms. Each one has to pay attention to these symptoms.
- **Understand the source of emotions:** Understanding the source of feelings will help to figure out the best ways to handle them.
- **Accept emotions:** All emotions including those one regards as 'irrational', 'immature' or even 'inappropriate' need to be recognized and accepted. Give some time to recognize emotions and accept that these emotions are common, when other people are in your situation, they might react in the same way. Everybody is unique; accept your emotions as they are.
- **Express yourself in a healthy and constructive manner:** Emotions can be expressed in following healthy ways.
  - Writing a diary, a letter, poem, song, story
  - Taking a walk
  - Exercising/dancing/bowling/jogging
  - Taking a hot bath/cold shower
  - Singing out loud/painting/playing computer games

- Reading comics or watching a comedy and laughing aloud
- Crying out loud or going to a sad movie
- Talking to friends
- Participating in your favorite activities, hobbies

- **Build positive emotions:** Make a habit to focus on what is good in your life even the little things. Noticing the good things even when you are feeling bad can help you shift the emotional balance from negative to positive.

ROLE OF NURSING IN CARING FOR EMOTIONALLY SICK CLIENT

As the nurses spend more time in communicating and providing direct care to the patient than any other hospital personnel they are in a better position to assess the psychological reactions of patients. They can understand their emotional needs and plan for appropriate nursing interventions. A few nursing interventions are:

Spend Time with Patients

- Listen while the patient is describing his feelings.
- Try to identify what is frightening to the patient and offer appropriate explanations.

Facilitate Verbalization of Feelings

- Allow the patient to explore his emotions/feelings. Verbalization often brings about a tremendous relief of tension.

Handling the Emotions

- Verbalization of distress is often accompanied by tearfulness. Many women get great relief from a good cry. Men should not be denied too. It is just a manifestation. Any cry should be handled with care and privacy and support given until composure is regained.
- Show acceptance for patient's behavior even if the anger is directed at the nurse.
- Try to determine the cause for anger and then deal with it as realistically as possible.
- Recognize that a patient using denial protects himself from something he does not wish to face.
- Deal with denial carefully and in cooperation with other health personnel.
- Try to help the patient find ways to cope with depression such as engaging in some useful activity.
- Show respect for patient's feelings.

Orientation of Patient to Health Care Facility

Provide detailed explanation of the patient care services and of rationale behind various medical and nursing procedures that the patient has to undergo with constant reassurances all along. This will alleviate the fear of unknown in patients.

Identification of Learning Needs of Patients

Learning needs of patients have to be identified. For example, a patient before surgery may worry about prognosis, pain, ambulation, dependency, etc. Imparting knowledge on these aspects will satisfy the patients need to know about his condition and treatment thus reducing his anxiety.

Provide Diversional Activities

Encourage pleasurable and tension reducing diversional activities considering the patient's condition within permissible limits. Many chronically-ill patients do not recognize their need for recreation. Offer praise in a sincere and appropriate manner as the patients make progress towards independence.

Taking Care of Insomnia, Food and Fluid Intake, Elimination Pattern

- Employ measures such as low environmental stimuli, light meals in the night, engaging in daytime activities, reading books, listening to music at bedtime to promote sleep.
- Nurses need to ensure adequate fluid intake and nutrition. Many patients in depression have little interest in food and

their nutritional status can decline sharply. Offer food of good nutritional quality. Provide small attractively served portions frequently and allow enough time for the patient to consume it.

- Ensure regular elimination pattern as constipation is a common complaint in distressed patients.

Maintain Cheerfulness and Humor

Human emotions can be contagious. So truly patients tend to enjoy having persons who are cheerful and yet professionally competent and sincere about their work. Humor can often relieve anxiety, stress and anger and help to develop warm relationships when used appropriately.

Seek Help of Mental Health Professionals

Patients who experience serious and prolonged disruptions in their lifestyle and relationships with significant others due to their illness and emotional reactions should know that psychiatric interventions can offer relief. Nurses should provide information about the sources of mental health care in community.

STRESS AND ADAPTATION

Concepts of Stress

- Stress is a universal phenomenon. All people experience it.
- Stress can have both positive and negative effects.
- Stress is produced by a change in the environment that is perceived as a challenge, threat or danger.
- Stress affects the whole person, i.e., in all the human dimensions (physical, emotional, intellectual, social and spiritual). Perception of stress and the responses to it are highly individualized not only from person-to-person but also from time-to-time in the same person.
- Stress is a condition in which the human system responds to changes in its normal balanced state.
- When a person faces a stressor, responses are referred to as coping strategies, coping responses or coping mechanisms.

Definitions

- Stress is the 'non-specific response of the body to any kind of demand made upon it'.

  —Selye (1956)

- Stress is the arousal of mind and body in response to demands made upon them.

  —Schafer (2000)

STRESSORS

Stressor can be any stimulus that causes an individual to experience stress. Three major categories of stressors are:

1. Catastrophic events
2. Important life events (personal stressors)
3. Daily hassles (background stressors)

Catastrophic Events

A catastrophe is a large scale disaster that affects numerous people and causes extensive damage. Catastrophes include earthquakes, hurricanes, war, toxic waste contamination and nuclear accidents. Stress induced by catastrophic events is better shared with those who have also experienced the disaster. This permits people to offer one another social support.

Important Life Events

Major life events such as death of a family member have immediate negative consequences which usually fade with time. Other major life events are loss of one's job, diagnosis of a life-threatening illness, parent or relative in family getting very sick, breaking up with a close friend, moving to a new school or home, starting a new job, brother or sister getting married, etc.

Typically personal stressors produce an immediate major reaction. For example, stress arising from the death of a loved one tends to be greatest just after the time of death. However, people begin to feel less stressed and are better able to cope with the loss after passage of certain time.

Daily Hassles

These are the minor irritants of life that we all face time and again—traffic delays, noise, pollution, weather, social events, work demands, dissatisfaction with school or job, being in an unhappy relationship, people's irritating behavior, not having enough time, too many things to do, concerns about standards, too many responsibilities and so on.

Daily hassles by themselves do not require much coping on the part of the individual though they certainly produce unpleasant emotions and moods. Yet, daily hassles can add up and ultimately produce as great a toll as a single, more stressful incident. In fact, the number of daily hassles that people face is associated with psychological symptoms and health problems such as sore throat, flu and backaches.

Uplifts: These are minor positive events that make one feel good. Uplifts range from relating well to a companion to finding ones surroundings pleasing. Common uplifts are relating well with spouse or lover or friend, completing the task, feeling healthy, getting enough sleep, eating out, spending time with family, meeting responsibilities and so on. These uplifts are associated with people's psychological health in just the opposite way that hassles are; the greater the number of uplift experiences the fewer the psychological symptoms people later report.

STRESS CYCLE

Stress follows a cycle of events which circle around and around. Each step increases the severity of the next step **(Figure 7.15)**.

1. Stressor

Stressor can be any stimulus that causes an individual to experience stress. Stressors include either positive or negative life events, e.g., death, divorce, new job, marriage, etc. Stressors cause pressures, challenges or demands in life.

Ways to reduce stress: Avoiding or managing the stress, choosing what is important in life, time management, simple living, learning to say no, etc.

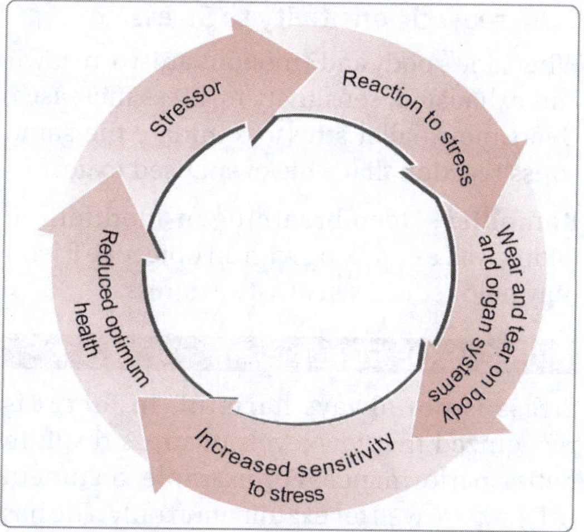

Figure 7.15: Stress cycle

2. Reaction to Stress

Once there is a stressor our body reacts to it. Reaction to stress relates to perception of the stress. When a person feels stressed due to the stressor, the body begins to release chemicals to confront it.

Reducing the reactions to stress: Asking God for help, spiritual practices, cognitive behavior therapy, reframing the problem, visualization of results.

3. Wear and Tear on the Body and Organ System

When a person becomes stressed and does not correct the stressor, the same stress reactions which helped cope in the beginning start to wear oneself down.

Remedies: Improving diet, regular exercises, yoga, meditation. All these activities reduce the emotional and physical effects of stress.

4. Reduced Optimum Health

After a sustained period of chronic stress the body wears down inviting more serious diseases like high BP, heart problems, diabetes, skin conditions, asthma, arthritis, depression and even cancer. Many diseases are associated with chronic stress.

Remedies: Consulting allopathic or homeopathy doctor or acupuncturist or naturopathy to make a plan for regaining health.

5. Increased Sensitivity to Stress

When one's body and emotions are worn down and exhausted, sensitivity to stress increases. Overtime smaller stressors initiate the same stress reaction that a big event used to get.

Remedies: Deep breathing or meditation, taking walks or talking with an objective friend may help reduce sensitivity to stress.

EFFECTS OF STRESS

Stress is not always harmful. In fact it is recognized that low levels of stress result in better performance. For example, a student will prepare well for examination only if he has some stress. However, excessive levels of stress are undoubtedly harmful.

- The body reacts to stressors by initiating a complex sequence of responses. If the perceived threat is resolved quickly the emergency responses subside. But if the stressful situation continues a different set of internal responses occur as the body attempts to adapt. Such attempts to adapt to the continued presence of a stress may deplete the body's resources making it vulnerable to illness. It results in wear and tear from chronic over activity of the physiological response to stress.
- Chronic stress can lead to physiological disorders such as ulcers, high BP and heart diseases. It may also impair the immune system thus reducing the body's ability to fight invading bacteria and viruses.
- Stress may affect health directly by creating chronic over arousal of the sympathetic division of the autonomic nervous system or the adrenal-cortical system or impairing the immune system.
- People under stress may not engage in positive health-related behaviors leading to illness. When under stress the individual is less likely to engage in healthy behaviors. For example, students taking exams stay up for most part of the night for several days, skip meals and snack on junk food.
- People under stress cease normal exercise routines and become sedentary. During stress some men consume excessive amount of alcohol and smoke excessively leading to cardiovascular diseases and emphysema. A high-fat diet contributes to many forms of cancer as well as cardiovascular diseases.
- People who do not regularly engage in a moderate amount of exercise are at an increased risk for heart disease and early death.
- Stress may indirectly affect health by reducing rates of positive health related behaviors and increasing rates of negative behaviors. People who engage in a healthy lifestyle—eating a low-fat diet, getting enough sleep and exercising regularly often report stressful events to be more manageable and being more in control of their lives.
- Thus, engaging in healthy behaviors can help reduce the stressfulness of life as well as reducing the risk or progression of a number of serious diseases **(Figure 7.16)**.

Three major types of consequences result from stress **(Flowchart 7.3)**:

1. Direct physiological effects
2. Harmful behaviors
3. Indirect health related behaviors

ADAPTATION TO STRESS

All of us face stress in our lives. Some psychologists believe that daily life actually involves a series of repeated consequences of perceiving a threat, considering ways to cope with it and ultimately adapting to threat with greater or lesser success. Although adaptation is often minor and occurs without our awareness, adaptation requires major effort when the stress is more severe or long lasting. Ultimately, our attempts to overcome stress can produce biological and psychological responses that result in health problems.

General Adaptation Syndrome (Hans Selye, 1945)

Homeostatic mechanisms are aimed at counteracting the everyday stress of living. If they are successful the internal environment

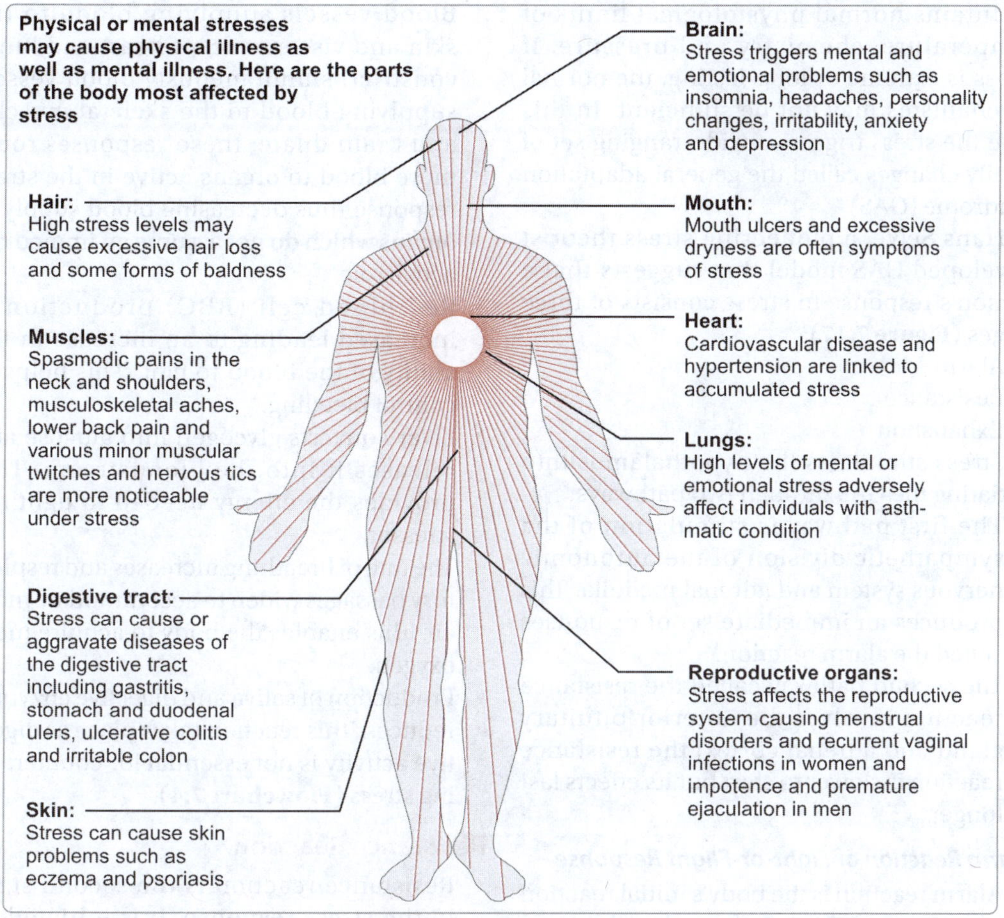

Physical or mental stresses may cause physical illness as well as mental illness. Here are the parts of the body most affected by stress

Hair: High stress levels may cause excessive hair loss and some forms of baldness

Muscles: Spasmodic pains in the neck and shoulders, musculoskeletal aches, lower back pain and various minor muscular twitches and nervous tics are more noticeable under stress

Digestive tract: Stress can cause or aggravate diseases of the digestive tract including gastritis, stomach and duodenal ulers, ulcerative colitis and irritable colon

Skin: Stress can cause skin problems such as eczema and psoriasis

Brain: Stress triggers mental and emotional problems such as insomnia, headaches, personality changes, irritability, anxiety and depression

Mouth: Mouth ulcers and excessive dryness are often symptoms of stress

Heart: Cardiovascular disease and hypertension are linked to accumulated stress

Lungs: High levels of mental or emotional stress adversely affect individuals with asthmatic condition

Reproductive organs: Stress affects the reproductive system causing menstrual disorders and recurrent vaginal infections in women and impotence and premature ejaculation in men

Figure 7.16: Effects of stress

Flowchart 7.3: Major types of consequences resulting from stress

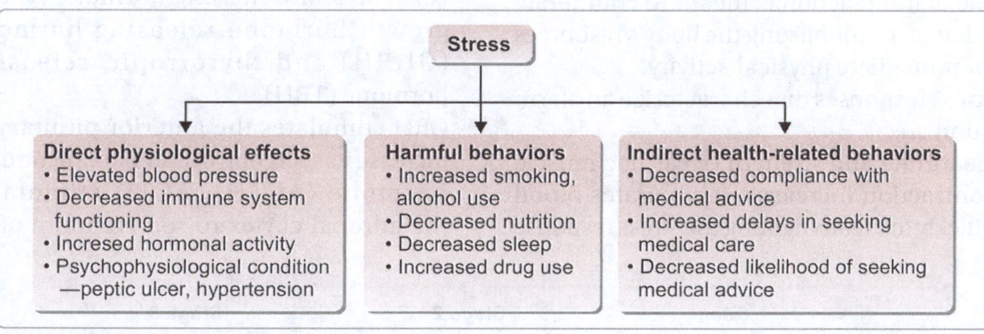

maintains normal physiological limits of temperature, chemistry and pressure. If stress is extreme or long-lasting, the normal mechanisms may not be sufficient. In this case the stress triggers a wide-ranging set of bodily changes called the general adaptation syndrome (GAS).

Hans Selye, a pioneering stress theorist developed GAS model that suggests that a person's response to stress consists of three stages **(Figure 7.17)**:

1. Alarm
2. Resistance
3. Exhaustion

Stress stimulates the hypothalamus into initiating the GAS through two pathways:

1. The first pathway is stimulation of the sympathetic division of the autonomic nervous system and adrenal medulla. This produces an immediate set of responses called the alarm reaction.
2. The second pathway called the resistance reaction involves the anterior pituitary gland and adrenal cortex; the resistance reaction is slower to start but its effects last longer.

Alarm Reaction or Fight-or-Flight Response

- Alarm reaction is the body's initial reaction to a stressor. It is a set of reactions initiated when the hypothalamus stimulates the sympathetic division of the autonomic nervous system and the adrenal medulla. The alarm reaction is meant to counteract a danger by mobilizing the body's resources for immediate physical activity.

Stress responses that characterize an alarm reaction are:

- Heart rate and strength of cardiac muscle contraction increases. It circulates blood quickly to organs fighting the stress response
- Blood vessels supplying blood to the skin and viscera except heart and lungs constrict; simultaneously blood vessels supplying blood to the skeletal muscles and brain dilate; these responses route more blood to organs active in the stress response thus decreasing blood supply to organs which do not assume an immediate active role.
- Red blood cell (RBC) production is increased leading to an increase in the ability of the blood to clot. This helps to control bleeding.
- Liver converts glycogen into glucose and releases it into the bloodstream. This provides the energy needed to fight the stressor.
- The rate of breathing increases and respiratory passages widen to accommodate more air. This enables the body to acquire more oxygen.
- Production of saliva and digestive enzymes reduces. This reaction takes place as digestive activity is not essential for counteracting stress **(Flowchart 7.4)**.

Resistance Reaction

- Resistance reaction is the second stage in the stress response. It is initiated by regulating hormones secreted by the hypothalamus and is a long-term reaction. These regulating hormones are corticotropin-releasing hormone (CRH), growth hormone-releasing hormone (GHRH) and thyrotropin-releasing hormone (TRH).
- CRH stimulates the anterior pituitary to increase its secretion of adrenocorticotropin hormone (ACTH). ACTH stimulates the adrenal cortex to secrete more of its

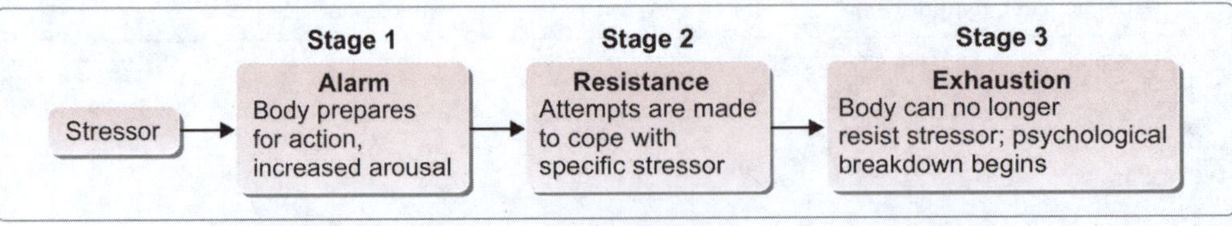

Figure 7.17: Three-stage model of general adaptation syndrome

Flowchart 7.4: Diagrammatic representation of alarm reaction

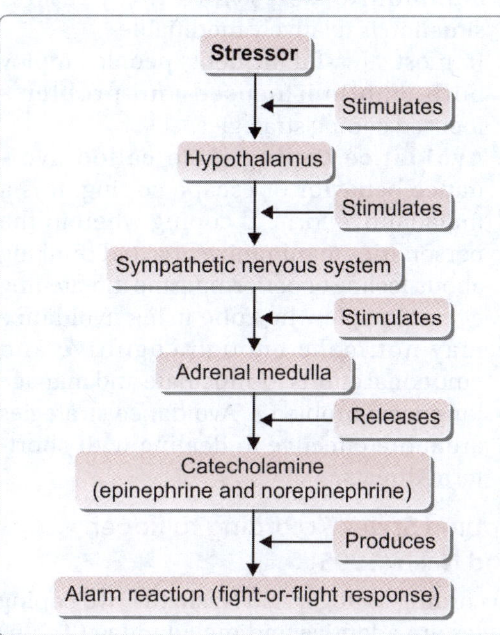

hormones. The action of these hormones helps to control bleeding, maintain BP, etc.

- GHRH stimulates the anterior pituitary to secrete human growth hormone (HGH). TRH causes the anterior pituitary to secrete thyroid-stimulating hormone (TSH). The combined actions of HGH and TSH help to supply additional energy to the body.
- The resistance reaction allows the body to continue fighting a stressor for a long time. It thus helps in meeting an emotional crisis, perform strenuous tasks, fight infection or resist the threat of bleeding to death.
- Generally, the resistance reaction is successful in helping the individual cope with a stressful situation and for the body to return to normal. Occasionally, it fails to fight the stressor especially if it is too severe or long-lasting. In such case the GAS moves into stage of exhaustion **(Flowchart 7.5)**.

Flowchart 7.5: Diagrammatic representation of resistance reaction

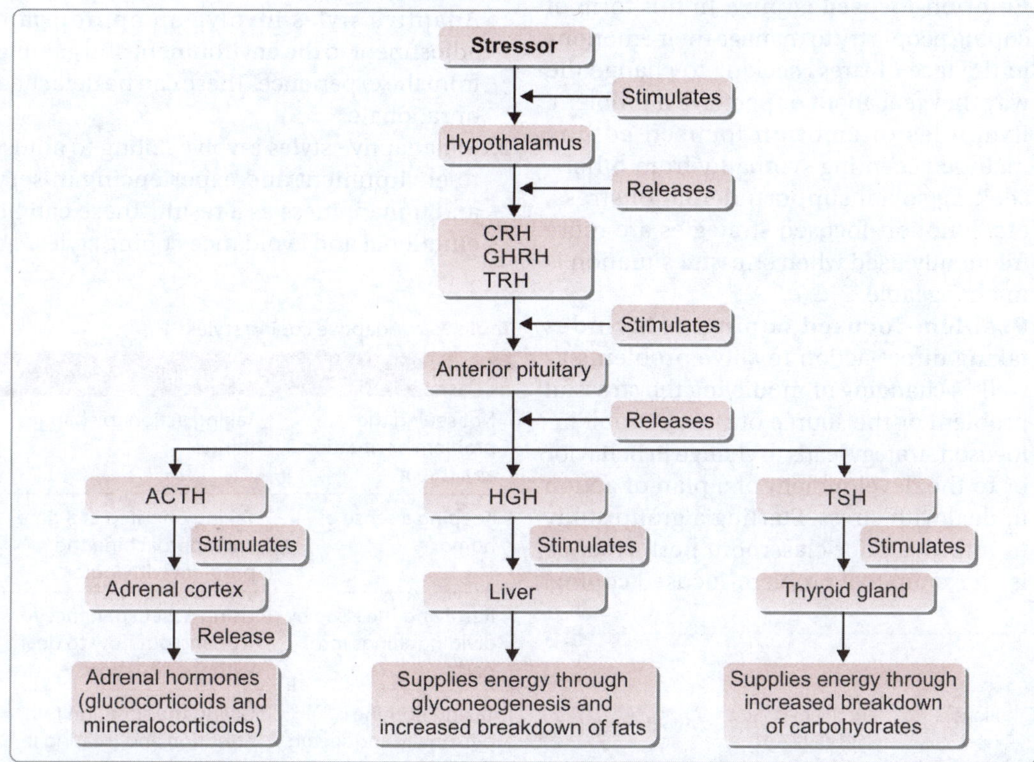

(CRH: corticotropin releasing-hormone; GHRH: growth hormone-releasing hormone; TRH: thyrotropin-releasing hormone; ACTH: adrenocorticotropin hormone; HGH: human growth hormone; TSH: thyroid-stimulating hormone)

Exhaustion Stage

In this stage the cells start to die and the organs weaken. A long-term resistance reaction puts heavy demand on the body particularly the heart, blood vessels and adrenal cortex which may suddenly fail under the strain. Under such situation the ability to handle stressors is determined to a large extent on the robustness of the general health.

Theorists have argued that Selye's model is limited because it does not give due importance to psychological factors.

COPING WITH STRESS

Coping refers to the thoughts and behaviors we use to handle stress or anticipated stress. Coping comprises of efforts to control, reduce or learning to tolerate threats arising out of stress. Effective coping depends on the nature of the stressor and the degree to which it is possible to control it. Coping strategies fall into three categories **(Figure 7.18)**:

1. **Emotion-focused coping:** In this form of coping people try to manage their emotions in the face of stress seeking to change the way they feel about or perceive a problem. Examples of emotion focused coping include accepting sympathy from others, seeking social support, denial of stress, etc. Emotion-focused strategies are more frequently used when stressful situation is unchangeable.
2. **Problem-focused coping***:* It includes taking direct action to solve problems as well as changing or modifying the stressful problem or the source of stress. Problem-focused strategy leads to change in behavior or to the development of a plan of action to deal with stress. Starting a group study to improve poor classroom performance is an example of problem-focused coping.

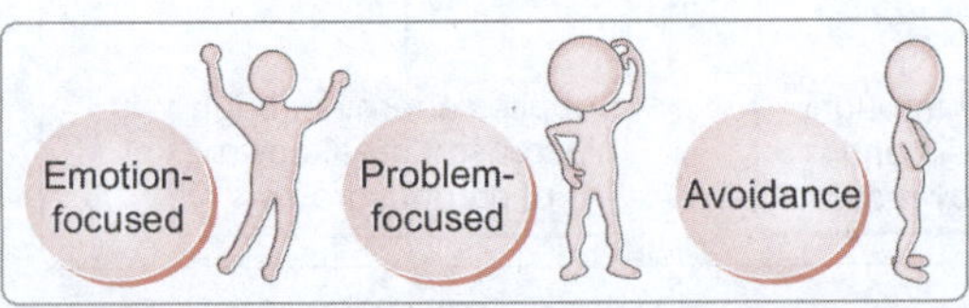

Figure 7.18: Types of coping strategies

Problem-focused approaches are more commonly used where the stressful situation is relatively modifiable.
In most stressful incidents people employ both emotion-focused and problem-focused coping strategies.
3. **Avoidance coping:** Also called avoidance behavior or escape coping, it is a maladaptive form of coping wherein the person tries to minimize or avoid thinking about, feeling or performing the threatening event. People who cope using avoidance may not make enough cognitive and emotional efforts to anticipate and manage long-term problems. Avoidance strategies are more effective in dealing with short-term threats.

Coping Styles According to Roger and Nash (1995)

According to Roger and Nash, the two coping styles are adaptive and maladaptive **(Tables 7.2 and 7.3)**.

1. Adaptive styles involve an appropriate adjustment to the environment and gaining from the experience. These can be detached or rationale.
2. Maladaptive styles involve failing to adjust to environment and experiencing misery and unhappiness as a result. These can be emotional and avoidance coping styles.

Table 7.2: Adaptive coping styles

Detached	Rationale
Not seeing the problem or situation as a threat	Taking action to change things
Keeping a sense of humor	Taking one step at a time and approaching the problem with logic
Resolving the issue by dividing things into parts	Using past experience for working out how to deal with the situation
Taking nothing personally and seeing the problem as separate from oneself	Giving the situation full attention and treating it as a challenge to be met

Table 7.3: Maladaptive coping styles

Emotional	Avoidance
◆ Feeling helpless, miserable, depressed and angry ◆ Showing frustration on other people ◆ Preparing for the worst possible outcome and seeking sympathy from others	◆ Pretending like nothing ever happened ◆ Sitting idle and hoping it all goes away ◆ Thinking about something else and talking about the matter as little as possible ◆ Trusting in fate and believing things will sort themselves out

Classification of Coping Strategies According to Cohen and Lazarus (1979)

- **Direct action response:** The individual tries to directly change or manipulate the stressful situation such as coping with or removing it.
- **Information seeking:** The individual tries to understand the situation better and predict future events related to the stressful event.
- **Inhibition of action:** Doing nothing.
- **Intrapsychic or palliative coping:** The individual reappraises the situation (use of psychological defense mechanisms) or changes the internal environment (through drugs, alcohol, relaxation or meditation).
- **Turning to others:** Seeking others help or emotional support.

ATTITUDE

Attitude is a specific mental state of an individual towards something according to which his behavior towards it is molded. Attitude is a way we perceive, think, feel and react more or less permanently in relation to something.

Definitions

- An attitude can be defined as an enduring organization of motivational, emotional, perceptual and cognitive processes with respect to some aspect of the individual's world. —**Krech and Crutchfield (1948)**
- An attitude may be defined as a learned and more or less generalized and an effective tendency or predisposition to respond in a rather persistent and characteristic manner, usually positively or negatively (for or against in reference to some situation, idea, value, material object or class) of such objects or person or group of persons. —**Young K**

NATURE OF ATTITUDE

- **Attitudes are not innate:** Attitudes are formed or learnt by the individual.
- **Attitudes are more or less lasting**: Attitudes are enduring.
- **Attitudes imply a subject-object relationship:** Attitudes are always formed in relation to certain persons, groups or institutions. Thus attitudes are not just internal factors without any relationship to the environment.
- **Attitudes are related to images, thoughts and external objects:** For example, upon hearing of the enemy attack on Indian territory every Indian developed a negative attitude towards the aggressors. Here the attitude involved is related to the thought that by attacking India, enemy has made the most unjustified and immoral move. In this attitude some imaginary concepts concerning the aggressors are formed in the mind of the individual based upon his knowledge of the enemy attack. Because of this attitude the individual is persuaded to contribute a portion of his wealth to the national defense fund in order to help expel the aggressor from the country.
- **Attitudes guide the behavior of the individual in one particular direction:** For example, due to negative attitude towards the aggressors the individual was prepared to do his best to help the Indian soldiers who were fighting them. Since attitudes direct the activities of an individual his reaction can be predicted by knowing his attitudes.

- Various kinds of affective experiences are also attached to attitudes.
- The unconscious motive is an important factor in the creation of attitudes. At times even the individual himself is unaware of the motive for his attitude towards a particular person or object as it is present in the unconscious.
- Attitudes are related to the person's needs and problems.

Formation and Development of Attitude

- Heredity may only play a small role in the development of attitude. It is mainly the environmental factors that are responsible for development of attitudes. These include parents, peers, school, cultural norms, personal motives, emotional conflicts, mass media, etc.
- Attitudes are formed in the context of an individual's wants, information, group affiliation and development of responsibility. The individual in trying to satisfy his wants develops favorable attitudes towards people and objects that aid in satisfying those wants. He develops unfavorable attitudes towards people and objects that block the satisfaction of his wants and prevent him from achieving his goals. What attitudes we select for adoption depends upon the needs, motivations and personality that we have cultivated.
- Family is the first place for formation of attitudes. Parents are exceedingly important in the formation of attitudes. They control rewards and punishments. Their smiles are a sign of approval and their frowns a sign of disapproval of the child behavior. It is the parents who establish the initial categories of good and bad. Their approval and disapproval of certain activities lays the foundation for formation of favorable and unfavorable attitude towards that activity in the child. Attitudes shape the information to which the individual is exposed. Parents are a source of information for the child as regards social and national groups, religion, rules of conduct, rules of thinking, etc.
- Group affiliations help in the formation of individual's attitudes. The peer group is a very important source of attitude formation especially in the young population. They learn the attitudes of their peer groups in order to be accepted by them. Attitudes originated in the family are further strengthened when they are appreciated by peers and playmates.
- Attitudes are also influenced by mass media, e.g., newspapers, journals, books, movies, etc.
- Many of our attitudes are acquired by us as a result of the pressure from others or may be the outcome of some experience. For example, an unhappy experience in a hospital alters our attitude towards hospitalization in general and also about the said hospital in particular.
- Attitudes may be formed as a result of learning. This is the process of growing up and learning. For example, male supremacy may be developed inside a house when much attention is given to sons than to daughters.
- Attitudes may also be formed as a result of various experiences. Experiences become more distinct and patterned as we grow up. One example for this is education. We develop attitudes that are favorable when we experience success in school or when we realize how much society values education.
- We may also develop attitudes through a single traumatic experience. Molested children may feel bad when given something that reminds them of the person who molested them.
- Also, attitudes may be formed through imitation. This is done by imitating readymade attitudes or prejudiced attitudes towards various objects or people. Racism is an attitude that some people imitate from others.

BEHAVIOR AND ATTITUDE (EFFECTS OF ATTITUDES ON BEHAVIOR)

- Attitudes are the motivating forces behind human social behavior. It is because of attitudes that the individual's behavior exhibits consistency. In the absence of a permanent organization the individual would be a new person in every situation. For example, if an individual has a negative attitude towards communism he will always be seen opposing the communist party.

- Attitudes also influence an individual's abnormal behavior. For example, some people believe in the existence of ghosts, witches, etc. Consequently they develop specific attitudes towards certain objects encouraging them to indulge in various religious rituals.
- An individual not only formulates attitudes towards external objects but also possesses attitudes about himself. These attitudes are very important for his social adjustment. His behavior may become abnormal if he forms a wrong attitude towards himself. For the individual's behavior to be desirable his attitude towards self and external objects should be favorable.
- Attitudes are our expressions of the likes and dislikes towards people and objects. They determine or guide our behavior in social situations.
- An individual's entire personality structure and behavior may be thought of as organized around a central value system comprised of many related attitudes.

The major reason for studying attitudes is the expectation that they will enable us to predict a person's future behavior. In general, attitudes have been found to predict behavior best when:

- **They are strong and consistent:** Strong and consistent attitudes predict behavior better than weak or ambivalent ones. When the affective and cognitive components of an attitude are not consistent, ambivalence and conflict can arise from within the individual making it difficult to predict behavior. In general, when the components of an attitude are clear and consistent they better predict behavior. For example, when we like something that we know is bad for us it is often difficult to predict the behavior.
- **They are specifically related to behavior being predicted:** For example, in one study students were asked about their general and specific attitudes towards nuclear war. Specific attitudes were much better predictors of activist behavior such as writing a letter to a newspaper or signing a petition than mere general attitudes (Newcomb, Rabow and Hernandez, 1992).
- **They are based on person's direct experience:** Attitudes based on direct experience predict behavior better than attitudes formed from reading or hearing about an issue.
- **The individual is aware of his or her attitudes:** There is evidence that people who are more aware of their attitudes are more likely to behave in ways that are consistent with those attitudes.

ATTITUDINAL CHANGE

Once the attitudes have been formed they have a tendency to persist or continue. It is therefore difficult to change the attitude that has been established. However, it is necessary to modify unhealthy or irrational attitudes for learning new things. In order to change attitudes we should:

- Change perceptions by new experiences and factual knowledge. Provide information to the individual who harbors a negative attitude towards an object/person; provide information that contradicts the attitude without any comments, suggestion, persuasion, etc. It allows the individual to take a decision all by himself without any pressure leading to a more favorable attitude towards the object/person concerned.
- Seek group support.
- Provide an opportunity for much closer contact with the object/person concerned. Let the person learn through it and modify his own attitude.

Health Education and Attitude Change

Health education means imparting knowledge and information in order to achieve and maintain health. Teaching helps the patient to cope with disease. Very often attitudes interfere with health and well-being of the patient. The initial step of a health educator is to eradicate negative attitudes that a person may hold towards himself, his illness and his future life. Through health education cognitive component of an attitude is altered leading to emotional component being altered parallelly.

FACTORS AFFECTING ATTITUDINAL CHANGE

- Attitudes can be changed through reducing cognitive dissonance. Cognitive dissonance is a state of unpleasant psychological tension that motivates us to reduce our cognitive inconsistencies by making our beliefs more consistent with each other (Atkinson et al., 1990). People experience dissonance when they do something that threatens their image of being decent, kind and honest especially if there is no way they can explain away this behavior as due to external circumstances. There are ways to reduce, lessen or minimize cognitive dissonance. One can add or change beliefs. One can add a new belief or change the old one he is holding so as to make it consistent with the behavior he is holding.
- Counter attitudinal advocacy is a process by which individuals are induced to state publicly an opinion or attitude that runs counter to their own private attitudes. For example, one can help smokers change their attitude towards smoking by letting them make a speech about the negative effects of smoking.
- Self-perception theory says that first we observe and perceive our own behavior and then change our attitude.
- Although these dissonance techniques are powerful they are difficult to carry out on a mass scale. In order to change as many people's attitudes as possible one can use persuasive communication.

ROLE OF ATTITUDE IN HEALTH AND SICKNESS

Attitudes related to health may be based on factual information or misinformation, common sense or myths, reality or false expectations. Attitudes influence health behaviors which in turn can affect a patient's level of health positively or negatively.

As far as health is concerned there are favorable and unfavorable attitudes which determine the outcome of illness. Attitudes related to some illnesses are:

- One cannot regain normalcy after brain damage.
- Chickenpox is caused due to the curse of Goddess.

Attitudes Towards Treatment

- Rural folk have a favorable attitude towards herbal and traditional medicines.
- Christians have a favorable attitude towards modern medicine as they are westernized.
- Muslims have a favorable attitude towards Unani medicine as it is a part of their culture.
- Those influenced by Gandhian thoughts have favorable attitude towards naturopathy.
- Generally educated people have more favorable attitude towards Allopathy system of medicine.

To most people illness comes as an unwelcome intrusion into their lives potentially denying them of their preferred pursuits and involving pain or discomfort. Despite this, some regard illness as a challenge. Their efforts to overcome illness and disability may lead to greater achievements. Some people on recognizing permanent impairment of their lower limbs may compensate by engaging in sports and activities where the use of their arms is at a premium. Some people use the time of illness as an opportunity to develop new interests.

Suffering helps many people find a new faith in religion or discover a new purpose in life. Illness can in this way be viewed positively even leading to great personal fulfillment. Some illnesses bear a stigma despite the efforts of health education and attitude change. For example, people suffering with mental illness, epilepsy and venereal diseases may still be treated as outcasts.

In some cultures, ill-health is regarded as shameful and wicked. Children in particular may regard illness as some form of punishment. As it is common for people to adopt an attitude of guilt and shame towards their own pain and suffering they find it impossible to discuss the illness even with a doctor or a nurse. While assessing the patient the nurse needs to assess his beliefs and attitudes that will influence his receptivity to nursing and medical care. Patient attitude to his own sex and the opposite sex, to youth, adulthood and old age will all have a bearing on his relationship with staff and other patients.

Nurses should understand patient's attitudes and values about health and illness so as to provide effective care. One of the great tasks for a nurse is to grasp any opportunity to modify harmful attitudes. Behavior resulting from negative attitudes not only militates against reaching an early diagnosis of the disorder, but may severely and unnecessarily disadvantage the sufferer by delaying the medical and nursing intervention.

Nursing Implications of Attitude (Importance of Positive Attitude for a Nurse)

Attitudes influence the behavioral responses of the individuals. Importance of study of attitudes for nurses can be related to the following factors:

Patient Care

- Any negative attitude towards race, community or a disease results in a prejudiced behavior adversely affecting patient care. Many a times stereotypic beliefs which the nurse might have developed in earlier sociocultural milieu may not be based on rational scientific reasoning. Due to these she may behave inappropriately causing interference with her professional competence.
- The nurse should recognize her attitudes and prevent them from interfering with nursing care.
- The nurse should try to understand patient's attitudes. While some visit the hospital with a positive attitude others do not mostly because of their previous hospital experience. It is mostly because of this that a patient with negative attitude may not co-operate with healthcare personnel.
- The nurse should explore the causes for such unfavorable attitudes and change them into favorable ones as it can help in treatment and recovery. A nurse can do this by providing efficient care, better experience and give adequate explanations where necessary.
- The nurse needs to develop and cultivate professional attitude which will contribute to her success at work.

Formation of Attitudes of Peers or Juniors

Senior nurses have a significant impact on the formation of opinion concerning health related issues. These attitudes could be cultivated by peer nurses, student nurses and other hospital staff associated in health care. One has to be careful about the negative attitude of one person generating similar attitude among other group members. Her attitude should be in conformity with the rules and regulations of the profession for which she is preparing.

Acceptance of New Technology

Present times are witness to many new innovations in techniques, equipment and methods of health care delivery. Our attitudes can bias our acceptance towards new technology and high profile specialties.

Curriculum Planning

While planning a new curriculum or revising an existing curriculum in educational courses one needs to identify the attitudes of students and teachers. Accordingly attitude change for altered behavior patterns can be sought and incorporated in the curriculum. For example, to plan a course on acquired immunodeficiency syndrome (AIDS) one may study the attitudes on nursing care of AIDS patient. Misconception or areas that need attitude change can be planned and incorporated. This would enhance the competency in dealing with AIDS patients.

Effects of Attitudes on Meaningful Learning and Retention

It is being recognized that besides cognitive factors, positive or negative attitudinal bias has differential effect on the learning of controversial material. With favorable attitude one is highly motivated to learn, put greater effort and concentrate better while analyzing new material. Negative attitude leads to a close minded view leading to impaired learning. Attitude structure exerts an additional facilitating influence on retention that is independent of cognition and motivation. A nurse with favorable attitude on learning will be highly motivated to learn, put greater effort and concentrate better.

Thus, a nurse should be aware of the correct attitudes required in her profession. List of correct attitudes for a successful and efficient nurse put forward by Kempf and Averill are:

- Ambition to do her task well
- Conformity with the rules and regulations of the profession for which she is preparing
- Willingness to work with effectiveness
- Cheerfulness and optimism
- Interest in the problems and difficulties of other people
- Co-operativeness, industriousness, respect for the opinion and judgment of others
- Interest in increasing the fund of knowledge underlying effective nursing care
- Determination to grow professionally
- Maintenance of poise and self-control in all professional situations
- Maintaining a consistent pride in their profession
- Rising to the unexpected without undue panic
- Determination to make the patient comfortable by giving attention to small details.

In order to succeed in her profession the nurse should develop the above attitudes and change her former attitudes accordingly.

Importance of Positive Attitude for a Nurse

Positive attitude is important for a nurse because of the following reasons:

- Knowledge of attitude formation and change is very essential for nurses as it helps the nurses to identify both positive and negative attitudes, i.e. those which are helping for effective nursing care and those which are affecting adversely.
- A nurse with a positive attitude towards her work will stay motivated and interested facilitating better performance. It will also enable her to achieve the ultimate goal in health care. However, with negative attitude she may neglect her duties, become careless and be inattentive leading to many dangerous consequences.
- Positive attitude will also reduce accidents or unintentional incidents. If the nurse is not focused she is likely to give less-than-your-best care. This can lead to errors, injury or even accusations.
- A nurse with a positive attitude is better able to handle job stress and is more constructive in approaching difficult situations.
- Finally, positive attitude can make a big impact on her career and success. It will aid in increasing the probability of optimum and consistent performance.

The nurse is ultimately in control of her attitude and can choose to be either an optimist or a pessimist. Understanding the attitude of patients is equally important as it is the patient's attitude towards the hospital, doctors, nurses and the treatment that will make him accept and co-operate. A negative attitude of the patient will result in not heeding medical advice resulting in non-cooperation with the treatment regimen.

Hence, the nurse should try to understand the attitudes of patients and attempt to change them, if negative. This requires the nurse to develop a friendly, warm and sober attitude towards her duties and patients.

PSYCHOMETRIC ASSESSMENT OF MOTIVATION, EMOTIONS AND ATTITUDES

Psychometric Assessment of Motivation

The important methods used to measure motivation are projective techniques, personality inventories and situational tests.

Projective Techniques

Most commonly used projective technique to measure motives is Thematic Apperception Test (TAT). In this test subjects are shown a series of ambiguous pictures and asked to narrate a story about what is going on in each picture. The assumption is that while narrating stories, the subject projects his or her own needs into the behavior of the character. The psychologist then identifies the needs being projected and judges from the number of related items in the story as to how strong each need is.

Personality Inventories

These are pencil and paper questionnaires made up of true-false or multiple choice questions about a person's habits, likes and ambitions. Examples are: Edwards Personal Preference Schedule—measures human social needs; Taylors Manifest Anxiety Scale—measures anxiety level.

Situational Tests

These involve the subjects being put into real life situations and witnessed by an observer. For example, a child's aggressiveness can be measured by letting it play with dolls and observing the number of times he is aggressive or does something destructive with them.

Psychometric Assessment of Emotions

Measurement of emotion is important in understanding the physiological basis of emotion. The following methods are used to measure emotions:

Galvanic Skin Response

Galvanic skin response (GSR) test measures the activation of sweat glands during emotional arousal resulting in lowering of electrical resistance of the skin.

Electrocardiography or Electrocardiogram

Electrocardiography (ECG) test measures changes in the rate and rhythm of the heart during emotional arousal.

Electroencephalogram

Electroencephalogram (EEG) test measures the brain rhythmic activity during emotional arousal.

Other Tests

They include recording the changes in muscle tension, breathing rate and BP during emotional arousal.

Psychometric Assessment of Attitudes

Measurement of Attitudes

Attitude is measured using attitude scales like the Likert scale, the semantic differential and the sociometry. These scales attempt to measure how a person or a group feels about something. The most commonly used among these is the Likert scale. It is a unidimensional scale which the researchers use to collect respondents' attitudes and opinions. It is the sum of responses of several likert items. A likert item is simply a statement which the respondent is asked to evaluate using any of the options: strongly agree, agree, do not know, disagree or strongly disagree.

Attitudes cannot be directly observed but are inferred from overt behavior, both verbal and non-verbal. Attitudes can be measured by the following tools:

- **Opinion surveys (public opinion polling) and self-report methods:** These surveys are concerned with replies to specific questions in which people are asked to respond to questions by expressing their personal evaluations. Answers to such questions are separately tabulated in an effort to identify sources of particular opinion.

  In the self-report method a questionnaire or a list of statements related to the attitudinal objects are given to the respondent. The response format is either fixed, i.e., categories for the responses are named such as agree-disagree, like-dislike, favorable-unfavorable; or left open ended where respondents can use their own words.
- **Attitude scales*:*** Attitude scales generally yield a total score indicating the direction and intensity of an individual's attitude towards an object, event or class of stimuli, e.g., Thurstone attitude scale, Likert scale, Guttmans scalogram and Osgood's semantic differential type.

- **Voluntary behavioral methods:** These involve the use of physiological measures. GSR and size of the pupil of the eye were earlier being used as an indicator of arousal to measure attitudes. These have not been very successful as only extremity of attitudes could be measured and also there was no indication on the direction of attitude. Recently electromyography recordings from the major facial muscles are being used to measure attitudes though it has not been successfully established.

ROLE OF NURSING IN CARING FOR EMOTIONALLY SICK CLIENT

Nurses spend maximum time with the patients than any other hospital personnel and therefore are in a better position to assess the psychological reactions of the patients. They can understand their emotional needs and plan for appropriate nursing interventions. A few nursing interventions are:

Spend Time with Patients

- Listen while the patient is describing his feelings.
- Try to identify what is frightening to the patient and offer appropriate explanations.

Facilitate Verbalization of Feelings

Allow the patient to explore his emotions/ feelings. Verbalization often brings about a tremendous relief of tension.

Handling the Emotions

- Verbalization of distress is often accompanied by tearfulness. Many women get great relief from a good cry. Men should not be denied too. It is just a manifestation. Any cry should be handled with care and privacy and support given until composure is regained.
- Show acceptance for patient's behavior even if the anger is directed at the nurse.
- Try to determine the cause for anger and then deal with it as realistically as possible.
- Recognize that a patient using denial protects himself from something he does not wish to face.
- Deal with denial carefully and in co-operation with other health personnel.
- Try to help the patient find ways to cope with depression, such as engaging in some useful activity.
- Show respect for patient's feelings.

Orientation of Patient to Healthcare Facility

Provide detailed explanation of the patient care services and of rationale behind various medical and nursing procedures that the patient has to undergo with constant reassurances all along. This will alleviate the fear of unknown in patients.

Identification of Learning Needs of Patients

Learning needs of patients have to be identified. For example, a patient before surgery may worry about prognosis, pain, ambulation, dependency, etc. Imparting knowledge on these aspects will satisfy the patients need to know about his condition and treatment thus reducing his anxiety.

Provide Diversional Activities

Encourage pleasurable and tension reducing diversional activities considering the patient's condition within permissible limits. Many chronically-ill patients do not recognize their need for recreation. Offer praise in a sincere and appropriate manner as the patients make progress towards independence.

Taking Care of Insomnia, Food and Fluid Intake, Elimination Pattern

- Employ measures such as low environmental stimuli, light meals in the night, engaging in daytime activities, reading books, listening to music at bedtime to promote sleep.
- Ensure adequate fluid intake and nutrition as patients suffering from depression exhibit little interest in food thereby recording a sharp decline in their nutritional status.
- Offer food of good nutritional quality.
- Provide small attractively served portions frequently and allow enough time for the patient to consume it.

- Ensure regular elimination pattern as constipation is a common complaint in distressed patients.

Maintain Cheerfulness and Humor

Human emotions can be contagious. So truly patients tend to enjoy having persons who are cheerful and yet professionally competent and sincere about their work. Humor can often relieve anxiety, stress and anger and help to develop warm relationships when used appropriately.

Seek Help of Mental Health Professionals

Patients who experience serious and prolonged disruptions in their lifestyle and relationships with significant others due to their illness and emotional reactions should know that psychiatric interventions can offer relief. Nurses should provide information about the sources of mental health care in community.

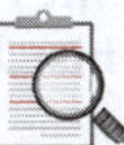

SYNOPSIS

- Needs are general desires.
- Drive is an aroused state resulting from need.
- Drives are influenced and guided by incentives.
- A need gives rise to one or more motives.
- A motive is an energetic force or tendency within the individual to compel him to act for the satisfaction of his basic needs.
- Abraham Maslow classified human motives as physiological, safety, love/belonging, esteem and self-actualization.
- The needs at one level must at least be partially satisfied before those at the next level become important determinants of action.
- Motives act as an immediate force to energize behavior.
- Emotion is a stirred up state of an organism. It plays an important role in human life.
- Stress is the non-specific response of the body to any kind of demand made upon it.
- Stress follows a cycle of events—stressor, reaction to stress, wear and tear on the body, reduced optimum health, increased sensitivity to stress.
- The low levels of stress result in better performance as excessive levels of stress are harmful.
- Homeostatic mechanisms are aimed at counteracting the everyday stress of living.
- According to Hans Selye the person's response to stress consists of three stages—alarm, resistance and exertion.
- Coping comprises of efforts to control, reduce or learn to tolerate threats arising out of stress.
- Attitude is a way we perceive, think, feel and react more or less permanently in relation to something.

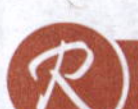

Review Questions

Long Essays

1. Explain the concepts and theories of motivation.
2. Define motivation. Explain social motives.
3. What is an emotion? Explain theories of emotions.
4. Explain Maslow's theory of motivation.
5. Distinguish between primary and secondary drives. Describe briefly the physiological drives that determine our daily behavior.
6. What is motive? Classify different motives. Describe in detail the physiological motives.

Short Essays

1. Psychometric assessment of emotions and attitudes
2. Maslow's need theory
3. Stress and adaptation

4. Explain two theories of emotion
5. Development of attitude
6. Coping with stress
7. Emotions and health
8. Theories of emotion in brief
9. Theories of motivation
10. Characteristics of emotions
11. Discuss Maslow's self-actualization theory
12. What is a motive? Explain the biological motives hunger and thirst
13. Clarify need, drive and motives
14. Explain Abraham Maslow's theory of motivation
15. Explain biological and social drives with one example for each
16. Explain why it is important for a nurse to form good habits?

Short Notes

1. Adaptation and coping
2. Stress
3. Social motives
4. Biological motives
5. Personal motives
6. Emotions and health
7. Types of emotions
8. Explain development of attitudes
9. Hunger drive
10. Need
11. Maternal drive
12. Self-actualization
13. Motivational cycle

Multiple Choice Questions

Motivation

1. Forces that govern the initiation and persistence of behavior are called:
a. Emotions
b. Motives
c. Intellectual capacities
d. Personality attributes

2. Primary drives are those which:
a. Are based on expectation
b. Are biologically based
c. Are satisfied last
d. Are based on knowledge

3. Motives whose satisfaction is essential for life are called:
a. Primary motives
b. Secondary motives
c. Accessory motives
d. All of the above

4. An individual fighting to climb the career ladder is striving to satisfy his:
a. Primary motives
b. Personal motives
c. Biological motives
d. Secondary motives

5. A person joining a variety of social clubs and having wide variety of friends is likely to be:
a. High in the need for affiliation
b. Low in the need for achievement
c. Low in the need for affiliation
d. High in the need for solitude

6. A couple attends an anniversary party hoping that the couple being honored will attend their future party. This motivation is best understood by invoking the:
a. Drive-reduction theory
b. Instinctive theory
c. Incentive theory
d. Cognitive theory

7. According to Maslow, which of the following is the highest-order need?
a. Esteem
b. Physiological
c. Safety
d. Belongingness

8. A person who works hard to increase his wealth is satisfying his:
a. Social motives
b. Personal motives
c. Biological motives
d. None of the above

9. Physical, security and safety, belongingness, self-esteem and self-realization needs are:
a. Needs of the learner
b. Maslow's hierarchy
c. Needs of teacher
d. None of the above

10. The hierarchy of needs according to Abraham Maslow is:
a. Physiological needs → safety needs → love needs → esteem needs → self- actualization
b. Safety needs → physiological needs → esteem needs → love needs → self- actualization
c. Self-actualization → esteem needs → physiological needs → safety needs → love needs
d. Physiological needs → self-actualization → safety needs → esteem needs → love needs

11. The concept of unconscious motivation is one of the cornerstones of:
a. Social theory
b. Psychoanalytic theory
c. Incentive theory
d. Humanistic school

12. The body's tendency to maintain a constant internal environment is called:
a. Thermostat
b. Homeostasis
c. Need
d. Aggression

13. Which of the following theories of motivation might be described as the 'push theories of motivation'?
a. Social learning theory
b. Drive theories
c. Incentive theories
d. Opponent process theory

14. Opposition of one motive by the other motive results in a:
a. Set
b. Habit
c. Conflict
d. Psychosis

15. A state that results when a motive is blocked can be referred to as a:
a. Mental conflict
b. General tension
c. General stress
d. None of the above

16. An individual who is unable to choose between a job and higher education is experiencing:
a. Problem of adaptation
b. Motivational conflict
c. Personality problem
d. Negative emotion

17. _______are forces that guide a person's behavior in a certain direction.

18. Biologically determined inborn patterns of behavior are known as _____.

19. By drinking water after running a marathon, a runner tries to keep his or her body at an optimal level of functioning. This process is called _____.

20. According to Maslow, a person with no job, home and friends can become self actualized - True or False?

21. Mr Balachandar is a type of person who constantly strives for excellence. He feels intense satisfaction when he is able to master a new task. Balachandar most likely has a high need for _______.

Emotional Processes

1. Emotions are different from feelings because:
a. They do not occur in normal people
b. They do no good for one's health
c. They can cause physiological changes in the body
d. All of the above

2. The word emotion etymologically means:
a. To stir up
b. To test
c. To express
d. To cry

3. The General Adaptation Syndrome (GAS) was described by:
a. Hans Selye
b. Hull
c. Gerald Caplan
d. Carl Rogers

4. The organ in the body which triggers GAS is:
a. Anterior pituitary
b. Adrenal gland
c. Liver
d. Hypothalamus

5. GAS is a response to:
a. Poor intelligence
b. Wrong perception
c. Stress
d. Poor nutrition

6. The set of reactions occurring as a result of the first stage of GAS can be termed as:
a. Resistance reaction
b. Exhaustion reaction
c. Stress reaction
d. Fight-or-flight response

7. Who among the following proposed that emotional states are a function of the interaction of cognitive factors and a state of physiological arousal?
a. William James
b. S Schachter
c. A Maslow
d. Carl Rogers

8. The stages of general adaptation syndrome progress in which of the following order:
a. Resistance → exhaustion → alarm
b. Alarm → exhaustion → resistance
c. Alarm → resistance → exhaustion
d. Exhaustion → alarm → resistance

9. Which of the following activities is aimed at reducing anxiety?
a. Aerobic exercises
b. Yoga
c. Meditation
d. All of the above

10. The immediate bodily reaction to short- term stress is likely to be:
a. Aches and pains in diverse locations throughout the body
b. Arousal in the sympathetic autonomic nervous system
c. Denial; refusal to confront and accept the stressor's reality
d. Illness resulting from failure of the immune system

11. Disorders that occur due to severe stress are called __________.

12. ________ is a state of heightened susceptibility to the suggestions of others.

13. ______ is a learned technique for refocusing attention to bring about an altered state of consciousness.

14. Emotions are always accompanied by a cognitive response - True or False?

15. The ______ theory of emotions states that emotions are a response to instinctive bodily events.

16. According to the ______ theory of emotions both an emotional response and physiological arousal are produced simultaneously by the same nerve stimulus.

17. What are the six primary emotions that can be identified from facial expressions?

18. ______ is defined as a response to challenging or threatening events.

Attitude

1. A predisposition to respond in a certain way is:
a. Prejudice
b. Attitude
c. Bias
d. Trait

2. **Attitudes are:**
   a. Innate b. Unlearned
   c. Acquired d. Learned
3. **Components of attitude are:**
   a. Cognitive, affective, conative
   b. Id, ego, superego
   c. Imagination, thinking and reasoning
   d. None of the above
4. **Which of the following methods like most other attitude measurement techniques relies on the self-report of respondents?**
   a. Physiological measures
   b. Public opinion polling
   c. Interview
   d. Case study
5. **Which factors play an important role in development of attitudes?**
   a. Heredity b. Environment
   c. Health d. Illness
6. **A procedure which measures the electrical resistance of skin is:**
   a. EMG b. GSR
   c. EEG d. ECG
7. **Measurement of attitudes is carried out by:**
   a. Opinion surveys
   b. Self-report methods
   c. Likert's method of summated ratings
   d. All of the above
8. **An intuitive attempt to infer the causes of behavior is:**
   a. Attitude b. Attribution
   c. Will d. Character
9. **What causes do we require to explain behavior?**
   a. Situational causes
   b. Dispositional causes
   c. Attitudes
   d. Both a and b

ANSWER KEY

MOTIVATION					
1. b	2. b	3. a	4. b	5. a	6. c
7. a	8. b	9. b	10. a	11. b	12. b
13. b	14. c	15. a	16. b	17. Motives	18. Instincts
19. Homeostasis	20. False, lower-order needs must be fulfilled before self-actualization can occur		21. Achievement		
EMOTIONAL PROCESSES					
1. c	2. a	3. a	4. d	5. c	6. d
7. b	8. c	9. d	10. a	11. Psycho-physiological disorders	12. Hypnosis
13. Meditation	14. False, emotions may occur without a cognitive response		15. James–Lange	16. Cannon–Bard	17. Surprise, sadness, happiness, anger, disgust and fear
18. Stress					
ATTITUDE					
1. b	2. c	3. a	4. b	5. b	6. b
7. d	8. b	9. d			

CHAPTER

8 Psychological Assessment and Tests

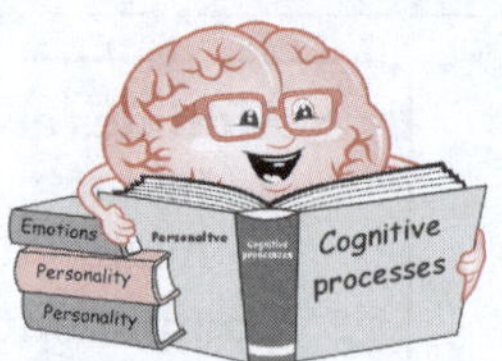

CHAPTER OUTLINE

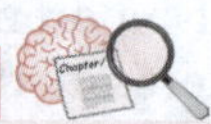

- Psychological tests—types, development, characteristics, principles, uses, limitations, interpretations
- Role of nurse in psychological assessment

Psychology has a long tradition of scientific research on human behavior and personality. Through this research a multitude of psychological assessment scales have been developed to measure objectively and precisely the various aspects of psychological functioning and personality characteristics.

Psychological assessment is the attempt of a skilled professional usually a psychologist to evaluate thinking, learning and behavior of a person be it general or specific. It uses standardized tools and techniques to measure intelligence, development, personality, attitudes and cognitive, social or emotional functioning. These are also used by clinicians to diagnose disorders. Psychological assessments may take the form of a questionnaire, interview or observational method. Example, paper-pencil test, Beck depression inventory. 'Psychometrics' is a technical term synonymously used for psychological testing.

TYPES OF PSYCHOLOGICAL TESTS

Psychological tests can broadly be categorized based on: (1) how they are constructed and administered and (2) skills and abilities that they are designed to measure.

Classification based on Construction and Administration

- **Individual and group tests:** Individual tests involve one to one consultation and are administered one person at a time. Group tests are administered to a group of persons at the same time. These are cheaper and usually include multiple choice items.
- **Speed and power tests:** Speed tests have a fixed time limit at which point everyone taking the test must stop. Test items are of uniform difficulty with individual differences being evaluated entirely on the speed of the performance. Power tests on the other hand have no time limit with applicants being allowed as much time as needed to complete the test. These tests assess the underlying ability of the individual by allowing them sufficient time.
- **Computer-assisted tests:** These are a means of administering psychological tests to large groups of applicants wherein an applicant's response determines the level of difficulty of succeeding items. In this form of testing the individual does not have to waste time answering questions below his level of ability. The computer program begins with a question of average difficulty and with the individual clicking

the correct answer proceeds to questions of greater difficulty. If not it poses less difficult questions.
- **Paper-pencil and performance tests:** Paper pencil tests are administered using printed forms with answers recorded on standard answer sheets. However, such test formats are not appropriate for carrying out performance tests as they are meant to assess complex skills, such as word processing and mechanical ability.

Classification based on Skills and Abilities they are Designed to Measure

Based on tests of knowledge, skills and abilities psychological tests can be classified as under:

- **Achievement tests:** These tests attempt to measure achieved knowledge and are mostly employed in educational or employment settings. For example, term ending examinations.
- **Aptitude tests:** These tests measure specific abilities such as mechanical or clerical skills. These include measurement of perceptual speed and accuracy, attention detail, capacity to visualize and manipulate objects in space, principles of mechanical operation, ability to operate computers, etc. For example, General Aptitude Test Battery (GATB), Differential Aptitude Test (DAT).
- **Intelligence tests:** These tests attempt to measure intelligence, i.e., basic ability to understand the world around. For example, Stanford-Binet Intelligence Scale (SB), Army Alpha Test, Army General Classification Test (AGCT).
- **Interest tests:** These psychological tests assess a person's interests and preferences and are primarily used in career counseling. For example, interest inventory.
- **Neuropsychological tests:** These tests measure deficits in cognitive functioning (ability to think, speak, reason, etc.). The deficit may result from some sort of brain damage such as a stroke or a brain injury. For example, Cambridge Neuropsychological Test Automated Battery (CANTAB), Benton Visual Retention Test, Wechsler Adult Memory Scale (WMS).
- **Occupational tests:** They attempt to match interests with that of people in known careers. For example, McQuaig Occupational Test (MOT).
- **Personality tests:** They attempt to measure basic personality style. For example, Minnesota Multiphasic Personality Inventory (MMPI), Rorschach ink blot test.
- **Specific clinical tests:** They attempt to measure specific clinical matters such as current level of anxiety or depression. For example, Hamilton Rating Scale for Depression (HRSD), Brief Psychiatric Rating Scale (BPRS).

DEVELOPMENT OF PSYCHOLOGICAL TESTS

Several steps are involved in development of a psychological test. These include:

- **Analysis of the situation:** The first step involves a detailed analysis of the psychological processes required for successful performance of the task in question.
- **Tentative selection of the test items:** Following the analysis, selection of tests from those already available is done by the psychologist. However, he may also device a test which he feels will measure the processes.
- **Development of standardized procedures:** Psychological tests are administered and scored in the same way for every individual tested in order to obtain consistent results.
- **Administration of the test to a representative group:** Psychologist administers the test to a representative group of subjects to see if they score the way expert judgment or other evidence suggests. Accordingly, the psychologist is able to determine the effectiveness of the test.
- **Final selection of the test items:** Many test items are either discarded or revised so as to contribute more directly to the overall purpose of the test. This procedure is called

item analysis. The final selection of items is based on empirical findings.

- **Evaluation of the final test:** Effectiveness of the final test is evaluated in terms of a specified criterion.

CHARACTERISTICS OF PSYCHOLOGICAL TESTS

Carefully developed and researched psychological tests have several characteristics **(Table 8.1)**:

- **Standardization:** It refers to the consistency or uniformity of the conditions and procedures for administering a test. To achieve standardization people must be tested under uniform conditions.
- **Objectivity:** It refers primarily to the scoring of test results. The scoring process must be free of subjective judgment or bias on the part of the scores.
- **Test norms:** To interpret the results of a psychological test, a frame of reference or point of comparison must be established to compare the performance of one person with that of the other. This is accomplished by means of test norms. The distribution of test scores of a large group of people is similar in nature to the individual being tested. For example, a science graduate applies for a job that requires mechanical skills and achieves a score of 83 on a test of mechanical ability. This score alone does not suggest anything significant about the level of applicant's skill. However, if the score of 83 is compared with the test norms and the distribution of scores on the test from a large group of science graduates, some meaning can be ascribed to the individual score. If the mean of the test norms is 80 and the standard deviation 10, it can immediately be inferred that the applicant who scored 83 has only an average or moderate mechanical ability. With this comparative information one can objectively evaluate the applicant's chances of succeeding on the job relative to the other applicants tested.
- **Reliability:** It refers to the consistency of a person's scores. For example, a boy takes a cognitive ability test and achieves a mean score of 100 followed by a mean score of 72 in a repeat test after a week. This would suggest the test as unreliable as it yields inconsistent measurements.
- **Validity:** It refers to the test's accuracy in measuring what it is supposed to measure. For example, if a test is a valid measure of intelligence, people's scores on that test should strongly be correlated with their grades in school.

Table 8.1: Characteristics of psychological tests

Characteristics of psychological tests				
Standardization	Objectivity	Test norms	Reliability	Validity

PRINCIPLES OF PSYCHOLOGICAL TESTS

- Psychological tests should have three components, viz. standard, content and procedure that make it possible for anybody to administer it anywhere, anytime.
- Tests should have norms to allow comparison of an individual test score with that of a known group who have taken the test.
- Test items are of high technical quality prepared by experts, pretested and selected on the basis of difficulty, discriminating power and relationship to a clearly defined rigid set of specifications.
- Directions for administrating scores are precisely stated so that procedures are standard for various test users.
- A test manual and other accessory material is provided as a guide for administering, scoring, evaluating its technical qualities and interpreting and using the results.

USES OF PSYCHOLOGICAL TESTS

- It is easier to gather information through tests rather than from a clinical interview.
- Information gathered through tests is considered scientifically more consistent than that from a clinical interview.
- They assist in diagnosis. For example, Rorschach inkblot test.

- They assist in the formulation of psychopathology and identification of stress and conflict areas. For example, thematic apperception test.
- They help in determining the nature of deficits present. For example, cognitive neuropsychological assessments.
- They help in assessing severity of psychopathology and response to treatment. For example, Hamilton rating scale for depression, brief psychiatric rating scale.
- They help in assessing general characteristics of the individual. For example, assessment of intelligence, assessment of personality. Personality tests help us understand an individual's interpersonal style, basic personality traits and emotional functioning. In addition to clinical measures for conditions like depression, mood disorders or anxiety, such tests may also help identify general personality traits such as introversion vs extroversion, dominance vs submissiveness, leadership style, etc. These personality factors relate to a wide variety of issues in one's life such as school or work performance, marital or family concerns and overall happiness.
- These tests are also used in forensic evaluations, litigation, family court issues and criminal cases.
- These tests besides assessing level of functioning or disability and treatment outcome, also help in direct treatment.

LIMITATIONS OF PSYCHOLOGICAL TESTS

- No psychological test is ever completely valid or reliable because the human psyche is just too complicated to know anything about it with full confidence. That is why there can be uncertainty about a case even after extensive testing.
- Many applicants experience considerable test anxiety.
- Negative attitude towards psychological tests may also lower an applicant's motivation to perform well on the tests which in turn reduces its predictive validity.
- Administration and interpretation of the test can only be done by qualified psychologists.

INTERPRETATION OF PSYCHOLOGICAL TESTS

Integration of test findings into a comprehensive, meaningful report is probably the most difficult aspect of psychological evaluation. Inferences from various tests must be related to one another in terms of clinicians' confidence in them and of a patient's presumed level of awareness that consciousness is being tapped.

Most clinicians follow a general outline while preparing a psychological report which includes test behavior, intellectual functioning, personality functioning (reality testing ability, impulse control, manifestation of depression and guilt, manifestations of major dysfunction, major defenses, overt symptoms, interpersonal conflicts, self-concept, affects), inferred diagnosis, degree of present overt disturbances, prognosis for social recovery, motivation for personality change, primary assets and weaknesses, recommendations and summary.

ROLE OF A NURSE IN PSYCHOLOGICAL ASSESSMENT

- Nurses should become familiar with the many standardized psychological tests that are available to enhance each stage of the nursing process.
- These tests help in providing care and so also measurable indicators of treatment outcome. For example, if a nurse is caring for a patient with depression, it would be helpful to use one of the depression rating scales with the patient at the beginning of care/treatment to establish a baseline profile of the patient's symptoms and help confirm the diagnosis. The nurse might then administer the same scale at various stages during the course of treatment to measure patient progress.
- A nurse should have complete knowledge of all the psychological tests enabling her to clarify the various doubts that a patient or

his relative might express while undergoing them.

- The nurse should reassure the patient on safety of the tests and confidentiality of the observations of the psychologist. Psychological tests are another source of data for the nurse to use in planning care for the patient.

SYNOPSIS

- Psychometrics is a technical term synonymously used for psychological testing.
- Psychological assessment is the evaluation of thinking, learning and behavior of a person.
- The main characteristics of psychological tests are standardization, objectivity, test norms, reliability and validity.
- A nurse should have complete knowledge of psychological tests for planning care for the patient.

Review Questions

Short Essays

1. Characteristics and uses of psychological tests.
2. Types of psychological tests.
3. Development of psychological tests.
4. Role of nurse in psychological assessment.

Multiple Choice Questions

1. **Following are the characteristics of psychological tests, *except:***
   a. Standardization
   b. Appropriateness
   c. Reliability
   d. Validity
2. **Which of the following is the first step in development of psychological tests?**
   a. Analysis of situation
   b. Selection of test items
   c. Administration of test
   d. Evaluation of test
3. **Which of the following tests is designed to be administered one person at a time?**
   a. Group test
   b. Power test
   c. Paper-pencil test
   d. Individual test
4. **Specific abilities are measured by:**
   a. Achievement tests
   b. Aptitude tests
   c. Intelligence tests
   d. Occupational tests
5. **Standard measure devices that assess behavior objectively are called:**
   a. Factor analysis procedures
   b. Psychological tests
   c. Temperament assessment scales
   d. Behavioral assessment tests
6. **______ is the consistency of a personality test, while ______ is the ability of a test to actually measure what it is designed to measure.**
7. **______ are the standards used to compare scores of different people taking the same test.**

ANSWER KEY

1. b	2. a	3. d	4. b	5. b	6. Reliability, validity
7. Norms					

CHAPTER

9 Application of Soft Skill

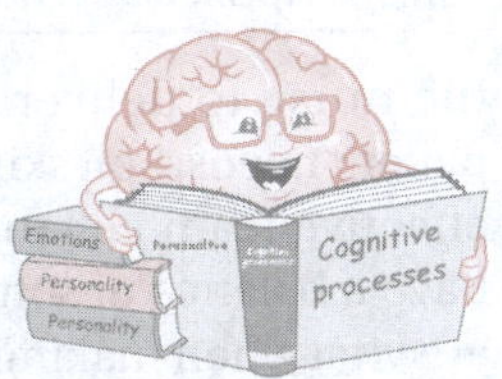

CHAPTER OUTLINE

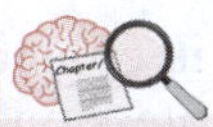

- Soft skills—concept, components and uses
- Communication skills—types, components, importance of communication in nursing
- Building relationship with patient and society
- Interpersonal relationships—types, purposes, techniques, barriers, strategies to overcome
- Time management for nurses
- Coping with stress
- Resilience—contributing factors, development of resilience
- Work-life balance—importance, strategies
- Presentation skills, social etiquette, telephone etiquettes, motivational skills, team work

Soft skills are personal traits required to establish and maintain interpersonal relationships with others in an organization. These are a combination of personal attributes, attitude and qualities. Also termed as social skills, personal skills or emotional intelligence, they define the ability to interact harmoniously with others. Though not related to any specific task or position these skills describe one's approach to life, work and relationship with other people.

DEFINITIONS

- Soft skills are the intangible behavior traits that enhance or endorse knowledge or skills in the workplace.

  —Sharma and Sharma (2010)

- Soft skills are interpersonal qualities and personal attributes that one possesses.

  —Heckman and Kautz (2012)

CONCEPT OF SOFT AND HARD SKILLS

There are two types of skills that any professional needs to develop: hard skills and soft skills.

Hard skills are the individual specific abilities required to perform a given task. Also termed as occupational skills these are usually taught as a part of academic curriculum that can be learned and perfected over a period of time. Example of hard skills are technical knowledge and skills required to perform a task or procedure efficiently. In nursing, these skills refer to the technical/procedural skills that a nurse learns through hands on training or in clinical laboratories or real life ward settings. Every nurse is expected to master these hard skills without which she can neither provide effective patient care nor progress in her career.

On the other hand soft skills are personal traits required to establish communication and interaction with others. These are difficult to learn and measure but yet as important and valuable as the hard skills. Examples of soft skills are personality traits, workplace etiquette, communication style, interpersonal skills, optimistic attitude and dependability. Also termed as emotional intelligence quotient (EQ) it is difficult to acquire and once acquired difficult to change. In nursing these skills include empathy, understanding, active listening, behavioral competence, good bed side manners and other interactive skills. These skills provide the necessary tools for the nurse to deliver quality care and meet patient needs. Soft skills are also important for effective team collaboration. Nurses should have a balance of soft and hard skills as both are vital when making patient care decisions.

COMPONENTS OF SOFT SKILLS AND THEIR APPLICATION

Important components of soft skills include ability to communicate, adaptability, critical thinking, empathy, flexibility, problem solving ability, professionalism, taking initiative, teamwork and networking, tolerance and conflict resolution, work ethics and commitment. These skills can be extensively applied in nursing profession **(Table 9.1)**.

Use of Soft Skills in Nursing

- A nurse is considered to be successful in her profession only if she can provide

Table 9.1: Application of soft skills to workplace and society

Soft skill component	Description	Application in nursing
Ability to communicate	Establishing, maintaining and improving contact with others	Ability to communicate effectively allows a nurse to interact with the patient, their family members, friends and other healthcare team members. This improves patient satisfaction and results in better health outcomes.
Adaptability	Agreeable to learn, adapt new techniques and follow latest guidelines	Nurses should readily accept the introduction and implementation of new procedures and techniques. They should also be agreeable to follow the changes in policies and guidelines.
Critical thinking	Analyze and evaluate the problem, interpret the result	Nurses should display analytical thinking while making patient care decisions. Applying both logic and creativity in resolving patient related issues is highly valued.
Empathy	Ability to understand and feel what the patient is going through	An empathetic nurse can understand patient's problems, needs and feelings. This helps her to approach the patients in a kind and generous manner.
Flexibility	Willingness to adjust to the work schedules	Nurses should be willing to adjust their working hours, do extra shifts or put in few more hours when required.
Problem-solving ability	Identify the problem, determine various alternatives and select suitable solution	When nurses encounter problems in their day-to-day activities they are expected to assess the situation, understand the problem and determine the course of action for each problem.
Professionalism	Knowledge, skills, values and beliefs that guide the profession	It enables the nurse to provide high standards of practice and care at all times.
Taking initiative	Exhibiting eagerness	Nurse should exhibit willingness and eagerness to manage the work situation without being told to do so.
Teamwork and networking	Two or more people interacting independently towards a common goal	Being a member of the health team she needs to co-ordinate with other healthcare professionals to provide best possible patient care.
Tolerance and conflict resolution	Coping with stressful situations	Nurses should have the ability to face critical situations in a calm and composed manner.
Work ethics and commitment	Moral principles related to work	Nurses should be honest, trustworthy, diligent and have a strong work commitment to meet professional requirements.

safe patient care and maintain healthy work environment. This can be achieved by a combination of soft skills and job related proficiencies. Soft skills are a crucial component in nursing as they promote collaborative and efficient workforce.

- At times patients struggle to comprehend the diagnosis and treatment modalities leading to utter confusion. In such situations the nurse must show confidence in patient's abilities and help him understand the disease condition and intervention being followed. Only a nurse with soft skills can communicate with the patient and their caregivers effectively enabling them to take appropriate patient care decisions.
- She is also able to interact with co-workers and other health team members thus promoting team work. Under certain circumstances soft skills may seem more effective and satisfying than the technical or procedural skills.
- Good critical thinking skills and ability to think out of the box make her more competent.
- Good coping and tolerant skills allow a nurse to handle stressful situations without losing focus on the task.
- Soft skills make a nurse more flexible and adaptable allowing her to take the day-to-day challenges in her stride while remaining positive. This keeps the patient comfortable.
- As a part of the curriculum the nurse needs to be taught soft skills alongside technical skills so as to take patient care to next level.

COMMUNICATION SKILLS

Communication is the fundamental aspect of human interaction that permits individuals to establish, maintain and improve relations with others. It is a broad soft skills category. The word communication originates from 'communis' a Greek word meaning 'to make common'. Communication is a process by which people exchange ideas, facts, feelings or impressions in a way that each gains a 'common understanding' of the meaning, intent and use of a message.

In general, communication refers to the giving and receiving of information, ideas, facts, opinions, beliefs, feelings and attitudes through verbal or non-verbal means between people. It includes listening and understanding with respect as well as expressing views and ideas and passing information to others in a clear manner. It is a means by which people influence the behavior of another. Thus, good communication skills constitute the ability to not only speak confidently but also listen, empathize and present well whenever necessary.

It is a vehicle used to establish a therapeutic relationship involving three elements: sender, message and receiver. The sender prepares or creates a message when a need occurs and sends the message to a receiver or listener who then decodes it. The receiver may then return a message or give feedback to the sender or initiator of the message **(Figure 9.1)**.

Types of Communication

Communication takes place on two levels: verbal and non-verbal.

1. Verbal communication takes place through spoken or written words.
2. Non-verbal communication occurs through gestures or behaviors that do not involve spoken or written words. Various types of non-verbal communication include vocal cues, gestures, physical appearance, space, posture, touch and facial expression.

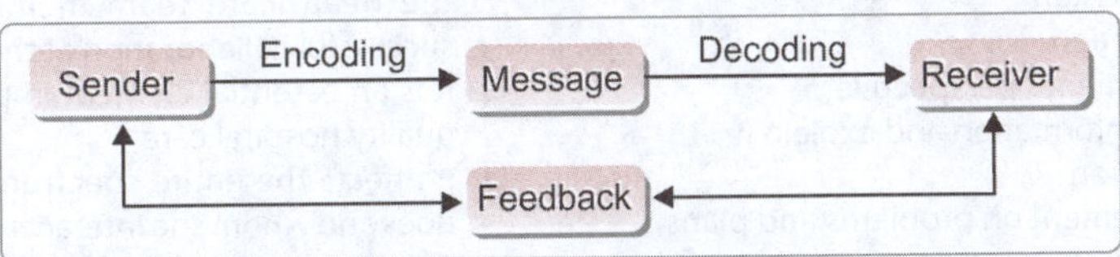

Figure 9.1: Communication process

Non-verbal communication may more accurately reveal patient feelings than verbal communication.

Components of Communication

Better communication between the nurse and the patient builds confidence and improves compliance with treatment. While subject knowledge and practical skills constitute the science of nursing practice, communication skills constitute the art of nursing practice. The key components for establishing communication with patient are presented in **Box 9.1**.

Importance of Communication in Nursing

Effective communication is a core skill for all healthcare professionals, nursing staff in particular as they play an important role in patient care across various healthcare settings. It is also because the nurses spend more time with patients and caregivers than any other healthcare professional.

A dynamic profession like nursing requires professionals to be vocal. The ability to communicate effectively is crucial when dealing with the patient, patient caregiver, co-workers and superiors. This is a field where communication is vital and clear communication style a must.

It is the backbone over which various aspects of patient care rest such as establishing therapeutic relationship with patient, assessing patient problem, counseling a patient, explaining disease condition, providing health education and taking informed consent, etc. Nurse's communication skills have a significant impact on patient satisfaction, compliance with treatment and better health outcomes. The quality of care provided depends upon the quality of communication existing between the nurses and their patients.

Without communication a therapeutic nurse-patient relationship is impossible. It is essential that nurses develop and maintain communication skills to meet patient needs. Therefore, every point of contact can be an opportunity to improve patient care and relationships using effective communication. Good communication skills are a critical component of nursing practice. Importance of good communication in nursing is highlighted in **Box 9.2**.

Box 9.1: Key components for establishing communication with patient

- ❑ Open the discussion
- ❑ Gather information
- ❑ Understand patient's perspective
- ❑ Comprehend information and explain it
- ❑ Share information
- ❑ Reach an agreement on problems and plans
- ❑ Be able to listen

BUILDING RELATIONSHIP WITH PATIENT AND SOCIETY

Nurses are responsible for total patient care as it includes physical care, performing technical procedures, creating safe and comfortable environment, formal and informal teaching, counseling, and acting as a patient's advocate. To perform all these tasks the nurse needs to build a therapeutic relationship with the patient. This therapeutic relationship forms the foundation for nursing care throughout the spectrum of health and illness continuum. The main purpose of building a relationship with the patient is to support and promote healing process, and enhance illness recovery.

Box 9.2: Importance of good communication in nursing

- ❑ It generates trust between nurse and the patient
- ❑ It provides professional satisfaction and improves patient wellbeing
- ❑ It helps to promote managerial skills and provides a basis for leadership action
- ❑ It provides a means for coordination with the healthcare team members and fosters successful collaboration at the work place
- ❑ It is an essential element in patient safety and quality hospital care
- ❑ It affects the entire spectrum of what a nurse does and whom she interacts with including the patient experience

Box 9.3: Qualities required for a nurse to build therapeutic relationship

- Competence in knowledge and skill
- Competence in soft skills and communication skills
- Honesty/genuineness
- Trust
- Empathy
- Confidentiality
- Showing respect and caring attitude

The following elements or qualities help a nurse to build therapeutic relationship with the patient **(Box 9.3)**:

1. **Competence in knowledge and skill:** It is the ability to perform activities effectively and efficiently. Nurses should have adequate knowledge and skills in performing their roles and responsibilities. By being knowledgeable and skillful in nursing practice the nurse begins to gain patient's trust and confidence making him feel more secure.
2. **Competence in soft skills and communication skills:** To establish a good relationship with the patient and his care givers the nurses are required to have effective communication skills. These skills include being aware of verbal and non-verbal cues of patients, active listening to patient without interruption, giving information, having a non-judgmental approach, paraphrasing, summarizing and clarifying information. All these techniques help build a trusting relationship with the patient.
3. **Honesty:** Honesty in nursing simply means doing the right thing in a right way, coming to work on time, not skipping on patient care, admitting to mistakes made and facing the consequences, not gossiping about the patients and being true to ones beliefs. Nurses are expected to work with honesty and integrity to maintain patient and public trust and uphold the reputation of the profession. An honest approach will allow the patient to develop respect and a belief that the nurse is acting in his best interest.
4. **Trust:** Oxford English Dictionary defines trust as a firm belief in the reliability, truth or ability of someone or something. Trust is the main element of all interpersonal relationships. Some of the nursing activities which facilitate trust are active listening (patient feels understood), respecting (patient feels valuable), being honest and consistent in activities (patient feels the nurse is trustworthy), and having an acceptable attitude (patient is comfortable in sharing information). If the patient develops trust on the nurse they are more likely to share and disclose information. Performing roles in an ethical way is essential to building a trusting relationship with the patient.
5. **Empathy:** It refers to the nurse's understanding of what the patient is experiencing from his own perspective. This process allows the nurse to see the suffering from patient's own point of view without experiencing the emotional content. This understanding allows the nurse to identify the patient's problems more precisely, set goals for the patient, provide specific interventions and evaluate patient outcomes.
6. **Confidentiality:** It refers to the duty of an individual to refrain from sharing confidential information with others and respecting privacy. Nurses have the moral obligation of keeping the patient information confidential and not sharing it with others except in specific circumstances. In nursing, confidentiality indicates maintaining privacy in a physical setting while dealing with sensitive issues concerning the patient. It also includes closing the room door or at least using the separation screen when sharing sensitive information. Keeping the patient information confidential includes not speaking about the patient and his condition in public places where it could be overheard. It also includes strictly limiting or removing mobile phones from patient

areas to avoid malicious or accidental recording of private records or information. If the patient is certain that his personal information is kept confidential he may be more forthcoming about his problems.

7. **Showing respect and caring attitude:** In nursing these refer to introducing one self, calling the patient with his/her formal name, treating the patient with dignity, arranging for patient comfort and privacy at all times, preparing the patient before any procedure, encouraging the patient to make choices regarding his care, being compassionate, spending appropriate time with patient, helping and advising the patient to resolve his problems and demonstrating active listening. These activities improve professional relationship with the patient.

INTERPERSONAL RELATIONSHIPS

A relationship is defined as a state of being related or a state of affinity between two individuals.

Interpersonal relationship (IPR) is an interaction between two or more people who communicate, exchange their opinions and values.

Interpersonal relationship is a close association between two or more individuals with varying duration. These relationships are formed in the context of family, work, neighborhood or other social interactions. These are often regulated by customs, agreements or societal norms.

In nursing, interpersonal relationship is a process by which the nurse establishes a rapport with the patient by employing her professional knowledge and skills so as to help the patient physically, psychologically and socially.

In healthcare system the nurse establishes interpersonal relationships with a goal to assist the patient in utilizing his own resources for healing. It also includes association with the health team members.

Types of Relationships

For an individual in a interpersonal relationship to share common goals and objectives with other member/s he or she should more or less be from a similar setting and possess similar thoughts and interests. Honesty and transparency are the key factors for establishing and maintaining an interpersonal relationship. There are three types of relationships (**Figure 9.2**):

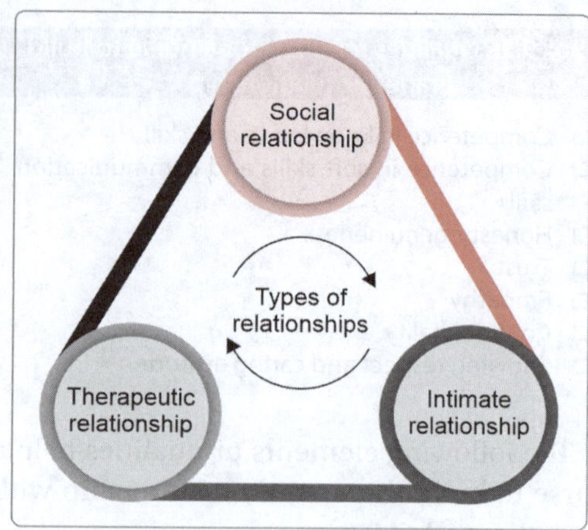

Figure 9.2: Types of relationships

Social Relationship

It is a relationship that is primarily established with the purpose of meeting mutual needs which may range from friendship, socialization, enjoyment to accomplishing a task. In this relationship participants share ideas, feelings and experiences. For example, relationship between friends, individuals working in the same organization or for a similar motive.

Intimate Relationship

An intimate relationship develops between two individuals who have an emotional commitment to each other. In such a relationship each member reacts naturally and cares for the other person to meet his/her life goals. It is more often seen in marital relationships. For example, relationship between a man and a woman (love or marriage), relationship with immediate family members or relatives.

Therapeutic Relationship

This relationship differs from a social or an intimate relationship. It usually occurs between a nurse and a patient wherein the nurse utilizes her knowledge of human behavior, personal strengths and communication skills to fulfill the patient needs. The focus of relationship is on patient ideas, experiences and feelings **(Box 9.4)**. For example, relationship between a nurse and a patient, nurse and a patient care giver. Differences between therapeutic and social/intimate relationship are presented in **Table 9.2.**

Purposes of Interpersonal Relationship in Nursing

- Good nurse-patient relationship helps in building trust between the nurse and the patient resulting in better co-operation for the treatment
- It helps in collecting patient information
- Effective communication helps the patient in taking correct decisions
- It enhances patient and nurse satisfaction
- It reduces stress, promotes wellbeing and improves overall quality of life among nurses
- Effective interpersonal skills help in building trust, improve co-operation and mutual understanding between nurse and patient; nurse and nurse; nurse and health team members; nurse and patient relatives.

Box 9.4: Goals of therapeutic relationship

- ❑ Facilitating communication of distressing thoughts and feelings
- ❑ Assisting the patient with problem solving
- ❑ Helping patients examine self-defeating behaviors and test alternatives
- ❑ Promoting self-care and independence

Interpersonal Skills

Interpersonal skills refer to an ability to build rapport with the individuals. Nurses need to develop these skills to establish good interpersonal relationships with patients. These are:

- Attentive listening
- Meaningful talk
- Non-judgmental approach
- Empathetic understanding
- Unconditional positive regard
- Genuineness in approach
- Accepting constructive criticism
- Respecting others
- Good communication skills

Techniques to Improve Interpersonal Skills

In nursing, communication refers to fundamental practical skills required to establish a therapeutic relationship, explore patient problems, understand patient perspective and guide them towards improving their health. Quality of information obtained by the nurse during consultation is closely associated with the communication skills of the nurse and the patient.

Research literature has shown that the ability of a nurse to actively listen, empathize, and explain have a profound effect on the patient's

Table 9.2: Differences between therapeutic and social/intimate relationship

Component	Therapeutic relationship	Social/Intimate relationship
Nature	Planned	Occurs with mutual interests
Objective	To help the patient	To satisfy the needs of one another
Duration	Limited	Varies; may last for years
Accountability	Nurse is accountable for achieving the goals of relationship	Both members are responsible and accountable
Acceptance	Nurse accepts the patient as he/she is without any personal or emotional attachments and interests	Personal/emotional attachments and interests are involved
Termination	Planned and generally discussed with the patient in advance	Relationship may terminate gradually or continue to exist over a lifetime

health status and functioning as well as on their satisfaction regarding health care received.

Some techniques to improve interpersonal skills are:

- Interact with patient and health team members more often
- Communicate in a clear, complete and concise manner
- Be courteous while interacting with others
- Learn the art of listening
- Develop positive attitude
- Seek feedback regarding communication skills being employed
- Be empathetic towards the patient

Barriers in Interpersonal Relationship and Strategies to Overcome

Barrier is anything that prevents, restricts, or impedes the conveyance of meaning by words or gestures between two or more persons in a social setting (Tofoya, 1976). These barriers cause unsuccessful communication. Barriers to interpersonal relationship are presented in **Box 9.5**.

Box 9.5: Barriers to interpersonal relationship

- ❑ Physiological barrier
- ❑ Environmental barrier
- ❑ Psychological barrier
- ❑ Social barrier
- ❑ Cultural barrier
- ❑ Semantic barrier
- ❑ Organizational barrier
- ❑ Communication process related barrier

1. *Physiological Barriers*

In the context of nurse patient relationship, communication largely depends on physical condition of the patient. If the patient is in pain or having sensory deficits he can neither convey nor receive information effectively **(Table 9.3)**.

2. *Environmental Barriers*

Environment is anything that surrounds or interacts with the patient providing a unique habitat for each person. Environmental factors influence the three elements of communication, viz., sender, message and receiver **(Table 9.4)**.

Table 9.3: Physiological barriers and strategies to overcome them

Physiological barriers	Strategies to overcome
◆ Lack of attention ◆ Discomfort due to illness ◆ Hearing problem ◆ Poor listening skills ◆ Lack of retention due to poor memory	◆ The nurse should ensure that the patient is paying complete attention during the communication process ◆ Before initiating communication the nurse should ensure patient comfort ◆ While initiating communication the nurse should consider retention and recollection abilities of the patient ◆ The nurse should avoid information overload while interacting with the patient ◆ While interacting the nurse should ensure intactness of patient's sensory perception ◆ While communicating due regard should be given to the difference in gender

Table 9.4: Environmental barriers and strategies to overcome them

Environmental barriers	Strategies to overcome
◆ Loud noise ◆ Poor lighting ◆ Uncomfortable setting ◆ Unhygienic surroundings and bad odor ◆ High or low room temperature ◆ Distance factor ◆ Lack of privacy	◆ Before establishing communication the nurse should ensure comfortable position, adequate room temperature and lighting for the patient ◆ Patient environment must be clean and free from bad odors ◆ For communication to be effective both nurse and the patient should maintain optimum distance ◆ Maintain privacy in physical setting when sharing sensitive issues concerning the patient. This may include using a separate room or a screen

3. Psychological Barriers

Communication between nurse and the patient largely depends upon the mental condition of the patient. If the patient is overwhelmed with emotions he cannot receive or convey the information effectively **(Table 9.5)**.

4. Social Barriers

Societal norms play an important role in the process of communication. These norms decide the appropriateness of a conversation which may again depend on the setting, context and people involved. For example, although discussing patient information with healthcare members may be acceptable, discussing the same in another forum may not be appreciated **(Table 9.6)**.

Table 9.5: Psychological barriers and strategies to overcome them

Psychological barriers	Strategies to overcome
• Shyness or embarrassment in sharing information • Distressing emotions • Misperception and misunderstanding • Prejudice	• Nurse should acknowledge patient emotions and use appropriate communication techniques such as clear and simple words • Nurse and the patient should not have preconceived negative ideas or stereotyped views of the other person • Nurse and the patient should be free from fear, anxiety and confusion • The nurse should use therapeutic communication techniques to encourage the patient in sharing his views • The nurse should assess misconceptions and misunderstandings of the patient on a periodic basis and clarify them with proper facts

Table 9.6: Social barriers and strategies to overcome them

Social barriers	Strategies to overcome
• Differences in social norms and values • Differences in social strata	• Nurse needs to respect social norms and values • Social strata need to be considered while communicating with the patient

5. Cultural Barriers

Customs, traditions and cultural background greatly influence the style of communication. If the patient is from a different cultural background it becomes difficult for the nurse to communicate **(Table 9.7)**.

Table 9.7: Cultural barriers and strategies to overcome them

Cultural barriers	Strategies to overcome
• Ethnic, religious and cultural differences • Traditions, customs and cultural beliefs	• As perception greatly depends on the cultural background of any individual, a nurse should duly understand the cultural differences and traditional values of the patient while providing care

6. Semantic Barriers

Semantics refers to the study of meaning in a language which can be applied to a single word or the complete text. The choice of words, their meaning, pronunciation, dialects may be interpreted differently by different individuals as the same word may have various meanings in various contexts. This may lead to conveying the message in a distorted way or in a way not intended by the sender **(Table 9.8)**.

7. Organizational Barriers

Organizational policy, procedures and style of functioning also play a vital role in the communication process. These factors influence the mode of communication and enhance the interpersonal relationship among the employees **(Table 9.9)**.

Table 9.8: Semantic barriers and strategies to overcome them

Semantic barriers	Strategies to overcome
• Language, jargon (terminology) • Faulty language translations	• The nurse should preferably communicate in the same language as used by the patient and avoid needless translation • The nurse should ensure that the patient is attentive while conveying any kind of information • The language used should be simple and include minimum technical jargon

Table 9.9: Organizational barriers and strategies to overcome them

Organizational barriers	Strategies to overcome
• Organizational policy, rules and regulations • Complexity in organizational hierarchy • Size of the organization	• Organizational policy, rules and regulations must be pro communication • Organizational structure must be simple and non-complex for smooth communication • Decentralization in an organizational structure promotes effective communication

8. Communication Process-Related Barriers

Communication process includes sharing of ideas, information, opinions, feelings, emotions, etc. among individuals. It includes four elements, viz., sender, message, receiver and feedback. Disturbance in any of these elements can create distortion in communication **(Table 9.10)**.

Table 9.10: Communication process-related barriers and strategies to overcome them

Communication process-related barriers	Strategies to overcome
• Unclear and conflicting messages • Use of inappropriate channels • Lack of or poor feedback	• The nurse should communicate in clear, simple language with the patient • The nurse should select appropriate channel for communication • The nurse should ensure proper feedback from the patient

Interpersonal skills are essential for a nurse to discharge her duties effectively and also progress in her career.

SURVIVAL STRATEGIES

Survival strategies are specific stress responses which include specific adaptive and maladaptive, biological, psychological and social constituents. They form four complimentary pairs—rescue and attachment, assertiveness and adaptation, fight and flight and competition and cooperation. These help to explain the great variety of post-traumatic symptoms. Hence survival strategies alert us to a great variety of emotions, physiological responses and social outcomes.

1. **Rescue/caretaking:** People in disasters always try to find their loved ones first to ensure their safety, and frequently apply life preserving measures to others who are helpless.
2. **Attachment:** It is the complementary strategy to rescue/caretaking. Secure attachment leads to contentment and a sense of belonging.
3. **Assertiveness/goal achievement:** It is a frequent prerequisite to achievement of survival goals, such as food, shelter and territory. It requires will, strength, control and a sense of potency.
4. **Adaptation/goal surrender:** Adapting to new circumstances requires surrendering old goals and grieving losses. Inability

to adapt can lead to unresolved grief, depression, and feelings of hopelessness and despair.

5. **Fight:** The purpose of fight is to defend life, property and territory. Successful fight provides a sense of relief and security.
6. **Flight:** Successful escape is associated with a sense of relief. Inability to escape is associated with a sense of being trapped, about to be engulfed and crushed.
7. **Competition/struggle:** Competition is a contest for hierarchical levels or status. Dominant ones have the advantages of first access to food, better shelter, more sex.
8. **Cooperation/love:** In cooperation people bond in mutual trust, generosity and reciprocity without regard to hierarchy. It is the opposite survival strategy to competition.

TIME MANAGEMENT

"Time isn't the main thing. It's the only thing."

—Miles Davis

"It is not enough to be busy... The questions is: what are we busy about?"

—Henry David Thoreau

"Lack of direction, not lack of time, is the problem. We all have twenty-four hour days."

—ZigZiglar

Time management refers to the allocation of available time among specific activities based on certain priorities while giving preference to individual likes and dislikes. It is an important soft skill that can be applied in almost every job and almost for everybody. Good time management allows one to work smarter if not harder. It gets the individual to do more in less time and enhances the ability to function effectively even under time pressures. Some of the important benefits of time management are listed in **Box 9.6**.

Box 9.6: Benefits of time management

- ❑ Makes the individual more organized and confident
- ❑ Creates more opportunities for advancement in profession and reaching life goals
- ❑ Improves professional reputation
- ❑ Results in greater productivity and efficiency by cutting on poor work flow
- ❑ Reduces stress
- ❑ Allows greater control over job responsibilities

Building Time Management Skills

Mastering time management skills requires dedicated effort and practice. A few tips for improving time management skills are as under:

- **Prepare and follow a strict schedule:** Create a daily or weekly schedule outlining the tasks and commitments with specific time slots.
- **Set boundaries for yourself:** Set clear boundaries and learn to say no to tasks or activities that do not align with your priorities or goals.
- **Fix deadlines:** Assigning deadlines helps to create a sense of urgency and enables prioritization of work effectively. However, the deadlines should be realistic considering complexity and importance of each task.
- **Set long-term and short-term goals:** Define the goals clearly and break them into small, actionable parts. It provides clarity and motivation. Review the progress regularly.
- **Manage your calendar effectively:** Use a digital planning tool to manage the tasks and deadlines. Review and update the work calendar regularly to stay on top of the commitments.
- **Prioritize your assignments:** Determining tasks which are most important and need immediate attention prevents from getting overwhelmed by less important tasks. Using techniques like Eisenhower Matrix can help to categorize tasks based on urgency and importance **(Figure 9.3)**.
- **Practice effective delegation:** Identifying and assigning tasks that can be done by someone else will help you to focus on higher priority tasks thereby improving productivity.
- **Minimize multitasking:** Though it might seem efficient, multitasking often leads to decreased productivity and lowers the quality of work.

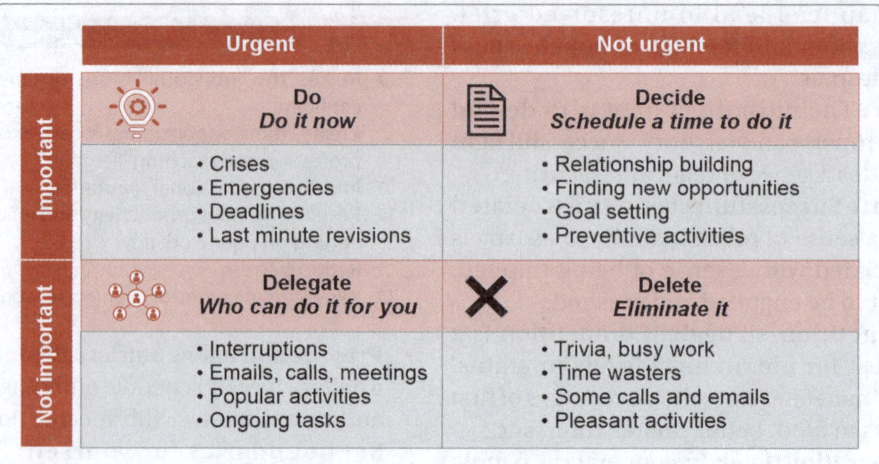

Figure 9.3: The Eisenhower Matrix

- **Take regular breaks:** Avoid long stretches of continuous work as it can lead to burnout and decreased productivity.
- **Learn from your experiences:** Engage in self-reflection to evaluate the progress. Focus on areas where improvements can be made. Assessing the productivity pattern and identifying habits that are having a bearing on time can help to refine the time management skills.

Improving time management skills is an ongoing process that requires self-discipline and commitment. By implementing these strategies consistently, one can achieve goals more effectively.

Time Management for Nurses

Nurses are an indispensable part of the fast changing healthcare scenario wherein they are required to meet the expectations of patients, peers and supervisors while managing their regular work schedule. They are also required to handle the emergencies along with their routine tasks. Continuous manpower shortage and pressures of the clinical setting have put a greater demand on the nurses to work smarter and harder. This calls for better time management skills which is crucial for their survival in busy shifts. Following strategies will allow a nurse to manage her time better:

- Plan, prioritize and delegate work
- Plan the patient care schedule
- Prioritize patient activities
- Set realistic goals
- Delegate non nursing activities to other staff
- Have a routine for regular ward activities
- Prepare for emergencies ahead of time
- Follow protocols and standards while providing care
- Maintain necessary records and reports
- Follow checklist for certain procedures
- Make use of time reminders, alarms
- Save precious time by gaining adequate knowledge, competence and confidence in performing procedures
- Spend right time for right activity
- Prepare activity logs

All these strategies allow the nurse to impart quality care and relive work related stress. It may also help them to relax and socialize at work without getting exhausted. A perfect balance between professional and personal life can only be achieved by good time management.

Time Management for Nursing Students

Not having adequate time to perform the set academic tasks is a frequently voiced phenomenon by many students. This is despite the fact that many are able to achieve much more than others under similar time constraints.

The answer lies in their ability to manage and utilize the available time more effectively. It is an important skill which applies to nursing students as well. As the nurse students graduate there is a greater need for them to cultivate time management skills among other life skills for the following reasons:

- Good time management skills facilitate the students in prioritizing their academic tasks.
- Students are able to plan ahead by setting aside the necessary time for projects and assignments.
- Becoming better at managing time makes the students more organized and confident.
- Following time management techniques leads to a healthy all round development.
- Exhibiting better time management skills while performing academic or clinical related tasks directly reflects on their levels of competence.
- It keeps them prepared for unexpected emergencies.
- A perfect balance between personal life and work/study can only be achieved by effective time management.
- Following proper time management techniques results in a marked reduction in unnecessary stress arising out of inappropriate planning.

A few time management techniques for students are listed in **Box 9.7.**

Box 9.7: Time management tips for students

- Prepare a time table for the routine
- Start early in the day
- Set goals for each study session
- Start working on assignments early
- Learn to differentiate between urgent and important
- Do not over commit
- Develop routines
- Work on one thing at a time
- Take short breaks during study hours
- Eliminate or minimize distractions
- Get adequate sleep
- Allow time for the unexpected
- Keep a track of learning
- Set reasonable time for each goal

COPING WITH STRESS

Stress is a universal phenomenon commonly experienced by most people. It is often defined as a state of emotional strain or tension resulting from adverse or demanding circumstances.

Stress affects the whole person across all dimensions, viz., physical, emotional, intellectual, social and spiritual. It comprises of three components: a stressor, perception of the event and the response. Stressor is the life change or extra demand which is the root of the problem. How an individual views the stressor and relates himself or herself to it is referred to as the perception of the event. Response is the way the body, behavior and thinking patterns change.

Coping includes efforts to control, reduce or tolerate the threats caused due to stress. There are three basic types of coping skills to deal with stress—physical, mental and social.

Physical/behavioral coping skills involve taking care of oneself and staying as healthy as possible. These coping skills involve strategies such as physical activity, yoga, stretching, healthy diet, adequate rest and sleep and relaxation exercises.

- Physical activities like walking, aerobic exercises, climbing stairs, cycling, gardening, swimming, house work, etc., reduce stress, improve mood and energy levels. These activities produce endorphins (a chemical in the brain) that relieve stress and pain and improve mood. WHO guidelines recommend that adults undertake moderate to vigorous physical activity for a minimum 150 minutes per week in bouts of ten minutes or more. Many research studies have shown that regular participation in aerobic exercises is instrumental in reducing overall stress levels, elevate mood, improve sleep and self-esteem.
- Yoga and stretching: Even daily sessions of yoga and slow stretching in durations as small as 5–10 minutes can promote relaxation and reduce stress.

- Diet rich in vegetables, fruits, whole grains, low fat dairy, lean meat, limited salt, sugar and saturated fats intake acts as a stress reducing agent. Eating a well-balanced diet, drinking plenty of water and emptying bowels everyday improves brain function, blood circulation, immunity, lowers blood pressure and eliminates toxins from the body.
- Adequate rest and sleep regulates the mood and helps the individual to cope with stressful situations.
- Relaxation techniques such as deep breathing exercises, progressive muscle relaxation, guided imagery meditation, mindful meditation, etc., slow breathing and heart rate, lower blood pressure and balance both the body and the mind.

Cognitive/mental coping skills involve using thoughts and the mind constructively to counteract negative effects of stress. These coping skills involve strategies such as following problem solving techniques, reappraising the situation, time management, being assertive and expressing emotions effectively, etc.

- When faced with a stressful situation follow the various steps in problem solving technique which include identifying the problem, determining various alternatives and selecting the suitable solution. These techniques help to choose the best alternative and also manage stress.
- Sometimes interpretation of a stressor can magnify its impact and make it feel more stressful than it really is. Reappraisal means reframing the meaning of the situation by changing the way one thinks about potentially emotion-eliciting events. It is an attempt to reinterpret an emotion-eliciting situation in a way that alters its meaning and changes its emotional impact. Reappraisal can modify emotional reactions to stressful situations and lead to emotional well-being. Do not blow things out of proportion.
- Effective time management allows individuals to maintain work-life balance, enhance sense of control, invest time on right things, better organize things, and improve efficiency. All these contribute to reducing stress precipitating factors.
- Assertiveness is the ability to express one's feelings and declare one's rights while respecting the feelings and rights of others. Being assertive helps to express one's own feelings and clarifies one's needs to the other person. This reduces stress as it makes the person feel he is in better control of the situation.
- A few other strategies that help in reduction of stress perception are positive thinking, positive attitude, trying to be reasonable, accepting that bad feelings are occasionally unavoidable, thinking of ways to make one self feel better, get an understanding of events that trigger sad feelings so that one can be prepared in advance and letting go of the past.
- Some activities that can effectively reduce stress by handling negative emotions are writing a diary, crying out, talking to a friend, participating in favorite activities, taking a hot bath or a cold shower.

Personal/social coping skills involve having social support networks, taking care of current relationships, exploring and developing personal interests.

- One of the best ways to reduce or control stress is to make happiness a priority, take a time out and make an extra effort to spend quality leisure time with friends and family. Friends and family members can prevent triggering of stress by reaching out before the situation goes out of control.
- Maintain regular contact with friends and relatives. Do not lose an opportunity to attend luncheons and gatherings in community halls. Social support is often mutual; relationships are maintained by reviewing, planning and nurturing.
- Develop hobbies and personal interests, enjoy nature and outing, go for a walk in a park, get away from routine life, relax when possible, love yourself by avoiding self-criticism, praise and support, be gentle and kind to yourself, take care of the body, connect with the inner self and volunteer

for community activities. All these activities can be rewarding and satisfying resulting in control and reduction of stress.

RESILIENCE

"Resilience is the process of adapting well in the face of adversity, trauma, tragedy, threats or even significant sources of stress."

— The American Psychological Association (2014)

Resilience refers to the ability to 'bounce back' by harnessing the inner strength after a setback or a challenge. Being resilient does not mean the individual is unaffected by the event or the problem or not experiencing anger, grief, distress, anxiety or pain. It just means that he has found a way to continue functioning both physically and psychologically and deal with it more quickly than others. Those who lack resilience are overwhelmed by unfavorable circumstances and usually turn to unhealthy coping mechanisms. Such individuals are slow to recover from the disaster and in the process experience greater psychological distress. Though resilience is often viewed as a trait, process or an outcome, it is ideal to view it on a continuum which may be present up to varying degrees in multiple life domains.

- Resilience though viewed as a personality trait can be learnt and developed as a skill over a period of time.
- Resilience does not do away with the problems or sense of loss but gives the ability to see beyond them.
- Resilience can help to cope and overcome mental health conditions like depression and anxiety.
- Resilience allows people to face difficulties head-on and emerge stronger than before.
- Resilience not only allows the affected individuals to carry on but provides an ability to offer emotional support to those affected by similar tragedies.

Factors Contributing to Resilience

All people do not react to a trauma or a tragedy in a similar fashion as it is determined by a combination of biological, psychological, social and cultural factors. It is the continuous interaction of these factors that determine how one responds to stressful experiences. Four factors contributing to resilience are presented in **Figure 9.4**.

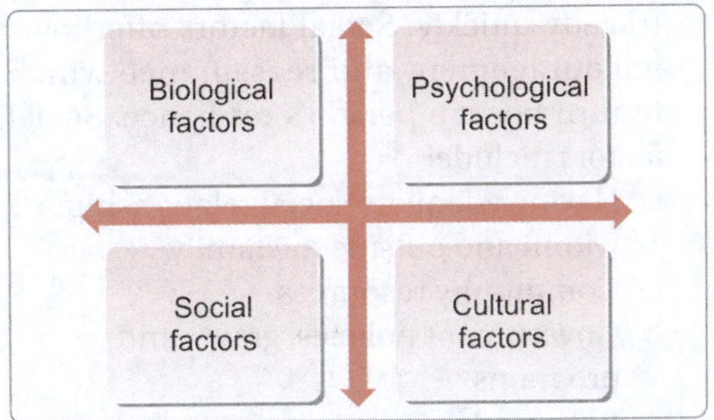

Figure 9.4: Factors contributing to resilience

1. **Biological factors:** These factors promote physical and mental health which in turn play a role in building and maintaining resilience. Biological factors include:
   - Good physical and mental health
   - Balanced diet
   - Healthy life style practices
2. **Psychological factors**: These factors help to build a proper perspective of the adverse situation and develop a capacity to manage strong negative feelings and impulses. This realistic perception of the event helps the individual to become more resilient. Psychological factors include:
   - Having realistic goals and ability to carry them out
   - High self-esteem, self-confidence and self-efficacy
   - Optimistic outlook and ability to adapt to change
   - Adequate problem solving abilities
   - Learning from past experiences
   - Being assertive and having adequate communication skills
   - Having high emotional intelligence
   - Securing childhood attachments
   - Adaptive coping mechanisms
   - Intelligence, temperament, sense of humor
3. **Social factors:** These factors support the individual during times of distress and aid in recovering from trauma or

tragedy quickly. Social factors offer love, encouragement and reassurance which in turn boost a person's resilience. Social factors include:
- Having adequate social relationships within and outside the family
- Community resources
- Government policies, grants and programs
- Role models, mentors

4. **Cultural factors:** Cultural parameters help an individual to develop coping strategies and allow better adjustment with the adverse situation. These factors decide how an individual connects with his friend and family members and shares his feelings. In an overall sense these allow better adjustment. Cultural factors include:
   - Belief systems
   - Cultural practices
   - Ethnic identification
   - Social class status
   - Cultural background (tradition, values, language, customs and norms)

Development of Resilience

Developing resilience is a personal journey. Learning to become resilient involves a dynamic process which requires lot of time, effort and commitment. A few tips to become more resilient are listed in **Box 9.8**.

Box 9.8: Tips to develop resilience

- Build a perception
- Leverage your strength
- Be positive
- Be proactive
- Be hopeful
- Be realistic
- Focus on progress
- Stay connected
- Care for self
- Make each day meaningful
- Learn from the past

- **Build a perception:** One of the foremost prerequisites to become more resilient is to build a perception of the adversity by looking at the individual situation in the bigger context which will determine its seriousness or the lack thereof. Look at the obstacle as a challenge rather than a hindrance.
- **Leverage your strength:** Knowing one's own strengths and values and listing them out provides a sense of direction and competence during times of distress. But if one is unaware of his strengths, a friend or family member's help may be sought to identify them.
- **Be positive:** Have a positive view of oneself (self-image) and confidence in one's own strengths and abilities (self-knowledge). This will help to get out of the negative mindset.
- **Be proactive:** Do not ignore or postpone the problems. No problem is impossible. Figure out the problems, make a remedial plan and act on it. Even a major loss or setback can be overcome when we work at it.
- **Be hopeful:** Accept the past and be hopeful about the future. Being open to changes makes it easier to adapt to new challenges which reduces anxiety.
- **Be realistic:** Make realistic plans and formulate achievable goals. Follow it up with action.
- **Focus on progress:** Monitoring the progress is crucial to strengthening the sense of resilience rather than focusing only on the goal. Reporting progress to family and friends or even physically recording it creates a sense of commitment to move towards the goal.
- **Stay connected:** Developing strong and positive relationships with friends and significant others provides the much needed support and acceptance both in good and bad times. Joining a spiritual community will help invent the feeling in an effective and healthy manner.
- **Care for self:** Meet your own needs and value your feelings. Participate in activities that bring joy. Eat healthy. Include physical activities in the daily routine. Get good sleep. Practice relaxation and stress reducing techniques.

- **Make each day meaningful:** Include activities in the routine that provide a sense of purpose and accomplishment. This will add a positive outlook to the future.
- **Learn from the past:** Recollect the skills and strategies that have helped to overcome past hardships. Identify behavioral patterns during the difficult times and learn from such experiences.

WORK LIFE BALANCE

Work life balance refers to effective management of dual role at work and family.

Work life balance means harmony between ones job and ones professional life. It means neither aspects of the life overtakes the other.

Work life balance is "the extent to which an individual is equally self-engaged and satisfied with his or her work role and family role."

—Greenhaus, Collins and Shaw (2003)

Work life balance refers to a state of wellbeing wherein one can find a healthy way to separate work responsibilities from personal life.

Importance of Work-life Balance in Nursing

Nursing is a demanding profession which requires scientific, interpersonal and emotional intelligence. It involves the use of multiple skills as patients with various disease conditions are cared for each day. Also nurses deal with long working hours, shift system and frequent job rotations. Other issues such as under staffing, minimal resources, outdated equipment, demands of sick patients, emotional strain of caregivers and patient attendants also put a lot of burden on her. These are some factors that expect a nurse to put extra attention on maintaining work life balance as compared to other professionals. Benefits that an individual and an organization can reap from work life balance are listed in **Box 9.9**.

Box 9.9: Benefits of maintaining work life balance

Individual benefits

- Develops self-esteem
- Maintains psychological wellbeing
- Helps in attaining contentment
- Helps to achieve harmony between work and life with minimum role conflict

Organizational benefits

- Reduced absenteeism
- Increased productivity
- Retention of skilled staff leading to reduction in training costs
- Reduced staff turnover
- Greater interest shown by skilled personnel to join the organization
- Continuous support from the employees

Individual Strategies to Maintain Work-life Balance

Some of the strategies for a nurse to maintain work-life balance are:

- Assess job areas that are most demanding
- Pay special attention to rest and relaxation while on night shift
- Build self-care activities in daily routine and follow practice relaxation techniques
- Talk to friends, family or counselor to overcome stressors
- Be flexible at both work place and home
- Accept that everything cannot be changed
- Learn to delegate work
- Do not feel guilty while seeking assistance at work
- Feel free to decline politely

Organizational Strategies to Maintain Work-life Balance

Some of the organizational strategies to help maintain work-life balance are:

- Reduce long working hours
- Allow flexible working hours where permissible
- Provide part time jobs with less hours and fewer shifts
- Make job sharing arrangements
- Make leave taking more flexible

- Allow staff to take extra leave by forgoing pay
- Provide access to child care
- Provide subsidies for childcare
- Allow receiving of urgent telephone calls or messages from family members while at work
- Offer programs for employees to return to work after extended leave

A nurse needs to prioritize both at professional and personal levels. Her inability to do so will lead to improper work life balance resulting in overstress. It will also lead to nurturing of negative thoughts and feelings making her susceptible to illness and early burn out. Burnt out nurses cannot connect with patients on an emotional level. They become apathetic and disinterested or detached from patients leading to medical mistakes. Thus a poor work life balance will result in higher turnover, staffing shortage and additional healthcare costs.

Workplace Rules for a Happy Life

World mental health day 2017 was observed with "Mental health in the workplace" as the central theme. The overall objective was to raise an awareness on mental health issues and mobilize efforts in support of better mental health. A few rules recommended by WHO in this direction are listed in **Box 9.10.**

Box 9.10: Workplace rules for a happy life

- Trust no one but respect everyone
- Never carry office gossips back home
- Enter office on time and leave on time
- Never make relationships at workplace
- Expect nothing
- Never rush for your position
- Never run behind office stuff
- Avoid taking everything on your ego
- Does not matter how people treat you
- Nothing matters except family

APPLYING SOFT SKILLS TO WORKPLACE AND SOCIETY

Presentation Skills

Nurses are responsible for conveying information to patients, doctors and other professionals in the healthcare system. To perform this role nurses must be able to communicate clearly and effectively even under stressful situations. Nurses with good presentations skills can provide quality care to patients.

Presentation skills are set of abilities that enable an individual to interact with the audience, transmit the messages with clarity, engage with audience in the presentation, interpret and understand the mindsets of the listeners. Effective presentation has been defined as an ability to communicate the message to an audience in a way that results in a change in understanding or opinion.

Steps in Effective Presentation

There are four effective steps to preparing an effective presentation—plan, prepare, practice and perform.

1. **Plan:** Define the purpose and list the aims and objectives of the presentation. Know the background of the audience, time duration, venue, number of audiences, availability of AV aids, such as computer for power point presentation, mikes, content of the topic, etc.
2. **Prepare:** Prepare visual aids, lecture notes, handouts well in advance. Structure the presentation.
3. **Practice:** Rehearse the presentation to examine facial expressions, body movements, etc. Rehearsals reduce anxiety and enable the presenter to look confident on the presentation day. Make sure to practice out loud as it enables to identify and eliminate errors more effectively.
4. **Perform:** Get a good start as it builds confidence. Arrange and test equipment and relax. Work logically through the presentation.
   - Introduce yourself
   - Explain aims and objectives of the presentation
   - Outline the order of presentation
   - Present information in a logical sequence
   - Interpret facts while explaining the complex concepts

- Conclude the session with a restatement of the main points
- Invite questions

Tips for Good Presentation

- Everyone experiences some nervousness when presenting. A good practice gives confidence. Practice presentation until comfortable with the content
- Prepare notes to stay on track
- Dress formally
- Make eye contact with the audience
- Pay attention to own body language
- Pause before and after important ideas
- Select language that will be understood by the audience
- Speak clearly and loud enough to be heard by all audience
- Practice relaxation to control nervousness

Importance of Presentation Skills for a Nurse

Nurses are required to give presentations frequently whether as part of a health education to a person/patient, job interview, case presentation, paper or poster presentation in a conference/workshop or as part of a professional development program. However, giving effective presentation is a skill everyone can learn.

- Nurses are increasingly being asked to present in formal and informal situations, such as conferences, poster presentations, job interviews, case reports and ward-based teaching. In order to share ideas, knowledge and opinions more widely, nurses need to either speak or write within the public arena. For all nurses, presentation skills are not just useful but essential.
- Good presentation skills allow nurses to not only share information and expertise but also communicate clearly with patients, their caregivers and other health professionals.
- Interaction with other healthcare professionals is a routine job for the nurses. Good presentation skills influence colleagues and enhance own growth opportunities.
- It grooms the personality of the presenter and elevates the level of confidence.
- Presentation skills are important for individual success as career growth in nursing necessitates presenting own ideas to others.
- Effective presentation skills reduce miscommunication, which is probably the biggest cause of work-related stress. Better presenters are usually better communicators.
- Every leader needs to deliver a clear and effective message as she is judged based on her presentation skills. Best presenters often make good leaders.

Presentation is an excellent opportunity for a nurse to show her own skills, knowledge, expertise and personality.

Social Etiquette

A nurse is an important member of the healthcare team. She must work in co-operation and harmony for providing best care to patients. Nurses should have professional relationships with all kinds of people in various settings. For smooth functioning and good interpersonal relationship with others the nurse should follow certain essential good manners.

Etiquette is a code of good manners. Social etiquette is the set of rules that controls accepted behavior in particular social groups. Social etiquette needs to be followed in social situations to be respectful and courteous towards everyone present.

Social etiquette relates to the norms of social behavior and interactions considered acceptable by everyone.

Basic Social Etiquette Rules

- Show basic courtesy and decency while interacting with others.
- Be punctual.
- Have personal space when interacting with others.
- Speak softly with warm gestures.
- Keep relationships formal in work place.
- Do not share any personal connections unnecessarily. Share information only when asked to do so.
- Be a reliable co-worker.
- Dress according to the situation. Keep the dress neat and tidy.
- Never gossip.

- Remember people's names as it is an excellent way to make a good impression.
- Limit cell phone usage when interacting with people. Pick only important calls.
- Be courteous to all. Be gentle and polite while talking to others.
- Address seniors, co-workers, patients, etc., with proper titles, such as sir, madam, mister, miss, etc.
- Greet seniors, co-workers and patients with appropriate salutations and in accordance with the time of the day.
- Stand up when people of higher rank enter the room.
- Maintain silence wherever and whenever necessary.
- Maintain eye contact and sit face to face when listening to someone.
- Excuse oneself before interfering with others engaged in talking or doing some work.
- Excuse oneself after sneezing.
- Say thank you or sorry when the situation demands.
- ABC of etiquettes are appearance, behavior and communication.

Importance of Social Etiquettes in Nursing

- Nursing is a career characterized by professional relationships with all kinds of people in various settings. They are involved in care of people of all ages in various communities. Hence nurses need to follow specific rules of social interactions to facilitate effective interpersonal relationships with other healthcare team members.
- Social etiquettes help nurses understand how they should behave in particular situations, guide in unfamiliar situations and help to know what to expect from others.
- As nurses move into top leadership positions it is certain that etiquette skills are a part of their power base.
- Social etiquettes are an important factor to succeed in healthcare career.
- Nurse's career advancements depend on effective professional etiquette.
- Social etiquettes project nurses as a kind and approachable person. This encourages others to interact with the nurses.
- Social etiquettes can help nurses initiate new relationships and improve established relationships.
- Social etiquette eases interactions between people by removing misunderstandings and lessens the confrontation that might arise out of such misunderstandings. This reduces conflict and promotes harmony with others.
- Communication is not only a spoken language but also the general behavior exhibited towards others. Good social etiquette communicates more about the person than his words.
- Good social etiquette is essential at workplace as it gives the nurse a professional outlook and projects a good impression of her.
- Understanding professional and social etiquettes are not an option for a nurse, but it is necessary to build confidence in the patients and foster positive interpersonal relations with co-workers.

Telephone Etiquette

Communication through telephone plays a significant role in any healthcare setting. Modernization and digitalization of health organizations has led to various channels of communication, such as mobile calls, video calls, automated answering machines, texting, emails, etc. Among all, telephone communication provides a personal touch, gives more clarity and a positive impression.

Telephone is one of the most important instruments of communication equipment in the hospital. When patients call the nurse, they expect certain etiquette.

Telephone etiquette refers to a set of rules that people should follow while calling and receiving calls from others. Telephone etiquette specifies the manners of using telephone communication which includes greeting the receiver, tone of voice, choice of words, listening skills, closure of the call etc. These are being respectful to the person whom we are talking to, showing consideration for the other person's limitations, allowing the person to talk, communicate clearly, etc.

Types of Incoming Calls

- Nurses encounter a wide variety of questions and requests when answering the telephone. Most incoming calls are from patients, physicians, laboratory personnel etc.
- Telephone calls from patients may have to do with appointment scheduling, billing inquires, request for medical or laboratory reports, questions about medications, progress information, advice or complaints.
- Nurses should keep the patient's information confidential and obtain authorization from the patient before disclosing any information to his family or friends.

Proper Telephone Etiquettes in Healthcare Setting

- The nurse needs to be courteous and helpful. She should give the caller her undivided attention and never try to perform other tasks while talking on the telephone.
- When the nurse deals with someone who is nervous or upset, she should communicate with empathy to show the caller that she understands their feelings.
- As most hospitals have multiple lines, the nurse will need strong multitasking techniques to transfer calls, leave voicemails and put calls on hold.
- Effective listening techniques by the nurse will allow her to understand whether a call is an emergency or not.
- A nurse should permit patients to complete their thoughts rather than anticipate what they are going to say.
- A nurse should also repeat back caller's request so that the caller knows that the nurse has properly listened to them.
- When concluding the call, the nurse should take a few seconds to summarize the important points of the call and thank the caller.
- An effective way to guide communication with doctors and other colleagues is to use a tool such as SBAR—situation, background, assessment and recommendation.
  - Situation: Mr John complaining severe headache.
  - Background: He is first day post-operative from a lumbar laminectomy.
  - Assessment: His vitals are stable, no numbness or tingling in his extremities.
  - Recommendation: Would you like to order something for him?

Before ending the conversation, repeat and clarify the medication order if doctor advices.

Telephone Voice Etiquette Techniques

- The nurse must keep an appropriate telephone voice using proper etiquette techniques including diction, pitch, tone, enunciation, volume, speed and pronunciation. The nurse must also be a good listener and answer the phone in a professional manner.
  - Diction: It relates to the proper pronunciation of words that allows others to understand clearly.
  - Pitch: It refers to the sound which may either be low and deep or high. It is always important to create a pleasing tone for the patient to be comfortable.
  - Tone: It refers to the quality of sound or the feeling conveyed in somebody's voice, especially while expressing a particular emotion.
  - Enunciation: It refers to the act of pronouncing words or parts of words clearly and precisely. This allows the listeners to understand what is being said.
  - Loudness: It refers to being strongly audible or having exceptional volume or intensity. A voice that is too loud or hard to hear can make a negative impression.
  - Speed: If the nurse speaks too fast the patient may miss a portion of the message.
  - Pronunciation: By pronouncing a name properly, the nurse can demonstrate respect for the patient.
- The nurse should use proper etiquette through pronunciation of words, keep the

pitch pleasant, speak with positive and respectful tone, sound intelligible, not be too soft or loud and speak at such a speed that the caller can understand the full message.

Importance of Telephone Etiquettes for a Nurse

- Mastering good communication skills is essential for all nurses at all career stages.
- Communicating with telephone manners always shows our professionalism as it makes the patient believe that their life is in good and safe hands.
- Impression that we create over telephone communication has a lasting effect.
- Telephone etiquette builds trust among patients and provides satisfaction.

Tips to Use Telephone

- Do not let a ringing phone interfere with work.
- Speak softly. When talking on cell phone do not annoy people around you. If possible, move away from others when using phone.
- Do not use a cell phone while driving.
- Always turn off cell phone during public performances, in worship areas, weddings, funerals and movie theatres.
- Answering the telephone in a professional manner involves answering within 2 or 3 rings.
- Always ask permission to place the caller on hold before doing so.
- Minimize background noise.
- Concentrate on listening and avoid multitasking.
- Schedule phone conversations to avoid playing phone tag.
- Smile when you talk as people love talking to happy people. Although it cannot be shown, a smile can be heard in the voice and the caller will be much more relaxed in their conversation with you.
- When you answer the phone, greet the caller warmly.
- Try and speak in a calm tone that will be easy to hear and understand.
- Speak clearly.
- Gestures, facial expressions, body language also have an impact while communicating on the telephone. A cheerful voice and a bright tone give the feeling to the receiver that you are relaxed and at ease. A professional body language gives a good impression.
- Tone of voice should be confident and show respect towards the caller.

Proper telephone etiquette is about making a good impression when speaking on the phone.

Motivation Skills

Motivation means encouragement. It is a driving force within the individual that influences or directs behavior. It may be learned or innate, working within the individual to attain a specific purpose.

There are two different types of motivation: intrinsic and extrinsic.

- Intrinsic motivation is an inner force that helps a person meet his personal goals, guide activity that he/she finds exciting.
- People who are intrinsically motivated have an internal drive which inspires them to meet responsibilities without any external effects.
- Internal motivation arises out of self-interest and without pressure from others.
- Internal motivation among nurses is defined as self-gratification or pleasure in carrying out responsibilities rather than working for external rewards.
- External motivation is an external force that helps the person meet personal and organizational goals, guide him in carrying out responsibilities using coercion or instruction to get rewards in return.
- People who are extrinsically motivated perform responsibilities to gain rewards, bonuses, pay and other benefits.
- Extrinsic motivation leads the nurses to achieve position, awards, incentives and other benefits.

Importance of Motivation Skills for Nurses

Motivation skills can be actions or strategies that elicit a desired behavior or response from a participant. Motivation skill is very important for a nurse to perform her task effectively, efficiently and on scheduled time. The source of motivation can be internal or external. While internal motivation comes from unsatisfied needs or desires, external motivation comes through rewards, pay, parents, spouse, etc. Motivation at work plays a vital role in the functioning of the nurse. Motivation skill:

- Reduces boredom in work
- Improves job satisfaction
- Helps to improve work efficiency
- Improves work output

Strategies to Improve Motivation Among Nurses

Nurse administrators should motivate nurses to perform their activities effectively using the following strategies:

- Help the nurses to perform their routine activities
- Provide positive feedback on their work
- Create a conducive environment for work
- Offer rewards or incentives based on their performance
- Provide supportive environment
- Encourage to participate in extra or co-curricular activities
- Appreciate hard work

Team Work

As the number of patients suffering from chronic conditions such as diabetes, cancer, arthritis, and kidney diseases, etc., is on a steady rise, patient care has become extremely complex and intricate. These illnesses by their complex nature require specialized care which has in turn resulted in sharp demand for multidisciplinary approach to treating patients. This approach refers to the collaboration between members of different disciplines who provide specific services to a patient. The multidisciplinary team includes doctors, nurses, nutritionist, physiotherapist and other healthcare professionals.

In multidisciplinary approach while nurses play the central role, they also co-ordinate with physicians and specialists to provide well-organized and comprehensive care to patients. Teamwork is essential to perform this role.

Team work is centered on the patient and focused on shared goals. Nurses constantly use teamwork skills in the work place by collaborating with other nurses and doctors to develop nursing care plans, track medication information and share information with the patients. Being proactive in improving teamwork at workplace can help a nurse to establish more efficient nursing practices and grow in her career.

Essential Components of Teamwork

- Communication, co-ordination and co-operation are the three essential components of teamwork.
- It is important that team members communicate clearly and effectively with one another in building a strong work relationship, share resources and solve problems.
- Team members should focus on patient-centered care by co-operating with one another.
- There should be a clear and effective exchange of information among members.
- Timely information should be provided to patients and other team members.
- All the available electronic resources should be well integrated.
- Each member of the team should have an understanding of his task and know how to work together collaboratively towards shared goals.

Advantages of Effective Team Work

Nurses are centrally positioned in the team which connects patients, doctors as well as administrative personnel. When nurses use teamwork successfully they can generate several benefits to patients and workplace organization. Some of these benefits include:

- Reduced morbidity rates
- Increased patient and healthcare worker satisfaction
- Team members support to make patient related decisions
- Effective accomplishment of following goals by working in a cohesive environment
    - Enhance patient safety
    - Reduce medical errors

- Improve clinical performance
- Raise efficiency and lower healthcare costs
- Decrease level of stress among patients and improve patient wellbeing

Importance of Teamwork in Nursing

Teamwork is an important aspect of nursing because it creates effective and open communication among healthcare professionals thus improving their ability to care for patients. Teamwork also results in:

- Greater job satisfaction: Working well as a team can help reduce stress and increase happiness at work. Nurses can thereby experience balanced workload and have the liberty to explore other aspects of nursing.
- Improved patient care: Teamwork ensures better standard of care to each patient. It enhances patient experience, encourages accountability and makes the treatment process safer.
- More efficient processes: When nursing professionals work together as a team not only can they delegate tasks effectively but also determine the most efficient way to accomplish their goals. Team work skills save time allowing serving of more patients while providing high quality care.
- Stronger professional connections: Communicating with various health care professionals provides nurses with mentorship opportunities, inspire career goals and share nursing expertise with others.

Strategies for Nurses to Promote Good Teamwork

- Volunteering for implementation of new ideas or solutions
- Being receptive when others offer suggestions
- Helping each other's strengths
- Focusing on what can be done, not on mistakes
- Encouraging sharing of thoughts and ideas among team members to improve patient condition
- Acknowledging contributions made by teammates

Tips to Improve Team Work Skills

- **Improve communication:** Use written or verbal communication to collaborate with other nursing and healthcare professionals so as to develop a team dynamic.
- **Be transparent:** Establish transparency by being honest and straight forward with colleagues and patients.
- **Clarify roles:** Classify and clarify roles to improve team collaboration. By establishing clear expectations for each member of a team, everyone accomplishes their assigned tasks without accidental overlap of responsibilities.
- **Promote adaptability:** Practice being flexible and adaptable. This can easily assist team members when they need help.
- **Follow-up:** Reach out to other healthcare providers and follow-up about patient care so as to improve accountability across the nursing team. Following up with colleagues and healthcare providers at other institutions can also help team stay organized and meet objectives on time.
- **Complete regular training:** Expand nursing skills by regularly attending professional development training opportunities with the team. Improvement in knowledge level and ability of each member of the nursing team contributes to collective strengths of the team.

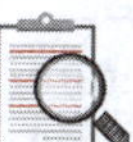

SYNOPSIS

- Soft skills are interpersonal qualities and the personal attributes that one possesses.
- Communication refers to the giving and receiving of information, ideas, facts, opinions, beliefs, feelings and attitudes through verbal or non-verbal means between people.
- Communication takes place at two levels: verbal and non-verbal.
- Interpersonal relationship is an interaction between two are more people who communicate, exchange their opinions and values.
- Time management refers to the allocation of time among specific activities based on certain priorities while giving preference to individual likes and dislikes.
- A perfect balance between professional and personal life can only be achieved by good time management.
- Coping includes efforts to control, reduce or tolerate the threats caused due to stress.
- Resilience refers to the ability to bounce back by harnessing the inner strength after a challenge or a set back.
- Learning to become resilient involves a dynamic process which requires a lot of time, effort and commitment.
- Work-life balance refers to effective management of dual role at work and family.
- The nurse needs to prioritize both at professional and personal levels.
- Presentation skills are set of abilities that enable an individual to interact with others.
- There are four steps in effective presentation, plan, prepare, practice and perform.
- Presentation is an excellent opportunity for a nurse to show her own skills, knowledge and personality.
- Social etiquettes is a set of rules that controls accepted behavior in particular social groups.
- Social etiquettes are related to the norms of social behavior.
- It is an important factor to succeed in healthcare career.
- Telephone etiquette refers to a set of rules that people should follow while calling and receiving calls from others.
- Mastering good communication skills is essential for all nurses at all cadres.
- Motivational skills can be actions or strategies that elicit a desired behavior.
- Team work is centered on the patient and focused on shared goals.

Review Questions

Long Essays

1. Explain components of soft skills and their application in nursing.
2. What is communication? List the key elements in communication process and describe various components to build relationship with a patient.
3. What is interpersonal relationship? List various purposes of interpersonal relationships in nursing. Mention IPR skills required for a nurse.
4. Enumerate in detail the barriers in IPR and strategies to overcome them.
5. Enumerate various coping strategies to manage stress.
6. Define resilience. Explain contributing factors.

Short Essays

1. Differentiate between soft and hard skills in nursing.
2. What are the uses of soft skills in nursing?
3. Benefits of time management in nursing.
4. List various strategies for time management in nursing.
5. Explain individual strategies to maintain work life balance.
6. Describe organizational strategies to maintain work life balance.
7. List the factors contributing to resilience.
8. Types of communication.

Short Notes

1. Elements of communication process
2. Communication

3. IPR
4. Barriers in IPR
5. Resilience
6. Stress

Multiple Choice Questions

1. Soft skills are:
   a. Interpersonal qualities
   b. Occupational skills
   c. Technical knowledge
   d. Skills required for performing a task

2. Ability to understand and feel what the patient is going through is called:
   a. Sympathy
   b. Empathy
   c. Acceptability
   d. Adaptability

3. Doing the right thing in a right way is called:
   a. Trust
   b. Honesty
   c. Empathy
   d. Sympathy

4. Which of the following strategies will reduce physiological barriers in IPR?
   a. Ensuring intactness of patient sensory perception before initiating communication
   b. Ensuring adequate temperature and lighting before initiating communication
   c. Maintaining privacy in physical setting before initiating communication
   d. Encouraging the patient to share his views using various communication techniques

5. Which of the following strategies will reduce environmental barriers in IPR?
   a. Ensuring intactness of patient sensory perception before initiating communication
   b. Ensuring adequate temperature and less noise before initiating communication
   c. Using clear and simple language
   d. Encouraging the patient to share his views using various communication techniques

6. Firm belief in the reliability, truth or ability of someone is called:
   a. Trust
   b. Honesty
   c. Empathy
   d. Sympathy

7. Communication process includes:
   a. Sender
   b. Message
   c. Receiver
   d. All of the above

8. In which of the following relationships does a nurse utilize her knowledge, behavior and professional strength to fulfill the patient needs?
   a. Social relationship
   b. Intimate relationship
   c. Therapeutic nurse patient relationship
   d. All of the above

9. Which of the following is a moral obligation of a nurse?
   a. Honesty
   b. Trust
   c. Confidentiality
   d. Respect

10. Allocation of available time for specific activities based on priorities is called:
   a. Work life balance
   b. Time management
   c. Structuring routine
   d. Mastering skills

11. Efforts to control, reduce or tolerate the threats caused by stress are:
   a. Mental mechanisms
   b. Physical mechanisms
   c. Coping mechanisms
   d. Social mechanisms

12. ____________ is the process of adapting well in the phase of adversity, trauma or stress.
   a. Coping
   b. Tranquility
   c. Spirituality
   d. Resilience

13. Management of dual role at work and family is called:
   a. Effective time management
   b. Efficiency
   c. Work life balance
   d. Resilience

14. Which of the following is an effective individual strategy to maintain work life balance?
   a. Assessing the job areas that are most demanding
   b. Be flexible at work place and home
   c. Both a and b
   d. Flexible working hours

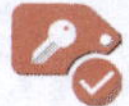

ANSWER KEY

1. a	2. b	3. b	4. a	5. b	6. a
7. d	8. c	9. c	10. b	11. c	12. d
13. c	14. c				

CHAPTER

10 Self-empowerment

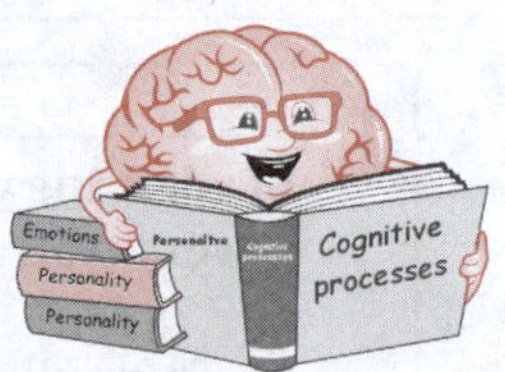

CHAPTER OUTLINE

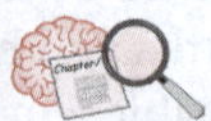

- Self-empowerment—dimensions, development, components, parameters and importance
- Patient empowerment—components, role of a nurse
- Professional etiquettes—need and aspects
- Professional grooming

The term empowerment has different meanings in different contexts. It is linked with concepts like gender, rights of weaker sections of society such as women, children and backward classes.

According to Webster's New World Dictionary (1982), the word 'empower' means to make or cause power. Power is the key term for empowerment. According to the International Encyclopaedia (1999), power means having the capacity and the resources to direct one's life towards desired social, political and economical goals or status.

The Oxford Dictionary 2016 defines empowerment as 'to give someone the authority or power to do something and to make someone stronger and more confident in controlling their life and claiming their rights.'

SELF-EMPOWERMENT

Empowerment is a process through which individuals in disadvantaged positions augment their access to knowledge, resources and decision making power. It raises their level of awareness and ability to participate in community activities thus attaining a level of control over their own environment.

According to Bandura 1986, empowerment is the process through which an individual gains efficiency and skills to control one's own environment.

According to Masi, et al. 2003 self-empowerment is an individual's ability to make decisions, have control over his or her personal life and characterize it by a sense of perceived control, competence and goal internalization. It combines personal efficacy and competence, a sense of mastery and control and a process of participation to influence decisions and institutions. It talks about the capacity of an individual to control both his environment and feelings.

Dimensions of Self-empowerment

- **Physical dimension**: Control over one's own mobility and physical condition including health.
- **Psychological dimension**: Level of self-confidence and self-esteem.
- **Cognitive dimension**: Awareness and understanding of one's own condition.
- **Economic dimension**: Ability to access resources, engage in productive activities and take independent decisions.
- **Political dimension**: Ability to set their own agenda, negotiate, lead and organize for altering the conditions.

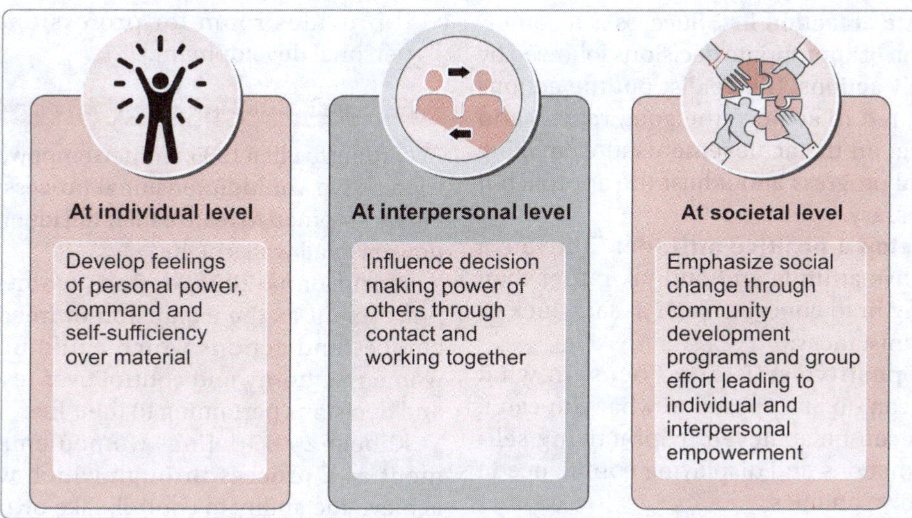

Figure 10.1: Phase of self-empowerment development.

Self-empowerment Development

Empowerment takes place over three phases —individual level, interpersonal level and societal level **(Figure 10.1)**.

Ways and Means of Achieving Empowerment

Empowerment can be achieved through education, organization, entrepreneurship, science and technology, information technology, microfinance institutions and law.

- Education plays the most important role in empowerment. It enables development of knowledge and skills for attaining self-independence.
- Organizations are the main source of power and strength for fighting collectively against age old practices such as dowry harassment, child marriage, domestic violence, *devadasi* system, etc.
- Entrepreneurship encourages individual's participation in the labor force besides augmenting his position in the society. Micro entrepreneurship on the other hand strengthens empowerment and reduces gender inequality.
- Science and technology can be effectively used to ease workload within and outside the house, involve individuals as equal partners, recognize their knowledge, experience and the significant role that they can play in sustainable development.
- Access to information is the key for empowerment as it provides various options to livelihood, education, health services and e-commerce.
- Microfinance programs play a dominant role in empowerment of low-income individuals as they grant access to various saving schemes, loans and other financial services.
- Law ensures protection of individual rights such as protection of underprivileged women from injustice, wrongful eviction, abuse and exploitation. It guarantees equal opportunities to individuals for accessing various resources.

Strategies to Promote Self-empowerment

Self-empowerment is an ongoing practice. By following the below steps one can develop self-esteem, initiative and other personal empowerment traits:

1. **Know yourself:** Understand your motivations, strengths and weaknesses.
2. **Improve your knowledge and competencies:** Focus on gaining expertise and improving skills or qualities that will allow us to reach our goals.

3. **Create an action list:** Success is a combination of appropriate decisions followed by timely actions. Hence, list out the actions required to achieve the goal, review and reflect on the achievements after making initial progress and adjust the approach if necessary.
4. **Develop a positive attitude:** Cultivate a positive attitude and outlook rather than giving in to concepts such as fate, luck or circumstances.
5. **Use positive self-talk:** Focus on what you can do as opposed to what you can't. This can be achieved by practicing self-affirmations and displaying confidence in our own abilities.
6. **Identify your goals:** Identify the most important aspects of your life where you can create a meaningful change and set measurable and achievable goals.
7. **Develop a strong community:** Seek friends and partners that share our values. Being in community with those who appreciate, affirm and constructively challenge our ideas and contributions can boost our confidence.
8. **Practice self-care:** It includes all activities such as eating right and exercising, scheduling time to relax and rejuvenate so as to make ourselves more productive. It also includes letting go of excessive negative thoughts. Being too result-oriented can at times make us feel disempowered.

Advantages of Practicing Self-empowerment

- It helps us to take decisions that are in our best interest.
- It allows us to follow our dreams and create the life we want to live.
- It allows us to take responsibility for our own happiness without relying on others.
- It gives us confidence and guides decision-making.
- It makes it easier to achieve our goals.
- It encourages skill development.
- It stops adversity from getting us down.
- It allows us to empower others.
- It provides room for professional and personal development.

WOMEN EMPOWERMENT

According to Pillai 1995, women empowerment is an active, multidimensional process which enables women to realize their full identity and powers in all walks of life.

World Bank 2001, defines women empowerment as the expansion of freedom of choices and actions which could increase women authority and control over resources and decisions pertaining to their life.

Kabeer 2001, defines women empowerment as a process through which women achieve the ability to control, take ownership over resources and make strategies concerning life choices.

Dimensions of Women Empowerment

Women empowerment is a multidimensional concept as it covers financial independence, social awareness and political consciousness of an individual. These elements can be categorized into social, economic and political empowerment **(Figure 10.2)**.

1. Social empowerment means an equitable social status for the women in the society. Some of the steps taken by the government to empower women socially are universalization of elementary education, promoting balwadis and crèches, encouraging distance and non-formal adult education, establishing women hostels and creating multipurpose institutions.
2. Economic empowerment means providing financial independence to women and

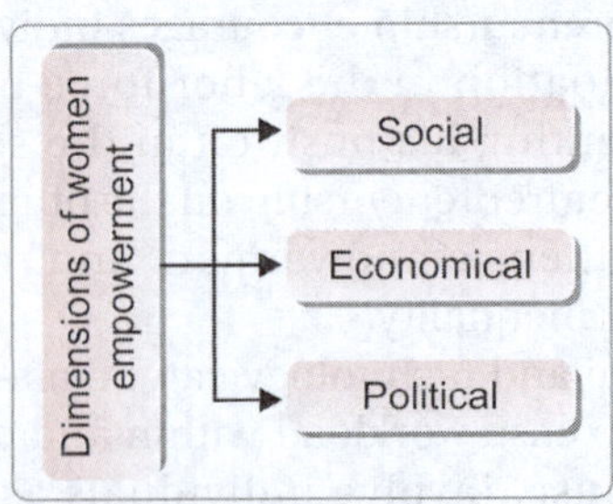

Figure 10.2: Dimensions of women empowerment

accounting their contribution by removing all gender specific barriers that prevent women from gaining access to their rightful share in every sphere of life.

3. Political empowerment for women means establishing their public presence by increasing their mobility and breaking their isolation from the decision making process. It improves their self-confidence and enhances self-image.

Components of Women Empowerment

- Awareness building on women's situation, discrimination and rights and opportunities as a step towards gender equality.
- Capacity building and skill development, ability to plan, take decisions, organize, manage and carry out activities to deal with people.
- Greater participation and control in decision making process at home, community and society.
- Action to bring about greater equality among men and women.

Parameters of Women Empowerment

- Self-esteem and self-confidence
- Positive image
- Ability to think critically and take decisions
- Opportunity for equal participation in the development process
- Access to legal literacy and their rights
- Level of knowledge and skill leading to economic independence

Importance of Women Empowerment in Society

Despite the considerable advancement in women's rights as well as gender equality there still are many obstacles and problems that prevent women from contributing to their fullest potential. Some of the strong arguments in favor of women empowerment for betterment of the society are:

1. **Gender equality:** Empowerment of women is necessary to achieve gender equality in terms of equal rights, opportunities and obligations. With empowerment social conventions, cultural practices as well as discriminatory attitudes that restrict women's rights and prospects can be overcome.
2. **Autonomy:** Empowerment enables women to acquire control over material assets, intellectual resources and ideology.
3. **Economic development:** With nearly half of the world's population comprising of women, economic sustainability can only be attained by providing them with equal opportunity for education, work and entrepreneurship.
4. **Education and knowledge:** Women with adequate education are more competent and self-assured which allows them to engage in social, economic and political spheres actively.
5. **Health and wellbeing:** Women's wellbeing and physical health are closely related to women empowerment. Being empowered puts them in a better position to take care of their health, seek medical attention when necessary and improve their wellbeing.
6. **Violence and discrimination:** Challenges to harmful practices such as domestic abuse, sexual harassment, human trafficking can only be made possible by empowerment of women.
7. **Leadership and decision making:** Gender parity in leadership roles is a must for creating effective policies and strategies. It is the only way to ensure that they have an equal voice in decision making at domestic and public level.
8. **Social and cultural change:** Women empowerment is probably the most logical way to challenge societal and cultural conventions that support gender inequality and prejudice, and advance a culture that honors and respects women's contribution.
9. **Realize full potential:** It enables women to inculcate a sense of self-confidence and independence thereby realizing their full potential and face challenges in various spheres of life.

Barriers to Women Empowerment

In the recent years while most societies are encouraging women empowerment, they are continuing to face problems in their daily lives. Even after being given equal rights and opportunities they suffer suppression and oppression. Some of the major barriers to empowerment of women are listed below:

1. **Lack of access to resources:** Around the world, women are significantly less likely than men to have access to productive resources such as land, finance and information.
2. **Discriminatory societal norms:** In most households there is a deep belief that women should not exist in many different contexts—in their homes, communities and workplaces.
3. **Unequal domestic responsibilities:** Around the world, women shoulder disproportionate responsibility for domestic work and unpaid care.
4. **Gender discrimination:** Women are considered as weaker section of the society and therefore given lesser importance. This has a bearing on women in areas such as nutrition, education, health, care, work and public life.
5. **Gender based violence:** Women workers across the world are at some instance or the other subjected to intimidation, hostile or humiliating work environment which not only limits their economic opportunities but also contributes to gender job segregation.
6. **Selective abortion and female infanticide:** It is a practice which involves abortion of the female fetus in mother's womb after fetal sex determination and sex selective abortion by medical professionals.
7. **Dowry and bride burning:** It is a problem which is more prevalent in low or middle class families during or after marriage.
8. **Disparity in education:** In the modern era though the level of women education is catching up with men education, female illiteracy continues to be higher in rural areas.
9. **Domestic violence:** No less than an endemic or widespread disease, it is mostly performed by the husband, family or relative.
10. **Child marriage:** It refers to the girls getting married even before they have attained the suitable age mostly to escape from the burden of dowry.
11. **Inadequate nutrition: Poor** nutrition in childhood affects the women in their later life especially those belonging to the middle class and poor families.
12. **Status of widows:** Considered as inauspicious and non-productive, widows are usually kept away from various cultural and family activities.
13. **Disparity in pay and treatment:** Compared to men, the women are paid and respected less for the same amount of work done. They are provided fewer opportunities despite having proved their strengths and capabilities.
14. **Lack of legal and political support:** Women usually enjoy limited legal and political support including limited representation in the Government and limited access to legal protection and services.
15. **Limited mobility:** Women are at times subject to greater restrictions when it comes to moving across places and getting access to various forms of transportation.

Only a co-ordinated effort from the Government, civil society and individuals can help to promote gender equality, improve access to education, provide economic opportunities and address violence and discrimination against women.

ROLE OF NURSE IN EMPOWERING OTHERS

Nurses play a vital role in empowering others, both patients and colleagues. They do this by providing education, support, and advocacy.

Nurses' Role in Empowering Junior Nurses

Being in a management or leadership role, it is important to empower your team or department to increase productivity. Some definite ways to empower others in workplace are:

- **Build trust:** It is crucial to trust the employees to complete certain tasks and achieve goals on their own. Demonstrating the trust in employees can empower them to perform at their optimum best.

- **Provide opportunities:** Allow the employees to learn from their mistakes and educate them on how to avoid committing similar mistakes repeatedly.
- **Proper communication:** Communicate your expectations clearly and ensure that the employees understand what to prioritize.
- **Implement feedback:** Introduce a feedback system wherein the employees can share their experiences and seek help and advice to be able to complete their tasks more quickly.
- **Provide encouragement:** It is important to let the nurses know that their opinions are valued and that their constructive feedback can be used to improve the work processes.
- Offer opportunities for professional development.

Nurses' Role in Empowering Student Nurses

Nurse educator has an important role to empower student nurses. Empowered students besides following professional etiquettes are well motivated, engaged and responsible for their own growth.

- **Know each students' interests:** Nurse educator should take time out to know interests, hobbies and goals of each student which will in turn help her to understand their innate abilities.
- **Provide consistent feedback:** Based on their capabilities set clear expectations, let the student know what you expect from them, and provide feedback on their progress. This will help them to stay motivated.
- **Provide positive reinforcement:** Praise students when they do well and provide constructive criticism when needed. Let the student know that you believe in them.
- **Be approachable:** Be available to students and let the student know that you are there to help them. This will create an atmosphere of trust and mutual respect.
- **Help students take responsibility for guiding their own learning:** Teacher should allow the students to display their learning in varied ways. By allowing variety, teachers can encourage the students' to develop extensive abilities and think in a broader way.
- **Build trust:** By trusting students, teachers create a trusting environment which in turn builds capabilities and empowers students to manage themselves.
- **Build positive teacher-student relationship:** Develop mentor and mentee group with periodic counseling facility to establish positive relationship between teacher and student.
- **Create innovative learning environment:** Use advanced class room technology, student focused teaching methods, engage students in reflection and critical thinking process.
- **Provide ample opportunities:** Provide ample opportunities to develop and mastering skills. Inform students about the opportunities to perform clinical procedures with supervision.
- **Enhance self-esteem:** Students' self-esteem can be enhanced by providing non-threatening learning environment, guiding, encouraging to form their own opinion, reinforcing positive behaviors.

Patient Empowerment

Patient empowerment is defined as helping the patient to discover and use his innate ability to gain mastery over his health problems. This empowerment process enables the patient to acquire knowledge, confidence, self-determination and gain greater control over decisions and actions affecting his health.

Components of Patient Empowerment

- Understanding of his or her role by the patient
- Acquiring sufficient knowledge and skills to be able to engage with their healthcare provider
- Developing necessary skills
- Presence of a facilitating environment

Role of a Nurse in Empowering Patients

A nurse plays an important role in empowering the patient. She contributes to patient empowerment in the following ways **(Box 10.1)**:

1. **Providing information:** Providing information is the fundamental process in patient empowerment. Patient is able to best decide about the course of treatment when he is provided adequate information. The nurse should provide accurate and relevant information by clearly communicating the available options and choices.
2. **Providing health and digital literacy:** Health literacy is defined as the degree to which individuals have the capacity to obtain, process and understand basic health information and services needed to make appropriate health decisions (National Library of Medicine). Digital literacy is defined as the ability to find, evaluate, utilize, share and create content using information technology and the internet. A nurse should educate the patient on disease condition and demonstrate needed skills to gain mastery over their health problems.
3. **Developing self-efficacy**: In the health context, self-efficacy is defined as the individual's ability to develop a sense of control on health issues and achieve health related goals. The nurse has to teach the patient specific care activities so as to be able to manage his health condition. She can even set goals for selected behaviors.
4. **Having mutual respect**: A nurse is the only healthcare professional who spends maximum time with the patient. Mutual respect between the nurse and the patient allows informed choices for patient treatment. Nurse activities that can improve mutual respect are: having a therapeutic relationship, seeing the patient as more than just a patient, involve in shared decision making regarding care and treatment, share knowledge and experience to set new goals and learn with and from each other.
5. **Involving the patient in shared decision making:** Many research studies have shown that health outcomes are better in patients who are more involved in decisions about their treatment. These may include decisions about the screening and diagnostic tests, medication, surgery and self-management. The nurse provides evidence based information about treatment options and describes their risks and benefits while the patient expresses his or her preferences and values. She assists the patient in weighing costs and benefits of various treatment options too.
6. **Providing a facilitating environment:** Providing a supportive environment is one of the key components of patient empowerment. The nurse has to not only educate but also support the patient in taking greater responsibility for his/her own health.

Box 10.1: Nurse's role in empowering a patient

- Providing information
- Providing health and digital literacy
- Developing self-efficacy
- Having mutual respect
- Involving the patient in shared decision making
- Providing a facilitating environment

PROFESSIONAL ETIQUETTE

Etiquette is a code of good manners, the polite rule of a society or a professional group. It refers to the various manners and behaviors that are prescribed and observed in social life. In the context of nursing, etiquette not only includes the nurse's behavior towards patients and colleagues but also the establishing of a relationship with patients, colleagues and supervisors.

Nurse is an important member of the healthcare team working in collaboration with other team members. She establishes a professional relationship among all the members in various settings. To ensure smooth functioning the nurse should follow certain professional etiquettes. It is good etiquette that leads to good interpersonal relationships besides strengthening professional life. First impressions and body language are of utmost importance while establishing relationships.

Need for Professional Etiquettes in Nursing

- Professional etiquette is an important first impression in building a rapport with the patient.
- Nurses are approached based on their ability to communicate, their body language and appearance.
- To establish interpersonal relationship with other healthcare members.

Aspects of Etiquette

For a nurse, etiquettes play an important role in her professional life. Some aspects of etiquettes are **(Box 10.2)**:

- **Posture:** Posture says much about the person and reflects his/her level of confidence, attitude and interests. Some of the posture etiquettes are:
  - Stand straight, do not lean against a desk or a cot.
  - Stand with hands by sides, not on hips or in pockets or arms crossed over the chest.
  - When sitting, put the knees together and do not cross the legs.
  - Show interest and demonstrate care
  - Use a sincere smile to convey warmth and friendliness.
- **Verbal communication:** It includes speaking and listening skills, ability to apologize, manner of addressing conflict and treating others. Some of the verbal communication etiquettes are:
  - Introduce self and explain one's role before providing care
  - Be courteous, gentle and polite while talking
  - Greet seniors, co-workers and patients appropriately and with a smile
  - Maintain silence where necessary
  - Convey thanks on receiving a favor
  - Maintain eye contact, show attention when listening
  - Excuse oneself when interfering with others already engaged in a talk or work
  - Convey thoughts clearly, practice effective communication
  - Use appropriate introductions such as Ms, Mr, Mrs, Dr, etc.
- **Word choice:** Selection of appropriate words is an important part of any communication.
  - Use polite and grammatically correct language
  - Select appropriate wording
  - Use clear voice, right tone and volume
- **Avoiding distracting behaviors:** Avoid certain behaviors and conditions while in a professional environment.
  - It is important not to have bad breath when working in close contact with others; practice proper oral hygiene.
  - Snack items should be consumed only during a formal break preferably at a designated place out of patient sight.
  - The food corner should be cleaned up after food or tea breaks.
  - It is highly offensive to smoke in a working environment.
  - Avoid appearing tired. When down with excessive fatigue find ways to cope with it.
  - Avoid constant yawning, resting head on table etc.
  - Keep the mobile phone in silent mode/switch it off while in a working environment.
  - Avoid streaming videos, playing music in work area.

Box 10.2: Aspects of etiquette

- Posture
- Manner of verbal communication
- Word choice/selection of words
- Avoiding distracting behaviors

Professional etiquettes are very important in the development of professional standards and delivery of quality care. It influences the public image of nursing.

PROFESSIONAL GROOMING

Grooming refers to the actions carried out to keep themselves clean and presentable. It is nothing but the art of keeping oneself clean and maintaining the body. It is important to feel good about ourselves, project a positive image of self and maintain a pleasing and attractive appearance. When we feel good about ourselves we naturally convey confidence and a positive attitude.

Professional grooming is important for all professionals. What we wear supports our professional image and sends a signal to others about how we see our self and want to be perceived by others. Professional appearance is also important for being respected at work place.

In nursing, grooming is all that more important as it impacts self, relationship with other health team members and patients. Grooming of the nurse is an essential factor as the patient judges her ability based on her appearance. Patients prefer the nurse to be well groomed and have a professional outlook. Personal grooming includes dress code, make up, jewelry, hair set up, etc.

Dress Code

Professionalism is generally conveyed by appearance, uniform being the major factor. Wearing a proper uniform not only shows respect for the patient but also for the nurse herself and the work she does. Nurse's appearance and uniform have a bearing on patient's judgment of nurse's level of confidence and competence. A good professional outlook allows the nurse to make a good first impression which makes the patient perceive that he is under the care of a capable healthcare professional.

Nurses have been wearing uniforms from the days of Florence Nightingale so as to differentiate them from other hospital staff and promote their professional image. Dress code for nurses includes the following:

- Uniform should be in accordance with the organization policy and occasion.
- Uniform clothing should be comfortable and fit well. It should allow free movement as the nurse is required to bend, stoop, reach and lift objects while discharging her duties.
- Uniform and apron should be clean and pressed well.
- Uniform skirts should not be too short.
- Uniform should not be of transparent fabric.
- Uniform fabric should not induce irritation or heavy sweating.
- Uniforms should be easily washable as they are subject to frequent spills and stains.
- Name tag or identity card should be visible and readable.
- Shoes should be clean and properly laced up.
- Open toed shoes should be avoided.
- Caps should be rightly placed on the head, not too far back or close to the front hairline.

Hair Set up

Hair set up is also an important component of professional grooming. Some of the dos and don'ts are:

- Hair should be clean, trimmed and neatly combed or arranged.
- It should be tied up according to the organization policy.
- When providing direct care hair should not be longer than shoulder length as it may interfere with patient care.
- Hair should not fall on the face as it obscures the eyebrows.
- Attractive rubber bands and pins should be avoided.
- Hair coloring must look natural.
- For men hair should be above the ears and not touch the neck collar.
- Moustache should be well groomed and not grown beyond the mouth corners.
- Beard should be trimmed and well groomed.

Jewelry

Though Jewelry may be a part of regular grooming it should be well within limits to project a professional outlook. Some important aspects are:

- Jewelry must be kept to a minimum and banned in some areas so as to safeguard from injury or transmission of infection.
- While in uniform large and dangling ear rings should be avoided.
- Necklaces should not show above the shirt line.
- Body piercing is not advisable except for ear rings for women.

Make-up

Though make-up is considered a part of personal grooming, the nurse should exercise care while using make up. Some instructions to be followed are:

- Make up should be used sparingly.
- When used it should blend with natural skin color and features.
- Lipstick color should be conservative and compatible with the individual.
- Artificial eyelashes should be avoided.
- Fragrance that smells from a distance or lingers even after leaving should be avoided.
- Scented body lotions, fragrances and colognes should not be used to excess in patient areas as it may cause irritation to patients.

Nails

As long finger nails have shown to harbour bacteria and transmit infection, nurses involved in direct patient care should follow below guidelines:

- Nails should be trimmed and not to exceed ¼ inch from the tip of the finger.
- Nail polish or artificial nails including nail art should be avoided to prevent transmission of infection.

Grooming process of a professional nurse should begin from the student period itself as poor professional grooming may lead to poor image.

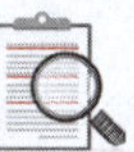

SYNOPSIS

- Empowerment is the process through which an individual gains efficiency and skills to control one's own environment.
- It can be achieved through education, organization, entrepreneurship, science and technology, information technology, microfinance institutions and law.
- Women empowerment is an active, multidimensional process which enables women to realize their full identity and powers in all walks of life.
- Patient empowerment refers to helping the patient to discover and use his innate ability to gain mastery over his health problems.
- Etiquette is a code of good manner, the polite rule of the society or a professional group.
- Professional etiquettes are important in the development of professional standards and delivery of quality care.
- Grooming refers to the actions carried out to keep themselves clean and presentable.
- Professionalism is generally conveyed by appearance.
- Grooming process of a professional nurse should begin from the student period itself as poor professional grooming may lead to poor image.

Review Questions

Long Essays

1. What is empowerment? Describe steps and importance of women empowerment in society.
2. What is patient empowerment? List the components and describe the role of a nurse in empowering a patient.
3. Define professional grooming. Explain aspects of professional grooming in nursing.
4. Define professional etiquette. Explain its various aspects.

Short Essays

1. Dimensions of self-empowerment.
2. Components of women empowerment.
3. Components of patient empowerment.
4. Factors involved in dress code of nursing.
5. Dos and don'ts of hair grooming in nursing.
6. Describe posture etiquette.
7. Explain verbal etiquette in nursing.
8. Explain ways and means of achieving women empowerment.

Short Notes

1. Women empowerment
2. Professional etiquette
3. Professional grooming
4. Patient empowerment

Multiple Choice Questions

1. **__________ is the process through which an individual gains efficiency and skills to control one's own environment.**
   a. Self-esteem
   b. Self-empowerment
   c. Self-control
   d. Self defense
2. **__________ is the process through which patient acquires knowledge, confidence and self-determination for his own health.**
   a. Patient empowerment
   b. Social empowerment
   c. Political empowerment
   d. Economic empowerment
3. **__________ is the process through which women achieve an ability to control life choices.**
   a. Women development
   b. Women literacy
   c. Women empowerment
   d. Social empowerment
4. **__________ is a code of good manners in a professional group.**
   a. Professional grooming
   b. Professional code
   c. Professional conduct
   d. Professional etiquette
5. **__________ refers to the actions carried out to keep themselves clean and presentable.**
   a. Personal grooming
   b. Personal conduct
   c. Professional grooming
   d. Professional etiquette

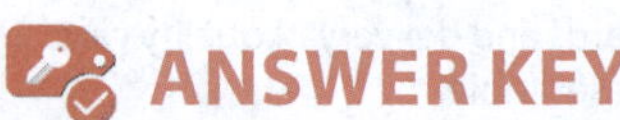

ANSWER KEY

1. b	2. a	3. c	4. d	5. c	

Glossary

A

Ability
A general term referring to the potential for acquisition of a skill; the term covers intelligence and specific aptitudes.

Abnormal Behavior
Behavior which deviates from what is considered normal; usually refers to maladaptive behavior.

Absolute Threshold
The smallest intensity of a stimulus that must be present for the stimulus to be detected.

Accommodation, Visual
A process by which the lens of the eye varies its focus. In Piaget's theory of cognitive development, it refers to the process by which an infant modifies a pre-existing schema in order to include a novel object or event.

Achievement Motive
An urge to succeed, to perform well or better than others.

Achievement Test
A test designed to determine a person's level of knowledge in a given subject area.

Adaptation
An adjustment in sensory capacity following prolonged exposure to stimuli.

Adolescence
The period of life ranging from puberty to completion of physical growth.

Alarm Reaction
The first stage of the general adaptation syndrome; consists of prompt responses of the body, many of them mediated by the sympathetic system, which prepare the organism to cope with stressors.

All-or-none Law
Principle that nerve fibers respond completely or not at all.

Altruism
Helping behavior that is beneficial to others but clearly requires self-sacrifice.

Amnesia
Generally, any loss of memory; often applied to situations in which a person forgets his or her own identity and is unable to recognize familiar people and situations.

Anal Stage
According to Freud, a stage from 12 to 18 months to 3 years of age, in which a child's pleasure is centered on the anus.

Antisocial Personality Disorder
A disorder in which individuals tend to display no regard for the moral and ethical rules of society or the rights of others.

Anxiety
A state of apprehension, tension and worry.

Approach-approach Conflict
Conflict in which a person must choose between two good things.

Approach-avoidance Conflict
Conflict in which the person feels both positively and negatively about the goal.

Aptitude
Specific ability indicative of one's potentiality to get desired future success.

Attention
Concentration of mental activity.

Attitudes
Learned predispositions to respond in a favorable or unfavorable manner to a particular person, behavior, belief or thing.

Attribution
A process by which we attempt to explain the behavior of other people. Attribution theory deals with the rules people use to infer the causes of observed behavior.

Autocratic Leadership
Autocratic leadership is a management style wherein one person controls all the decisions and takes very little inputs from other group members.

Avoidance-avoidance Conflict
A situation in which an individual is caught between two negative goals; as the individual

tries to avoid one goal, he or she is brought closer to the other.

B

Behavior

Anything a person or animal does that can be observed in some way.

Behavior Modification

Change in behavior brought about by operant conditioning techniques.

Beliefs

Cognitions or thoughts about the characteristics of objects.

C

Cannon–Bard Theory of Emotion

A belief that both physiological and emotional arousal are produced simultaneously by the same nerve stimulus.

Case Study

An in-depth, intensive investigation of an individual or small group of people.

Catharsis

A process involving the release of emotional tension through expression of emotion.

Central Nervous System (CNS)

The central nervous system is a part of the nervous system mainly comprising of the brain and spinal cord. It is the body's processing center wherein the components of the CNS work together to take in information and control how the body responds. It includes controlling the thoughts, movements, and emotions, as well as breathing, heart rate, hormones, and body temperature.

Central Traits

Major traits considered in forming impressions of others.

Cerebellum

Part of the brain close to the brainstem, responsible for body balance and co-ordination of body movements.

Cerebral Cortex

Cerebral cortex also called the gray matter is the brain's outermost layer. It has a wrinkled appearance from its many folds and grooves. It plays a key role in memory, thinking, learning, reasoning, problem solving, emotions, consciousness and functions related to senses.

Cerebrum

Cerebrum is the largest and uppermost portion of the brain which comprises of gray matter (the cerebral cortex) and white matter at its center. It consists of the cerebral hemispheres and accounts for two-thirds of the total weight of the brain. The left hemisphere is functionally dominant, controlling language and speech. The other hemisphere interprets visual and spatial information.

Character

It applies to the aggregate of moral qualities by which a person is judged apart from intelligence, competence or special talents.

Chromosomes

Rod-shaped structures that contain the basic hereditary information.

Chronological Age

Age in years or calendar age.

Classical Conditioning

A type of learning in which a neutral stimulus comes to bring about a response after it is paired with a stimulus that naturally brings about that response.

Clinical Psychology

A branch of psychology concerned with psychological methods of recognizing and treating psychological disorders and research into their causes.

Cognitive Approaches of Motivation

A theory suggesting that motivation is a product of people's thoughts and expectations—their cognitions.

Cognitive Development

Cognitive development is the process by which human beings acquire, organize, and learn to use knowledge.

Cognitive Psychology

A branch of psychology that focuses on the study of cognition.

Cognitive-behavioral Approach

An approach used by cognitive therapists that attempts to change the way people think through the use of basic principles of learning.

Cognitive-social Learning Theory

A study of thought processes that underlie learning.

Collective Unconscious

A set of influences we inherit from our own particular ancestors, the whole human race and even animal ancestors from the distant evolutionary past.

Communication
It is a process by which people exchange ideas, facts, feelings or impressions in a way that each gains a 'common understanding' of the meaning, intent and use of a message. In general, communication refers to the giving and receiving of information, ideas, facts, opinions, beliefs, feelings and attitudes through verbal or non-verbal means between people.

Community Psychology
A branch of psychology that focuses on the prevention and minimization of psychological disorders in the community.

Compliance
Conforming behavior that occurs in response to direct social pressure.

Concept
Concept is an idea or a group of ideas used to organize events and objects, often arranged in hierarchical order from general to more specific. Such categorization of ideas helps people to plan and understand new information.

Conditioned Response (CR)
The learned or acquired response to a stimulus that did not evoke the response originally.

Conditioned Stimulus (CS)
A previously neutral stimulus that comes to elicit a conditioned response through association with an unconditioned stimulus.

Conflict
Conflict means a painful emotional state which results from a tension between opposed and contradictory wishes.

Conformity
A change in behavior or attitude brought about by a desire to follow the beliefs or standards of other people.

Consciousness
An awareness of sensations, thoughts and feelings being experienced at a given moment.

Continuous Reinforcement Schedule
Reinforcement of behavior every time it occurs.

Control Group
A group that receives no treatment in an experiment.

Convergent Thinking
The ability to produce responses that are based primarily on knowledge and logic.

Coping
Efforts to control, reduce or learn to tolerate the threats that lead to stress.

Counseling
Counseling is a process of enabling the individual to know himself and his present and possible future situations in order that he may make substantial contributions to the society and solve his own problems through a face-to-face personal relationship with the counselor.

Creativity
The combining of responses or ideas in a novel way.

Crystallized Intelligence
The accumulation of information, skills and strategies learned through experience that can be applied in problem-solving situations.

D

Decay
The loss of information in memory through its non-use.

Declarative Memory
Memory for factual information: names, faces, dates and the like.

Defense Mechanisms
Strategies that people use to deal with anxiety, which are largely unconscious.

Dendrites
A cluster of fibers at one end of a neuron that receive messages from other neurons.

Dependent Variable
A variable that is measured and is expected to change as a result of changes caused by the experimenter's manipulation.

Developmental Psychology
A branch of psychology that studies patterns of growth and change occurring during the lifetime.

Difference Threshold
The smallest level of stimulation required to sense that a change in stimulation has occurred.

Discrimination
Negative behavior towards members of a particular group.

Displacement
A defense mechanism that involves an individual transferring negative feelings from one person or thing to another.

Dissociative Amnesia
A disorder in which the person has significant, selective memory loss.

Divergent Thinking
The ability to generate unusual yet appropriate responses to problems or questions.

Dominant Gene
A gene with the capacity to express itself wholly, to the exclusion of the other member of the gene pair.

Double Approach-avoidance Conflict
A conflict in which the person has both negative and positive feelings about either choice.

Down Syndrome
A congenital disorder arising from a chromosome defect causing intellectual impairment and physical abnormalities including short stature and a broad facial profile. It arises from a defect involving chromosome 21, usually an extra copy (trisomy-21).

Drive
Motivational tension or arousal that energizes behavior in order to fulfill some need.

Drive Theories
Theories of motivation that emphasize the role of internal factors.

E

Eclectic Approach to Therapy
An approach to therapy that uses techniques taken from a variety of treatment methods rather than just one method.

Ego
The part of the mind that mediates between the conscious and the unconscious and is responsible for reality testing and a sense of personal identity.

Egocentric Thought
A way of thinking in which the child views the world entirely from his or her own perspective.

Ego Integrity Versus Despair Stage
According to Erikson, a period from late adulthood until death during which we review our life's accomplishments and failures.

Emotional Intelligence
It is a form of social intelligence that involves the ability to monitor one's own and others' feelings and emotions, to discriminate among them, and to use this information to guide one's thinking and action.

Emotions
These are conscious mental reactions (such as anger or fear) subjectively experienced as strong feelings usually directed toward a specific object and typically accompanied by physiological and behavioral changes in the body.

Empathy
It refers to the nurse's understanding of what the patient is experiencing from his own perspective. This process allows the nurse to see the suffering from patient's own point of view without experiencing the emotional content.

Empowerment
It is a process through which individuals in disadvantaged positions augment their access to knowledge, resources and decision-making power.

Endocrine Gland
A ductless gland which secretes hormones into the bloodstream.

Episodic Memory
Episodic memory is a category of long-term declarative memory that involves the recollection of specific events, situations and experiences. In addition to the overall memory of the event itself, it also involves memory of the location and time that the event occurred.

Esteem Needs
It refers to the need for respect, self-esteem, and self-confidence. It is the basis for human desire that one has to be accepted and valued by others. In Maslow's theory, needs for prestige, success and self-respect are fulfilled after belongingness and love needs are satisfied.

Evolutionary Psychology
A branch of psychology that seeks to identify behavior patterns that are a result of our genetic inheritance from our ancestors.

Experiment
The investigation of relationship between two (or more) variables by deliberately producing a change in one variable in a situation and observing the effects of that change on other aspects of the situation.

Experimental Bias
Factors that distort the manner in which the independent variable affects the dependent variable in an experiment.

Experimental Group
Any group receiving a treatment in an experiment.

Experimental Manipulation
The change that an experimenter deliberately produces in a situation.

Explicit Memory
Intentional or conscious recollection of information.

Extinction
The decrease in frequency and eventual disappearance of a previously conditioned response; one of the basic phenomena of learning.

Extrasensory Perception (ESP)
The supposed ability of some people to gain knowledge about the world through avenues other than the sensory channels.

Extrinsic Motivation
Motivation directed towards goals, external to the person.

Extrovert
Jung's term to describe a personality that focuses on social life and the external world instead of its internal experience.

F

Figure-ground Relationship
Perception typified by one feature standing out against a larger background.

Fixation
In psychoanalytic theory it refers to failure of some personality characteristics to advance beyond a particular stage of psychosexual development.

Fixed Interval Schedule
In operant conditioning, a fixed-interval scheduling is a schedule of reinforcement where the response is rewarded only after a specified amount of time has elapsed.

Fixed Ratio Schedule
A schedule whereby reinforcement is given only after a certain number of responses are made.

Fluid Intelligence
Intelligence that reflects information processing capabilities, reasoning and memory.

Forgetting
Apparent loss of information that has been stored in long-term memory (LTM).

Fraternal Twins
Twins who develop from two different fertilized eggs, and who consequently are different in hereditary characteristics as ordinary brothers and sisters. Also called dizygotic (DZ) twins.

Free Association
A psychoanalysis technique in which the patient expresses whatever comes into his mind for revealing his unconscious.

Frustration
Blocking of goal-directed behavior.

Functional Fixedness
The tendency to think of an object only in terms of its typical use.

G

Galvanic Skin Response
A change in electrical resistance of the skin that may occur during many emotions.

General Adaptation Syndrome (GAS)
A theory developed by Selye which suggests that a person's response to stress consists of three stages: alarm, resistance and exhaustion.

Generativity
According to Erikson, to take an interest in guiding the next generation.

Genes
It refers to parts of the chromosomes through which genetic information is transmitted.

Genital Stage
Genital stage is the fifth and final stage of Freud's theory of psychosexual development, which begins in puberty and continues to adulthood. During this stage, individuals start to become sexually mature and begin to explore their sexual feelings and desires more maturely and responsibly.

Gestalt (geh-SHTALLT) Psychology
An approach to psychology that focuses on the organization of perception and thinking in a 'whole' sense, rather than on the individual elements of perception.

Gestalt Laws of Organization
A series of principles that describe how we organize bits and pieces of information into meaningful wholes.

Gestalt Therapy
An approach to therapy that attempts to integrate a client's thoughts, feelings and behavior into a unified whole.

Grooming
It refers to the actions carried out to keep themselves clean and presentable. It is nothing but the art of keeping oneself clean and maintaining the body.

Group Therapy
Group therapy is a form of psychotherapy that involves one or more therapists working with a group of people at the same time. It aims to help people manage mental health conditions or cope with negative experiences and behaviors.

H

Health Psychology
A branch of psychology which investigates the psychological factors related to wellness and illness,

including the prevention, diagnosis and treatment of medical problems.

Homeostasis

A state of physiological equilibrium that is maintained by innate and automatic regulatory mechanisms.

Hormones

Chemicals that circulate through the blood and affect the functioning or growth of other parts of the body.

Humanistic Approaches to Personality

The theory that people are basically good and tend to grow to higher levels of functioning.

Hypnosis

A trance like state of heightened susceptibility to the suggestions of others.

I

Id

A concept in Freudian psychology that relates with unconscious, amoral and irresponsible personality. It functions on the pleasure principle and is the reservoir of instincts.

Identification

The process of trying to be like another person as much as possible, imitating that person's behavior and adopting similar beliefs and values.

Identity versus Role Confusion Stage

It is the fifth stage of Erik Erikson's theory of psychosocial development; occurs during adolescence between the ages of approximately 12–18. At this stage, adolescents are in search of an identity to determine one's unique qualities that will lead them to adulthood.

Implicit Memory

Implicit memory also known as unconscious or non-declarative memory is one of the two main types of long-term human memory. It is acquired and used unconsciously and can affect thoughts and behaviors. One of its most common forms is procedural memory, which helps people in performing certain tasks without conscious awareness of these previous experiences.

Incentive

A kind of reward that reinforces the behavior in its own right.

Incentive Approaches to Motivation

A theory suggesting that motivation stems from the desire to obtain valued external goals or incentives.

Independent Variable

A variable that is manipulated by an experimenter.

Inductive Reasoning

A type of reasoning that involves drawing a general conclusion from a set of specific observations.

Industrial Organizational (I/O) Psychology

A branch of psychology that focuses on work and job-related issues including productivity, job satisfaction, decision-making and consumer behavior.

Industry versus Inferiority Stage

According to Erikson, it is the last stage of childhood during which children (aged 6–12 years) either develop positive social interactions with others or feel inadequate and become less sociable.

Infancy

The period of development between the neonatal period and the appearance of useful language; the upper limit is about 18 months.

Integrity

According to Erikson, it is a state of fulfillment and completeness.

Intellectualization

A defense mechanism in which a person reduces anxiety by thinking of the anxiety producing situation in unemotional or abstract terms.

Intelligence

The ability to learn from experience, think in abstract terms and deal effectively with one's environment.

Intelligence Quotient (IQ)

A measure of intelligence. It is equal to a person's mental age divided by chronological age and multiplied by 100.

Intelligence Tests

Tests devised to identify a person's level of intelligence.

Interference

A phenomenon by which information in memory displaces or blocks out other information, preventing its recall.

Interference Theory of Forgetting

It refers to the learning of something new which causes forgetting of older material on the basis of competition between the two. It states that memory's information may become confused or combined with other information during encoding, resulting in the distortion or disruption of memories.

Intimacy versus Isolation Stage
According to Erikson, a period during early adulthood that focuses on developing close relationships.

Intrinsic Motivation
Desire to perform an activity for its own sake.

Introspection
A procedure used to study the structure of mind wherein subjects are asked to describe in detail what they are experiencing when exposed to a stimulus.

Introvert
A shy person who usually withdraws and prefers to be alone.

J

James–Lange Theory of Emotion
The theory states that the stimulus first leads to bodily responses and then the awareness of these responses constitutes the experience of emotion.

L

Laissez–Faire Leadership
Leadership in which the leader has poorly defined lines of authority and responsibility often allowing people to do as they please.

Language
Communication in which word symbols are used in various combinations to convey meaning.

Latency Period
According to Freud, it is the period between phallic stage and puberty during which children temporarily put aside their sexual interests.

Latent Learning
A form of learning in which a new behavior is acquired, but is not demonstrated until reinforcement is provided.

Learned Helplessness
A condition of apathy or helplessness created experimentally by subjecting an individual to unavoidable trauma such as shock, heat or cold.

Learning
Relatively permanent changes in the behavior of the learner brought about by experience or training.

Learning Theory Approach
The theory suggesting that language acquisition follows the principles of reinforcement and conditioning.

Libido
A concept in Freud's psychology denoting that basic sexual drive or instinct is responsible for every aspect of a person's behavior.

Life Review
A process in which people in late adulthood examine and evaluate their lives.

Limbic System
A group of closely interconnected structures at the core of the brain that works with the hypothalamus to control the emotions and motivational processes.

Long-term Memory
Long-term memory refers to the memory process in the brain that takes information from the short-term memory store and creates long lasting memories. These memories can be from an hour ago or several decades ago. This can hold an unlimited amount of information for an indefinite period of time.

M

Maturation
The changes in behavior of an organism resulting from physiological growth, the blueprints of which are provided by heredity.

Medulla
The part of the hindbrain that regulates breathing, heart rate and blood pressure.

Memory
The process by which we encode, store and retrieve information.

Memory Trace
A physical change in the brain that occurs when new material is learned.

Mental Age
The average age of individuals who achieve a particular level of performance in a test.

Mental Retardation
Having significantly below average intellectual functioning and limitations in at least two areas of adaptive functioning.

Midbrain
Area of the brain that controls auditory and visual responses.

Minnesota Multiphasic Personality Inventory (MMPI)
A pencil and paper version of a psychiatric interview that consists of more than 550 statements concerning attitudes, emotional reactions, physical and psychological symptoms and experiences. Test takers respond to each statement by answering, 'True', 'False' or 'Cannot Say'.

Modeling
A type of imitation in which one individual does what he/she sees his/her model doing.

Morale
A positive group feeling of satisfaction and enthusiasm for a task.

Motivation
Factors that direct and energize the behavior of humans and other organisms.

Motivational Cycle
A cycle including arousal of the motive, goal-directed behavior and satisfaction.

Motor (Efferent) Neurons
Neurons that communicate information from the nervous system to muscles and glands of the body.

Motor Area
Part of the cortex that is largely responsible for voluntary movement of particular parts of the body.

Multiple Approach-avoidance Conflict
A motivational conflict in which several incompatible positive and negative goals are involved; characteristic of many of life's major decisions.

Myelin Sheath
Specialized cells of fat and protein that wrap themselves around the axon, providing a protective coating.

N

Naturalistic Observation
A psychological method of studying behavior by observing the subjects in their natural settings.

Need
Deprivation caused by a lack of something necessary for survival or well-being.

Need for Achievement
A stable, learned characteristic in which satisfaction is obtained by striving for attaining a level of excellence.

Need for Affiliation
An interest in establishing and maintaining relationships with other people.

Need for Power
A tendency to seek impact control or influence over others and to be seen as a powerful individual.

Need Reduction
The satisfaction of one's biological or socio-psychological needs.

Negative Reinforcer
An unpleasant stimulus whose removal leads to an increase in the probability that a preceding response will occur again in the future.

Neo-Freudian Psychoanalysts
Psychoanalysts trained in traditional Freudian theory who later rejected some of its major points.

Nerve Fiber
An axon or dendrite of a neuron many of which together form a nerve thereby transmitting nerve impulses to and from the central nervous system.

Nervous System
Central control system of the body which organizes and co-ordinates functions of the organism.

Neural Stimulus
A stimulus which before conditioning does not naturally bring about the response of interest.

Neurotransmitters
Chemicals that carry messages across the synapse to the dendrite (and sometimes the cell body) of a receiver neuron.

Norm
A rule which guides behavior.

O

Obedience
Conforming behavior in reaction to the commands of others.

Observational Learning
Learning through observing the behavior of another person.

Oedipus Conflict
A child's sexual interest in his or her opposite-sex parent typically resolved through identification with the same sex parent.

Operant Conditioning
Learning in which a voluntary response is strengthened or weakened depending upon its favorable or unfavorable consequences.

Oral Stage
First stage in Freud's psychoanalytic theory of personality; during first 18 months of life in which intense pleasures are derived from activities that involve the mouth.

P

Parasympathetic System
The part of the autonomic nervous system which tends to be active when we are calm and relaxed; builds up and conserves the body's store of energy.

Paresthesia
A condition in which a person experiences false sensations.

Perception
A process of organizing environmental stimuli into some meaningful patterns or wholes.

Perceptual Constancy
A tendency to perceive the stimuli in the environment as unchanging though in reality there may be changes in shape, size or other characteristics.

Peripheral Nervous System
Part of the nervous system that includes the autonomic and somatic subdivisions made up of long axons and dendrites; branches out from the spinal cord and brain and reaches the extremities of the body.

Personality
Personality refers to the enduring characteristics and behavior that comprise a person's unique adjustment to life, including major traits, interests, drives, values, self-concept, abilities, and emotional patterns.

Personality Disorder
A mental disorder characterized by a set of inflexible, maladaptive personality traits that keep a person away from functioning properly in the society.

Personality Inventory
An inventory for self-appraisal consisting of many statements or questions about personal characteristics and behavior that the person judges to apply or not apply to him or her.

Persuasion
The act of giving information which causes a person to do or believe something.

Phallic Stage
According to Freud, a period beginning around age 3 during which a child's interest focuses on the genitals.

Phobias
Intense, irrational fears of specific objects or situations.

Pituitary Gland
Also called the 'master gland', it is a major component of the endocrine system which secrets hormones that control growth.

Pleasure Principle
A principle in Freudian theory emphasizing the immediate gratification regardless of the consequences, a function of the id.

Positive Reinforcer
A stimulus added to the environment that brings about an increase in a preceding response.

Positive Transfer
A type of transfer in which one learning helps facilitate the other learning.

Preconscious
Memories and thoughts of which a person is not aware of at a particular time but which may easily become conscious.

Prejudice
An unjustified attitude, fairly strong, usually in an unfavorable direction and not in line with the facts.

Proactive Interference
Forgetting caused by the prior learning of other material.

Projection
A defense mechanism in which conflict is dealt with ascribing one's own anxiety-provoking motives to someone else; blaming others; prominent in paranoid disorders.

Projective Personality Test
A test in which a person is shown an ambiguous stimulus and asked to describe it or tell a story about it.

Proximity
A principle of perceptual organization stating that nearness or closeness of objects leads the perceiver to perceive them in patterns.

Psychoanalytic Theory
Freud's theory that unconscious forces act as determinants of personality.

Psychodynamic Perspective
An approach based on the belief that behavior is motivated by unconscious inner forces over which the individual has little control.

Psychology
The scientific study of behavior and mental processes.

Psychosexual Stages
The five stages of psychological development as put by Freud in his personality theory.

Psychosocial Development
Development of individuals' interactions and understanding of each other and of their knowledge and understanding of themselves as members of society.

Psychosomatic Illness
A condition in which emotional stress causes physical illness.

Psychotherapy
Treatment in which a trained professional or a therapist uses psychological techniques to help someone overcome psychological difficulties and disorders, resolve problems in living or bring about personal growth.

Punishment
A stimulus which decreases the probability that a previous behavior will occur again.

R

Rationalization
A defense mechanism through which a person gives false reasons for his behavior.

Reaction Formation
A defense mechanism through which a person strongly expresses the reverse of what he feels.

Recall
The process of remembering without the aid of extra cues.

Recessive Gene
Gene whose hereditary potential is not expressed when it is paired with a dominant gene.

Recognition
The ability to look at several things and select one that has been seen or learned before.

Reflex
Involuntary, unlearned, immediate response to a stimulus.

Regression
A defense mechanism in which a person copes with anxiety by retreating to childish or earlier forms of behavior; often encountered in children and adults faced with frustration and motivational conflict.

Reinforcement
The process of strengthening a response with the help of an appropriate stimulus making it more likely to recur.

Reinforcer
Any stimulus that increases the probability that a preceding behavior will occur again.

Repression
A defense mechanism through which a person unconsciously forgets unpleasant experiences.

Resilience
It is the process of adapting well in the face of adversity, trauma, tragedy, threats or even significant sources of stress.

Retention
Storage of learned material in memory.

Reticular Activating System (RAS)
Nervous system structure running through the hindbrain and midbrain to the hypothalamus responsible for general arousal of the organism.

Retrograde Amnesia
Forgetting events one was exposed to in the past.

Role
A behavior pattern expected from a person in a certain social position.

Rorschach Test
A test developed by Swiss psychiatrist Hermann Rorschach that consists of showing a series of symmetrical stimuli to people and then asking them to state what the figures represent to them.

S

Schachter-Singer Theory of Emotion
The belief that emotions are determined jointly by a nonspecific kind of physiological arousal and its interpretation, based on environmental cues.

Schedules of Reinforcement
The frequency and timing of reinforcement following desired behavior.

Schemas
Organized bodies of information stored in memory that bias the way new information is interpreted, stored and recalled.

Scientific Method
The approach used by psychologists to systematically acquire knowledge and understanding about behavior and other phenomena of interest.

Self-actualization
According to Rogers, a state of self-fulfillment in which people realize their highest potential; the highest need in the hierarchical structure of needs proposed by Maslow that drives an individual to discover one's self and fulfill one's potential.

Self-concept
The general ideas and feelings that one acquires about himself as a unique individual of special significance.

Self-esteem
Self-esteem often seen as a personality trait is used to describe a person's overall sense of self-worth or personal value. It involves a variety of beliefs about the self such as appraisal of one's own appearance, beliefs, emotions and behaviors.

Semantic Memory
Memory for general knowledge and facts about the world as well as for the rules of logic that are used to deduce other facts.

Sensation
The process by which our sense organs receive information from the environment.

Sensory Memory
The initial momentary storage of information lasting only an instant.

Shaping
The process of teaching a complex behavior by rewarding closer and closer approximations to the desired behavior, a technique in operant conditioning.

Short-term Memory (STM)
Short-term memory refers to information that people can remember for a short period of time immediately after receiving it.

Skill
The ability to perform a specialized activity well.

Social Motives
Motives usually learned in a social group that require the presence or reaction of other people for their satisfaction.

Social Psychology
The study of how people's thoughts, feelings and actions are affected by others.

Soft-skills
Soft-skills are personal traits required to establish and maintain interpersonal relationships with others in an organization. Also termed as social skills, personal skills or emotional intelligence, they define the ability to interact harmoniously with others.

Somatoform Disorder
A behavioral disorder in which a person shows physical symptoms for which no physical cause can be found.

Somatotyping
Sheldon's system of classifying persons into certain body types according to the degree to which their somatic structure (body build) reflects certain physical characteristics.

Spontaneous Recovery
The recovery of part of the strength of a conditioned response sometime after it has been extinguished.

Stereotypes
Generalized beliefs and expectations about social groups and their members.

Stimulus
The physical energy or action which causes a response from an organism.

Stimulus Discrimination
A concept in the theory of conditioning emphasizing that an organism learns to react to differences in stimuli and to distinguish between them.

Stimulus Generalization
A concept in the theory of conditioning emphasizing that once an individual gets conditioned to respond to a specific stimulus, other similar stimuli bring the same response.

Stimulus Variability
Innate performance for change in environmental stimuli.

Stress
The response to events that are threatening or challenging.

Structuralism
Wundt's approach which focuses on the basic elements that form the foundation of thinking, consciousness, emotions and other kinds of mental states and activities.

Sublimation
A defense mechanism through which a person directs unacceptable desires into acceptable behavior.

Superego
According to Freud, the final personality structure to develop; it represents society's standards of right and wrong as handed down by a person's parents, teachers and other important figures.

Suppression
The act of consciously putting aside unacceptable feelings and desires.

Synapse
Fluid-filled space between the axon of one neuron and the receiving dendrite of the next that helps the flow of information through the nervous system.

T

Temperament
The hereditary emotional aspects of one's personality.

Temporal Lobes
Parts of the cerebrum at the sides of the head mainly responsible for hearing.

Thalamus
The egg-shaped part of the forebrain which relays sensory information and controls sleep and wakefulness.

Thematic Apperception Test (TAT)
A test consisting of a series of ambiguous pictures about which the person is asked to write a story.

Theories
Broad explanations and predictions concerning phenomena of interest.

Thinking
Thinking is the processing of information mentally or cognitively by rearranging the information from the environment and the symbols stored in the past memory.

Thyroid Gland
Endocrine gland located below the larynx that secretes thyroxin, which controls metabolism.

Trait
Particular feature of an individual's personality that seems to stand out and endure over a wide variety of situations.

Trait Theory
A model of personality that seeks to identify the basic traits necessary to describe personality.

Transactional Analysis (TA)
Altering one's state of consciousness by focusing on one's breathing while excluding all other thoughts.

Transduction
A process by which receptor cells transform physical energy into an impulse that the nervous system can carry.

Transference
In psychoanalysis, the process by which the patient transfers a variety of positive and negative reactions associated with parents and other childhood authority figures, directing these feelings towards the therapist.

Trust vs. Mistrust Stage
According to Erikson, the first stage of psychosocial development, occurring from birth to 18 months of age during which time infants develop feelings of trust or lack of trust.

Type A Behavior Pattern
A pattern of behavior characterized by competitiveness, impatience, tendency toward frustration and hostility.

Type B Behavior Pattern
A pattern of behavior characterized by co-operation, patience, non-competitiveness and non-aggression.

U

Unconditional Positive Regard
An attitude of acceptance and respect on the part of an observer no matter what the other person says or does.

Unconditioned Response (UCR)
A response that is natural and needs no training (e.g., salivation at the smell of food).

Unconditioned Stimulus (UCS)
A stimulus that brings about a response without having been learned.

Unconscious
A part of the personality of which a person is not aware and which is a potential determinant of behavior.

V

Variable-interval Schedule
A schedule whereby the time between reinforcements varies around some average rather than being fixed.

Variable-ratio Schedule
A schedule whereby reinforcement occurs after a varying number of reasons rather than after a fixed number.

Variables
Behaviors, events or other characteristics that can change or vary in some way.

Verbal Behavior
The use of spoken or written language in communicating with others.

Visual Acuity
Ability to distinguish fine details in the field of vision.

W

Withdrawal
A defense mechanism through which a person physically avoids unpleasant situations.

Working Memory
Memory that is stored for only a few seconds.

Z

Zygote
A new cell formed by the union of an egg and sperm.

Bibliography

1. Ann ZJ. Basic Psychology for Nurses in India. BI Publications Pvt Ltd: Chennai; 2003.
2. Bhatia BD, Margaretta C. Elements of Psychology and Mental Hygiene for Nurses in India. Orient Longman: Chennai; 2005.
3. Charles SE. Educational Psychology, 4th edition. Prentice-Hall of India Pvt Ltd: New Delhi; 1996.
4. David MG. Social Psychology, 6th edition. McGraw-Hill College: Boston; 1991.
5. Elizabeth HB. Developmental Psychology. A Lifespan Approach, 5th edition. Tata McGraw-Hill Edition: New Delhi, 2002.
6. Feldman RS. Understanding Psychology, 6th edition. Tata McGraw-Hill: New Delhi; 2004.
7. Helen SC, Josephine FN. Altschul's Psychology for Nurses, 7th edition. Bailliere Tindall: London; 1991.
8. Hilgard RE, Atkinson CR, Atkinson LR. Introduction to Psychology, 6th edition. Oxford and IBH publishing Co Pvt Ltd: New Delhi; 1975.
9. Jacob A. Psychology for Graduate Nurses, 4th edition. Jaypee Brothers: New Delhi; 2007.
10. Khan MA. Sociology for Nurses. Academa Publishers: Delhi; 2004.
11. Kuppuswamy B. An Introduction to Social Psychology. Media Promoters and Publishers Pvt Ltd: Mumbai; 1994.
12. Mangal SK. Advanced Educational Psychology, 6th edition. Prentice Hall of India Pvt Ltd: New Delhi; 2007.
13. Mangal SK. General Psychology. Sterling Publishers Pvt Ltd: New Delhi; 2006.
14. Margaret MW. Psychology, 3rd edition. Harcourt Brace College Publishers: Philadelphia; 1999.
15. Morgan CT, King RA, Weisz JR, et al. Introduction to Psychology, 7th edition. Tata McGraw-Hill Publishing Company Limited: New Delhi, 2004.
16. Nagaraja KR, Begum Shamshad B, Sudarshan CY. MCQs in Psychology for Nursing and Allied Sciences. Jaypee Brothers Medical Publishers Pvt Ltd: New Delhi, 2006.
17. Richard G, Nancy K. Psychology for Nurses and Allied Health Professionals. London: Hodder Arnold; 2007.
18. Shelley TE. Health Psychology, 6th edition. Tata McGraw-Hill Edition: New York; 2006.

Index

Page numbers followed by *b* refer to box, *f* refer to figure, *fc* refer to flowchart, and *t* refer to table

Q

R